Cochlear Implants: Adult and Pediatric

Guest Editors

J. THOMAS ROLAND Jr, MD
DAVID S. HAYNES, MD

OTOLARYNGOLOGIC CLINICS OF NORTH AMERICA

www.oto.theclinics.com

February 2012 • Volume 45 • Number 1

SAUNDERS an imprint of ELSEVIER, Inc.

W.B. SAUNDERS COMPANY
A Division of Elsevier Inc.

1600 John F. Kennedy Boulevard • Suite 1800 • Philadelphia, Pennsylvania 19103-2899

http://www.theclinics.com

OTOLARYNGOLOGIC CLINICS OF NORTH AMERICA Volume 45, Number 1
February 2012 ISSN 0030-6665, ISBN-13: 978-1-4557-1117-8

Editor: Joanne Husovski

Otolaryngologic Clinics of North America (ISSN 0030-6665) is published bimonthly by Elsevier, Inc., 360 Park Avenue South, New York, NY 10010-1710. Months of issue are February, April, June, August, October, and December. Business and Editorial Offices: 1600 John F. Kennedy Blvd., Suite 1800, Philadelphia, PA 19103-2899. Customer Service Office: 6277 Sea Harbor Drive, Orlando, FL 32887-4800. Periodicals postage paid at New York, NY and additional mailing offices. Subscription prices is $335.00 per year (US individuals), $628.00 per year (US institutions), $161.00 per year (US student/resident), $442.00 per year (Canadian individuals), $789.00 per year (Canadian institutions), $496.00 per year (international individuals), $789.00 per year (international institutions), $248.00 per year (international & Canadian student/resident). Foreign air speed delivery is included in all *Clinics'* subscription prices. All prices are subject to change without notice. **POSTMASTER:** Send address changes to *Otolaryngologic Clinics of North America*, Elsevier Health Sciences Division, Subscription Customer Service, 3251 Riverport Lane, Maryland Heights, MO 63043. **Telephone: 1-800-654-2452 (U.S. and Canada); 314-447-8871 (outside U.S. and Canada). Fax: 314-447-8029. E-mail: journalscustomerservice-usa@elsevier.com (for print support); journalsonlinesupport-usa@elsevier.com (for online support).**

Reprints. For copies of 100 or more of articles in this publication, please contact the Commercial Reprints Department, Elsevier Inc., 360 Park Avenue South, New York, NY 10010-1710. Tel.: 212-633-3812; Fax: 212-462-1935; E-mail: reprints@elsevier.com.

Otolaryngologic Clinics of North America is also published in Spanish by McGraw-Hill Interamericana Editores S.A., P.O. Box 5-237, 06500 Mexico D.F., Mexico.

Otolaryngologic Clinics of North America is covered in *MEDLINE/PubMed (Index Medicus), Current Contents/Clinical Medicine, Excerpta Medica, BIOSIS, Science Citation Index,* and *ISI/BIOMED.*

Printed and bound by CPI Group (UK) Ltd, Croydon, CR0 4YY
Transferred to Digital Print 2012

Contributors

GUEST EDITORS

J. THOMAS ROLAND Jr, MD
Mendik Professor and Chairman, Department of Otolaryngology–Head and Neck Surgery; Co-Director, New York University Cochlear Implant Center, New York University School of Medicine, New York, New York

DAVID S. HAYNES, MD
Professor, Department of Otolaryngology/Department of Hearing and Speech Sciences; Director, Division of Otology and Neurotology; Program Director, Neurotology Fellowship, Department of Otolaryngology–Head and Neck Surgery, Vanderbilt Bill Wilkerson Center, Vanderbilt University, Nashville, Tennessee

AUTHORS

TAMALA S. BRADHAM, PhD
Associate Director of Services, Department of Hearing and Speech Sciences, Vanderbilt Bill Wilkerson Center, Nashville, Tennessee

MATTHEW L. CARLSON, MD
Department of Otolaryngology–Head and Neck Surgery, Mayo Clinic School of Medicine, Rochester, Minnesota

DANIEL H. COELHO, MD
Assistant Professor, Department of Otolaryngology–Head and Neck Surgery, Director, Virginia Commonwealth University Cochlear Implant Center, Virginia Commonwealth University School of Medicine, Richmond, Virginia

MELINDA COHEN, MS
Genetic Counselor, Associate in Pediatrics, Division of Medical Genetics and Genomic Medicine, Vanderbilt University School of Medicine, Nashville, Tennessee

MAURA K. COSETTI, MD
Department of Otolaryngology, New York University School of Medicine, New York, New York

COLIN L.W. DRISCOLL, MD
Professor and Chairman, Department of Otolaryngology–Head and Neck Surgery, Mayo Clinic School of Medicine, Rochester, Minnesota

ANDREW J. FISHMAN, MD
Associate Professor of Otolaryngology and Neurosurgery, Otology-Neurotology Skull Base Surgery, Feinberg School of Medicine, Northwestern University, Chicago; Fellow of the Hugh Knowles Foundation, Department of Communication Sciences and Disorders, Northwestern University, Evanston, Illinois

HILLARY GANEK, MA, CCC-SLP, LSLS Cert. AVT
Department of Otolaryngology–Head and Neck Surgery, The Listening Center at Johns Hopkins, The Johns Hopkins University, Baltimore, Maryland

BRUCE J. GANTZ, MD
Professor and Head, Department of Otolaryngology, University of Iowa Hospital and Clinics, Iowa City, Iowa

RENÉ H. GIFFORD, PhD
Assistant Professor of Hearing and Speech Sciences and Director of Cochlear Implant Program, Department of Hearing and Speech Sciences, Vanderbilt Bill Wilkerson Center, Vanderbilt University, Nashville, Tennessee

DAVID S. HAYNES, MD
Professor, Otology-Neurotology and Skull Base Surgery, Department of Otolaryngology–Head and Neck Surgery; Professor of Neurosurgery and Hearing; Professor of Hearing and Speech Sciences; Otology Group of Vanderbilt, Department of Otolaryngology–Head and Neck Surgery, Vanderbilt Bill Wilkerson Center, Vanderbilt University, Nashville, Tennessee

SELENA E. HEMAN-ACKAH, MD, MBA
New York University School of Medicine, New York, New York

DANA KAN, MA, NBCT
Teacher of the Deaf and Hard-of-Hearing, Department of Hearing and Speech Sciences, Vanderbilt University School of Medicine, Nashville, Tennessee

CHARLES J. LIMB, MD
Department of Otolaryngology–Head and Neck Surgery, Peabody Conservatory of Muisic, Johns Hopkins University School of Medicine, Baltimore, Maryland

BRANNON MANGUS, MD
Otology Group of Vanderbilt, Department of Otolaryngology–Head and Neck Surgery, Vanderbilt Bill Wilkerson Center, Vanderbilt University, Nashville, Tennessee

SEAN O. MCMENOMEY, MD
Professor, Department of Otolaryngology–Head and Neck Surgery, Oregon Health and Science University, Portland, Oregon

THEODORE R. MCRACKAN, MD
Resident of Otolaryngology–Head and Neck Surgery, Vanderbilt University Medical Center, Nashville, Tennessee

SARAH E. MOWRY, MD
Fellow in Neurotology, Department of Otolaryngology, University of Iowa Hospital and Clinics, Iowa City, Iowa

JOHN K. NIPARKO, MD
Department of Otolaryngology–Head and Neck Surgery, The Listening Center at Johns Hopkins, The Johns Hopkins University, Baltimore, Maryland

JOHN A. PHILLIPS III, MD
David T. Karzon Professor of Pediatrics, Division of Medical Genetics and Genomic Medicine, Vanderbilt University School of Medicine, Nashville, Tennessee

ALEJANDRO RIVAS, MD
Fellow-Otology, Neurotology and Skull Base Surgery, Department of Otolaryngology–Head and Neck Surgery; Assistant Professor, Otology Group of Vanderbilt, Vanderbilt Bill Wilkerson Center, Vanderbilt University Medical Center, Nashville, Tennessee

AMY MCCONKEY ROBBINS, MS, CCC-SLP
Communication Consulting Services, Indianapolis, Indiana

J. THOMAS ROLAND Jr, MD
Mendik Professor and Chairman, Department of Otolaryngology–Head and Neck Surgery; Co-Director, New York University Cochlear Implant Center, New York University School of Medicine, New York, New York

JAY T. RUBINSTEIN, MD, PhD
Department of Otolaryngology–Head and Neck Surgery, Virginia Merrill Bloedel Hearing Research Center, University of Washington Medical Center, Seattle, Washington

WILLIAM H. SHAPIRO, AuD
Clinical Associate Professor, Department of Otolaryngology, NYU Langone Medical Center, Schwartz Health Care Center, New York, New York

UMA G. SOMAN, MED, LSLS Cert AVEd
Teacher of the Deaf and Hard-of-Hearing, Department of Hearing and Speech Sciences, Vanderbilt University School of Medicine, Nashville, Tennessee

ANNE MARIE THARPE, PhD
Professor and Chair, Department of Hearing and Speech Sciences, Vanderbilt University School of Medicine; Associate Director, Vanderbilt Bill Wilkerson Center, Nashville, Tennessee

BETTY S. TSAI, MD
Otology Group of Vanderbilt, Department of Otolaryngology–Head and Neck Surgery; Vanderbilt Bill Wilkerson Center, Vanderbilt University, Nashville, Tennessee

SUSAN B. WALTZMAN, PhD
Department of Otolaryngology, New York University Cochlear Implant Center, New York University School of Medicine, New York, New York

GEORGE B. WANNA, MD
Assistant Professor of Otolaryngology–Head and Neck Surgery, Division of Otology-Neurotology and Skull Base Surgery, Vanderbilt University Medical Center, Nashville, Tennessee; Otology Group of Vanderbilt, Vanderbilt Bill Wilkerson Center, Vanderbilt University, Nashville, Tennessee

ERIKA WOODSON, MD
Associate Staff, Head and Neck Institute, Cleveland Clinic Foundation, Cleveland, Ohio

Contents

of the implant incision and the methods used to secure the device and the electrode, the cochleostomy versus round window debate, and a discussion of the validity of intraoperative tests. Advanced technology, new surgical techniques, and refining established techniques are hallmarks of cochlear implant surgery. Advancements, including image-guided surgery, hearing preservation with full insertion, and telemetry-based advanced programming, are expected to be standard in the future.

Cochlear implantation (CI) is the standard of care for the treatment of children and adults with bilateral severe-to-profound sensorineural hearing loss. Because the ultimate and continuous goal of CI teams is to improve patient performance, a potential method is bilateral CI. The potential benefits of bilateral CI include binaural summation, squelch, equivalent head shadow for each ear, improved hearing in noise, sound localization ability, and spatial release from masking. The potential disadvantages include additional or prolonged surgical procedure, unproven cost/benefit profile, and the elimination of the ability to use future technologies and/or medical therapies in the implanted ear.

Implantation of the ossified and dysplastic cochlea presents many unique challenges to both the surgeon and programming team. Altered embryology and physiology of these labyrinthine dysplasias may result in forms and functions unfamiliar to those casually involved with cochlear implants. Remarkable developments in diagnosis, surgical technique, electrode design, processing strategies, and programming have all contributed to the ability to successfully implant patient populations previously excluded from this life-changing intervention.

Cochlear implants have become a viable treatment option for individuals who present with severe to profound hearing loss. While there are several parameters that affect the successful use of this technology, quality programming of the cochlear implant system is crucial. This review chapter focuses on general device programming techniques, programming techniques specific to children, objective programming techniques, a brief overview of programming parameters of the currently commercially available multichannel systems, and managing patient complaints and device failures. The chapter also provides what the authors believe the future may hold for new programming techniques.

The authors present a comprehensive review of the state of music perception with cochlear implant (CI) users. They discuss methods of assessment and results of studies of the aspects of music perception, melody, timbre, rhythm, and so forth in individuals with cochlear implants. They discuss neural mechanisms of music perception and the anticipation of broader acceptance of standardized tests for music perception in CI users.

A growing number of children with severe-to-profound hearing loss are receiving cochlear implants. This article provides information about the various educational and rehabilitation options for these children, emphasizing the need for a collaborative approach to rehabilitation planning and implementation. Decisions about such options should be individualized and are informed by several factors including age at implantation and family expectations and desires. A review of legislation affecting the education of children with hearing loss is also provided.

This article highlights variables that affect cochlear implant performance, emerging factors warranting consideration, and variables shown not to affect performance. Research on the outcomes following cochlear implantation has identified a wide spectrum of variables known to affect pos0timplantation performance. These variables relate to the device itself as well as individual patient characteristics. Factors believed to affect spiral ganglion cell survival and function have been shown to influence postoperative performance. Binaural hearing affects performance. Social and educational factors also affect postoperative performance. Novel variables capable of affecting performance continue to emerge with increased understanding of auditory pathway development and neural plasticity.

This article presents a focused review of language, speech, and comprehension outcomes in children with cochlear implants. Language acquisition with early-age implants and later-age implants are discussed, along with literacy and comprehension skills. A wide range of language outcomes is possible for children with cochlear implants, but many can achieve listening and spoken language skills at the same rate as their hearing peers. Appropriate auditory rehabilitation and parental guidance is vital for the development of listening and spoken language skills.

As cochlear implant technology has changed, so have implantation criteria. In addition to profoundly deaf individuals, candidacy has expanded to include those with significant remaining acoustic hearing. This article describes the devices that are now in clinical trial, discusses the rationale

RELATED INTEREST

Auris Nasus Larynx, December 2011 (Volume 38, Issue 6) Pages 739–742
**Safe use of Bipolar Radiofrequency Induced Thermotherapy (RFITT) for Nasal
Surgery in Patients with Cochlear Implants**
Walter Di Nardo, Alessandro Scorpecci, Sara Giannantonio, Gaetano Paludetti

THE CLINICS ARE NOW AVAILABLE ONLINE!

Access your subscription at:
www.theclinics.com

Cochlear Implants: An Evolving Technology

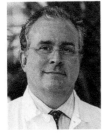 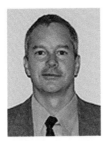

J. Thomas Roland Jr, MD   David S. Haynes, MD
Guest Editors

This edition of the *Otolaryngology Clinics of North America* is intended to provide the reader with an update on the dynamic field of the rehabilitation of severe to profound hearing loss with cochlear implants. Since the early 1980s, when the FDA first approved the multichannel cochlear implant for clinical use, cochlear implant candidacy, cochlear implant technology, surgical procedures, device programming, and expected and realized outcomes have changed dramatically.

The implementation of this miraculous technology requires a team approach unlike anything else in modern day medicine. Auditory scientists, speech therapists, audiologists, educators, engineers, and surgeons work together, each inspiring the others to achieve and make progress, and as a result of this collaborative endeavor, patients are achieving benefits that were unimaginable in the early days of cochlear implantation. Many of the authors in this volume were involved from the very beginning of clinical use of the device and each has contributed significantly to this work.

The editors' goal was to provide a comprehensive body of articles that experienced cochlear implant professionals as well as individuals new to the field can use and enjoy. The material contained herein should provide up-to-date overviews that might inspire others to make advances and contributions to this rapidly changing discipline. We are certain that the authors who contributed provided excellent, detailed information on each of their disciplines. We are indebted to all of them for the fine work.

J. Thomas Roland Jr, MD
Department of Otolaryngology
New York University Cochlear Implant Center
New York University School of Medicine
660 First Avenue, 7th Floor
New York, NY 10016, USA

David S. Haynes, MD
Otology Group of Vanderbilt
Department of Otolaryngology–Head and Neck Surgery
Vanderbilt Bill Wilkerson Center, Vanderbilt University
1215 21st Avenue South, 7209 Medical Center East
South Tower, Nashville, TN 37232, USA

E-mail addresses:
John.roland@nyumc.org (J.T. Roland)
david.haynes@Vanderbilt.edu (D.S. Haynes)

Otolaryngol Clin N Am 45 (2012) xiii
doi:10.1016/j.otc.2011.09.004

Imaging and Anatomy for Cochlear Implants

Andrew J. Fishman, MD[a,b,]*

KEYWORDS

• Cochlear implant • Malformed cochlea • Luminal obstruction
• Preoperative imaging

IMAGING AND ANATOMY CONSIDERATIONS FOR COCHLEAR IMPLANTATION

Radiographic imaging plays a major role in cochlear implantation with regard to preoperative candidacy evaluation, intraoperative monitoring, and postoperative evaluation, as well as research and experimental techniques. At a minimum, successful cochlear implantation requires that electrical impulses be delivered to a surviving spiral ganglion cell population, and that these impulses be transmitted to a functioning auditory cortex by an existent neural connection. Accordingly, imaging the auditory pathway of the implant candidate is necessary to screen for morphologic conditions that will preclude or complicate the implantation process. Increasing resolution of computed tomography (CT) and magnetic resonance (MR) imaging technology has provided the clinician with more detailed information about the integrity of the auditory pathway. As technologies evolve, a clear understanding of what information can be obtained as well as the limitations of various imaging modalities is essential to proper candidacy evaluation, and selection of the ear to be implanted in complex cases.

PREOPERATIVE IMAGING

Preoperative imaging is instrumental in determining the feasibility and facility of cochlear implantation. Analysis is preformed in a stepwise approach, answering of the following 3 questions. Are there cochleovestibular anomalies that preclude implantation? Is there evidence of luminal obstruction? Are there additional findings that may complicate the surgery or subsequent patient management? This section is not intended to review principles or techniques of image acquisition,

a Otology-Neurotology Skull Base Surgery, Feinberg School of Medicine, Northwestern University, Chicago, IL, USA
b Department of Communication Sciences and Disorders, Northwestern University, Evanston, IL, USA
* Department of Otolaryngology, 675 North Street, Clair Galter 15-200, Chicago, IL 60611.
E-mail address: ajfishman@mac.com

Otolaryngol Clin N Am 45 (2012) 1–24
doi:10.1016/j.otc.2011.08.014
0030-6665/12/$ – see front matter © 2012 Elsevier Inc. All rights reserved.

but to provide a platform for discussion between the implant team and the radiologist.

Are There Cochleovestibular Anomalies that Preclude Implantation?

Approximately 20% of patients with congenital sensorineural hearing loss have radiographically identifiable morphologic abnormalities of the inner ear.[1] In general, inner ear malformations can be associated with a wide range of hearing sensitivity.[2] These patients can manifest progression of hearing loss, though many may retain useful hearing into adult life. As a general rule, however, the more severe is the deformity, the worse the hearing.[2] Due to the variability and progressive nature of hearing loss in these disorders, most large implant centers are likely to evaluate several patients with a variety of malformations. Given the current technology, the minimum requirement for cochlear implantation is the presence of an implantable cavity in proximity to stimulable neural elements whose projections connect to the auditory cortex. Accordingly, the first question that must be answered is: are there any cochleovestibular anomalies that preclude implantation?

Embryology

To fully appreciate the wide variety of possible cochleovestibular malformations, it is helpful to first review the embryogenesis of the inner ear,[2,3] considering separately the formation of the membranous labyrinth, the bony otic capsule, and the cochleovestibular nerves and ganglia.

The development of the combined cochlear and vestibular membranous labyrinthine system begins with the formation of the otic placode as an ectodermal thickening, which forms on the surface of the neural tube in the third gestational week. The otic placode invaginates from the surface and forms the otocyst in the fourth gestational week. The otocyst develops 3 infolds in the fifth week. The resultant pouches represent: the primordial endolymphatic sac and duct; the utricle and semicircular canals; and the saccule and cochlea. Beginning in the sixth week, the cochlear duct grows from its primordial bud beginning from the basal region spiraling apically to reach its full two-and-a-half to two-and-three-quarter turns by the eighth to tenth week. The neuroepithelial end organs continue to develop beyond this period, with the organ of Corti completing its formation in the 25th week.

The semicircular canals begin their formation as 3 small folded evaginations on the primordial vestibular appendage. The canals develop as disklike outpouchings whose centers eventually compress and fuse to ultimately form the semicircular duct structure. By the sixth week of gestational life, this compression and fusion has taken place in first the superior and then the posterior canals. The 3 canals continue to enlarge and complete their formation to full adult size in sequence, beginning with the superior around the 20th week, followed by the posterior, and finally the lateral semicircular canals. Of interest, the endolymphatic sac and duct are the first to appear and the last to complete their development.

The osseous otic capsule eventually forms from a morphologically fully developed cartilage precursor model via 14 centers of ossification, beginning around the 15th gestational week, and is completed during the 23rd gestational week. The cartilage model and underlying membranous labyrinth continue to grow in the region of the posterior and lateral semicircular canals while other structures, which have previously attained their final shape and size, have begun ossifying. The cochleovestibular nerves and ganglia develop in concert with the membranous labyrinth and cochleovestibular end organs. These structures are of neural crest origin and migrate between the epithelial layer and basement membrane of the otic vesicle during the fourth gestational week.

Cochlear malformations

There is much confusion in the literature regarding the nomenclature of cochlear morphologic anomalies, especially regarding the term "Mondini malformation." In 1791, Carlo Mondini presented his findings on an anatomic dissection of a young deaf boy.[4] According to his writings, prior reports of human deafness were attributed to abnormalities of the external auditory canal and Eustachian tube, tympanic membrane, middle ear and ossicles, or compression of the auditory nerve. During his dissection on the posterior face of the petrous bone Mondini discovered significant vestibular aqueduct enlargement, and commented that the usual bony lip that "protects the vestibular aqueduct" was missing and was substituted by a membranous plate of dura. He noted that the vestibule was not deformed but was of greater than usual size. He also noted an increase in the size of the elliptical recess, though it was normal in shape. He commented that the semicircular canals appeared normal and that the positions of their openings into the vestibule were unremarkable. In observing the medial opening of the vestibular aqueduct, Mondini commented that it was quite enlarged and was larger than the size of the common crus. With regard to the cochlea, it was described to possess only one-and-a-half turns. He described the cochlea as ending in a cavity corresponding to the last spiral turn and described an incompletely formed interscalar septum. The more contemporary term "incomplete partition" is commonly used to describe this classic anomaly, and denotes this specific aspect of the deformity.[2,5] In this historic subject, the deformity was bilateral.

Because of its relative frequency as well as its historical significance, the term "Mondini malformation" is commonly used to describe all forms of cochlear morphologic abnormalities and not just the incomplete partition. The term Mondini dysplasia was used by Schuknecht[6] in an in-depth analysis of the histopathology and clinical features of cochlear anomalies. Schuknecht's treatise described a variety of malformations including one patient with "the normal $2^{1/2}$ turns but measur[ing] only 23 mm in length (normal: 32 mm)" and another with "Mondini dysplasia limited to the vestibular system," as well as several patients with cochleae possessing one-and-a-half turns, and other variant morphologies of both the cochlear duct and vestibular system. Schuknecht histologically described these malformations as isolated findings or in association with other named syndromes, namely Klippel-Feil, Pendred, and DiGeorge. His work detailed the clinical nature of these disorders as being unilateral or bilateral, and associated with acoustic and vestibular dysfunction, which is variable in severity, static, or progressive.

Phelps[7] reserves the term "Mondini deformity" for cochlea whose basal turns are normal and that possess a deficiency of the interscalar septum of the distal one-and-a-half coils. He differentiates these cochleae from those termed "dysplastic" owing to their widened basal turn being in wide communication with a dilated vestibule. According to Phelps, the significance lies in the clinical absence of spontaneous cerebrospinal fluid (CSF) leak and meningitis in patients with his strict definition of Mondini deformity, as opposed to those patients with dysplasia who did manifest these complications in a series of 20 patients studied.

Since the writings of Mondini, several investigators have documented a variety of inner ear malformations. Though not the first to describe or name these malformations, Jackler and colleagues[2] proposed a classification system in 1987 for the congenitally malformed inner ear based on the theory that a variety of deformities result from arrested development at different stages of embryogenesis. These investigators clearly stated that their classification could not describe all observable abnormalities but was meant to serve as a framework on which other describable anomalies could be added, which by their supposition would have resulted from aberrant, rather than arrested development.

This body of work deserves mention, as it is often cited and serves well as an initial systematic basis for the interpretation of images. Jackler and colleagues[2] formulated their classification system on review of polytomes and CT scans of 63 patients with 98 congenitally malformed ears, and provided the categorization listed in (**Box 1**). The disorders identified as having normal cochleae were subdivided solely for the purposes of Jackler's classification scheme. It is important to realize that disorders of the vestibule, semicircular canals, and vestibular aqueduct are also often found in conjunction with cochlear malformations. Inner ear deformities tend to occur bilaterally in 65%.[2] When bilateral, there is a 93% chance that they will be similar, although various combinations of morphologic classes have been documented.[2]

Complete labyrinthine aplasia, also called Michel deformity, could result from arrest prior to formation of the otocyst, resulting in complete absence of inner ear development.[2] This malformation is the rarest among those classified here (**Fig. 1**).

Cochlear aplasia is defined as absent cochlea with an intact but often variably deformed vestibular labyrinth. This cochlear malformation is the second rarest noted by Jackler and colleagues,[2] representing approximately 3% of identified cochlear malformations.

The term cochlear hypoplasia has been used to describe a range of abnormalities from a rudimentary cochlear diverticulum to an incompletely formed cochlear bud of several millimeters (**Fig. 2**). This group comprised 15% of cases reported by Jackler and colleagues,[2] was believed to represent arrested development during the sixth gestational week, and may be associated with either a normal or malformed vestibule and semicircular canals.

Incomplete partition is a term used by Jackler and colleagues[2] in their study, and it is pointed out that this is the closest to the malformation originally described by Mondini. This cochlear abnormality is the most commonly described, making up 55% of the study described. It is believed to represent arrest in development during the seventh gestational week, a time at which the cochlea would have completed one to one-and-a-half turns. Radiographically, these cochleae possess only one-and-a-half turns comprising a basal turn leading to the appearance of a confluent middle and apical turn, which may also be viewed and described as incomplete partitioning by a deficient interscalar septum.[2,5] These cochleae may also manifest varying degrees of abnormalities of the vestibular system and endolymphatic duct and sac (**Fig. 3**).

The term common cavity is used to denote confluence of the cochlea and vestibule into a common rudimentary cavity that usually lacks an internal architecture and is often associated with abnormally formed semicircular canals. This abnormality is

---

Box 1
Jackler's classification of congenital malformations of the inner ear

Absent or Malformed Cochlea

1. Complete labyrinthine aplasia

2. Cochlear aplasia

3. Cochlear hypoplasia

4. Incomplete partition

5. Common Cavity

Normal Cochlea

1. Vestibule—lateral semicircular canal dysplasia

2. Enlarged vestibular aqueduct

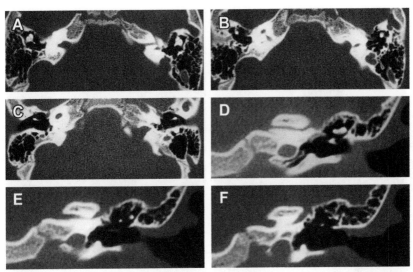

Fig. 1. Computed tomography (CT) scan of a patient with a common cavity deformity on the right and complete cochleovestibular aplasia on the left. Axial sections (*A–C*) are depicted from superior to inferior. Image *B* demonstrates the internal auditory canal on the right communicating with the common cavity. Image *A* demonstrates a narrow internal auditory canal on the left containing only a facial nerve. Coronal sections through the left temporal bone (*D–F*) demonstrate the absence of the otic capsule with only the carotid and facial nerve canals visible in the region. The tensor tympani muscle is seen in image *D*. This patient was successfully implanted in the right ear.

the second most common described, and comprised 26% of the study by Jackler and colleagues[2] (**Fig. 4**).

The classification scheme proposed by Jackler and colleagues is not all-inclusive. There are varieties of disorders that may be encountered that defy classification, as the investigators well noted. A very narrow internal auditory canal of a diameter 2 to 2.5 mm or less on either conventional tomography or CT has been reported in association with a normal inner ear as well as a variety of inner ear malformations.[8–11] This condition has been reported unilaterally and bilaterally, in association with a variety of other congenital anomalies and as an isolated disorder. The clinical significance of this finding with regard to preimplant evaluation is that there is a high likelihood that this represents the presence of only a facial nerve and the absence of the cochleovestibular nerve. A CT scan demonstrating an internal auditory canal of less than 2 to 2.5 mm is considered by many investigators to be an absolute contraindication to cochlear implantation.[8,9,12] Evaluation of the contents of the contents of the internal auditory canal using MR imaging may be warranted in selected patients, as increased experience is being gained with high-resolution scanning techniques.

There is also a particular form of X-linked deafness that has been both radiographically described and genetically identified.[9,13,14] It is seen in some severely deaf males who possess a deficiency of bone between the lateral end of bulbous internal auditory canal and the basal turn of the cochlea.[9] It has been detailed by both CT and MR imaging, and holds the clinical implications that there is an obvious large communication between the CSF-containing internal auditory canal and the cochlea. This situation also presents the concern that a multichannel electrode array may be introduced into the internal canal at the time of implantation.

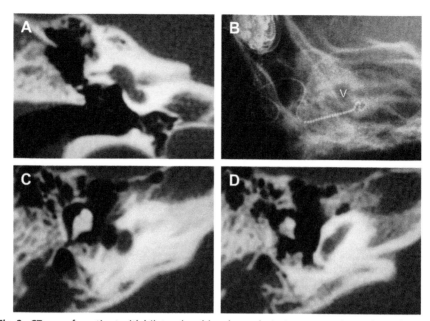

Fig. 2. CT scan of a patient with bilateral cochlear hypoplasia. Images are shown from the right temporal bone, which was successfully implanted. A coronal section (*A*) through the vestibule demonstrates the relatively normal formation of the vestibular apparatus as well as the presence of an oval window. The oval window and ossicles are also seen in axial image (*C*); these are useful surgical landmarks because they allow for the formation of a topographic roadmap when implanting abnormal cochleae. Only the proximal basal turn of the cochlea is present. (*D*) The middle or apical turns are absent. Image (*B*) is an intraoperative transorbital plain radiograph of the multichannel electrode array implanted in this patient; this is the expected appearance of the array placed into this small cavity. Note that the morphology is quite similar to the coronal section in image *A*. The vestibule (V) is marked for reference.

In summary, the specific terminology used is less important than the detail in which reported cases are described with regard to radiographic and histologic features of each element of the inner ear: specific cochlear morphology; size and relation to the vestibule; patency of the bony modiolus; and the nature of inner ear aqueducts. Jumping to conclusions regarding their association with various clinical features such as hearing, implantation outcome, and complications may in this way be avoided.

Patient evaluation
Initial radiologic evaluation of the cochlear implant candidate is typically performed with high-resolution CT scanning. Patients with a malformed inner ear or narrow internal auditory canal may undergo supplemental MR imaging. MR imaging of inner ear malformations requires different parameters to those commonly used in the evaluation of adult hearing loss. The acquisition of appropriate images requires higher resolution and magnets of greater strength.[15,16] Intravenous contrast is rarely used. The reasons for obtaining MR imaging in a patient with an inner ear anomaly are twofold: identification of nonosseous partitioning of the malformed cochlea and identification of the neural structures contained within the internal auditory canal (**Fig. 5**). CT and MR studies are only macroscopic evaluations of the cochleovestibular apparatus; form does not necessarily imply function. Evidence of the existence of

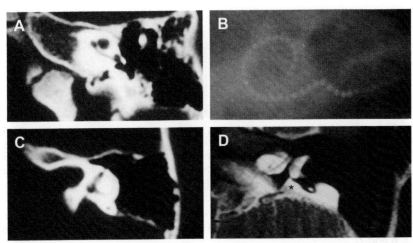

Fig. 3. Images from a patient with bilateral incomplete partition. Axial CT scan (*A*) clearly depicts an intact basal turn and confluent middle and apical turns. Note that a multichannel electrode array was implanted nearly a full turn with a few stiffening rings remaining outside the cochleostomy (*B*). This patient also has a wide vestibular aqueduct, as seen in the axial CT image (*C*) as well as in the T2-weighted magnetic resonance (MR) image (*D*) marked by an asterisk. Intraoperatively, egress of CSF was easily controlled with packing of fascia around the array at the cochleostomy.

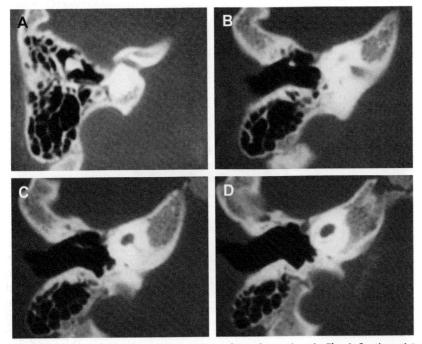

Fig. 4. Axial CT scan of the right temporal bone from the patient in **Fig. 1**. Sections *A* to *D* are depicted from superior to inferior. Note the labyrinthine facial nerve passing anteriorly and superiorly to the common cochleovestibular chamber. (*A*) In this patient the semicircular canals are absent. The bony cochlear aqueduct is visible in images *C* and *D*.

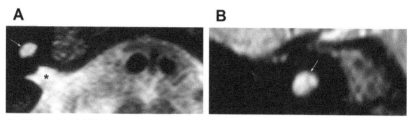

Fig. 5. T2-weighted MR images demonstrating nonosseous partitioning of a common cavity. These images are from the inner ear shown in **Fig. 4.** (*A*) Note the bright signal from fluid seen in the internal auditory canal (*asterisk*) and the cochleovestibular chamber in the axial section. There are low signal intensity septations visible within the common cavity on both the axial (*A*) and coronal (*B*) images that are not seen on CT scanning (*arrows*).

a stimulable auditory neural pathway, either by documentation of prior or residual hearing or by use of promontory stimulation testing, predict a more favorable outcome (**Figs. 6** and **7**).

A few cochleovestibular anomalies do preclude implantation. Complete labyrinthine aplasia would be an absolute contraindication for implantation on the affected side. The determination of cochlear aplasia should involve the careful differentiation from a common cavity deformity by a combination of MR imaging and promontory stimulation in selected patients, to evaluate the possible presence of an adjacent stimulable cochlear nerve ganglion cell population. The failure to identify a cochlear nerve by high-resolution MR imaging would also contraindicate implantation regardless of the presence of an implantable cavity.

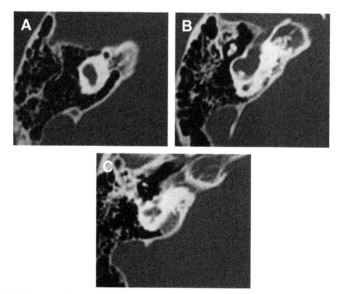

Fig. 6. Axial CT images in another patient with a common cavity deformity. Michel aplasia was present on the contralateral side. Sections *A* to *C* are depicted from superior to inferior. Note the formation of rudimentary semicircular canals (*B*). The internal auditory canal becomes apparent in section *C*. This patient demonstrated some preoperative subjective auditory sensations and language development. Moreover, promontory stimulation indicated the presence of auditory perception. She was successfully implanted with a multichannel device, and currently derives significant benefit from implant use.

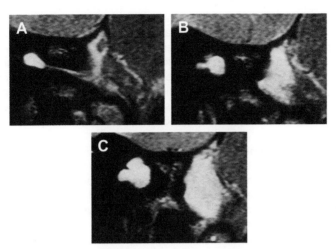

Fig. 7. T2-weighted coronal MR images of the inner ear depicted in **Fig. 6**. Images *A* to *C* are depicted from anterior to posterior. Note the narrow internal auditory canal leading to the fluid containing common cochleovestibular cavity (*A*). Images (*B*) and (*C*) demonstrate the formation of rudimentary semicircular canals that also contain fluid.

With careful patient selection and preoperative planning, using the various imaging and electrophysiologic testing modalities available, and employing experienced device programmers, many patients with a variety of cochlear malformations have been successfully implanted.[17–24]

Is There Evidence of Luminal Obstruction?

In the absence of morphologic contraindications to implantation, the next question that must be answered is: is there any evidence of luminal obstruction? Inner ear inflammation, abnormalities of bone metabolism or trauma, may ultimately result in luminal obstruction either by ingrowth of fibrous scar tissue or pathologic neo-ossification. The origin most commonly encountered, especially in pediatric cochlear implant candidates, is postmeningitic labyrinthitis ossificans. Other postinflammatory causes include suppurative labyrinthitis secondary to otitis media or cholesteatoma, and hematogenous infections (septicemia, mumps, rubella, or other viral infections). Metabolic bone disorders include otosclerosis and Paget disease. Common posttraumatic causes include labyrinthectomy and temporal bone fractures. Wegener granulomatosis and autoimmune inner diseases such as Cogan syndrome have also been reported to result in labyrinthine ossification.[25–28]

Bacterial meningitis is the most common cause of acquired severe sensorineural hearing loss in children.[29] In retrospective analyses some degree of hearing loss has been reported to develop in 7% to 29% of survivors of meningitis.[30,31] Deafness may follow bacterial meningitis in children in 2% to 7% of cases, with 1.5% being severe and bilateral.[29,32] The organisms commonly responsible for postmeningitic deafness are *Haemophilus influenzae* and *Streptococcus pneumoniae*. *Neisseria meningitidis* is also a causative organism, though is believed to result in a lower incidence of postinfectious deafness.[32,33] Although most series report *H influenzae* as the leading causative organism in most meningitic deafness, it is of note that a greater proportion of children surviving pneumococcal meningitis (33%) develop hearing loss, as opposed to *H influenzae* type b (9%) or meningococcal meningitis

(5%).[29,31,34] Pneumococcal meningitis, which presents a gram-positive exotoxin, is additionally associated with severe ossification, whereas the ossification associated with *Haemophilus* is generally less severe, owing to the effects of endotoxins that may be diminished by corticosteroids.[29,32] Some degree of cochlear neo-ossification may be encountered intraoperatively in as many as 70% of patients deafened by meningitis.[35] In series including all causes of deafness, some degree of basal-turn cochlear neo-ossification has been reported in approximately 15% of adult patients and in as many as 28% to 35% of pediatric patients.[36–38]

Pathophysiology of labyrinthine ossification

The cochlear aqueduct is a bony channel that connects the subarachnoid space of the posterior cranial fossa to the scala tympani. It opens adjacent to the round window and is lined with a loose network of fibrous tissue termed the "periotic duct," which is an extension of the arachnoid.[39] This location is believed to be the site of origin of the inflammatory process into the inner ear in cases of meningitis. Other possible routes include the internal auditory canal and modiolus, the middle ear windows secondary to otitis media, lateral canal fistulization secondary to chronic inflammatory processes, trauma, and hematogenous spread.[40,41] When encountered, ossification is nearly always most severe in the region of the round window and proximal scala tympani in the basal turn, adjacent to the opening of the cochlear aqueduct.[28] The middle and apical turns are less commonly affected and the scala vestibuli is often spared.[17] Because most cases of labyrinthitis ossificans are partial and the extent of obstruction commonly manifests asymmetrically within an individual patient, preoperative imaging plays an essential role in selection of which side to implant.[42] Total cochlear ossification may occur, and is more commonly seen in children than in adults.[17,43]

Cochlear ossification following meningitis is associated with a severe loss of cochlear hair cells as well as a decreased spiral ganglion cell population.[44] There is no clearly predictable relationship between the extent of ossification and the number of injured spiral ganglion cells.[45] Hinojosa and colleagues[46] studied the temporal bones of deaf patients with labyrinthitis ossificans, and found that the remaining neuronal cell population ranged from 6310 to 28,196 with a mean of 17,152; this in comparison with the total cochlear neuronal population of approximately 35,500 in the human infant.[47] Linthicum and colleagues[48] studied the postmortem effects of implants on neuronal population and found that benefit may occur with as few as 3300 neurons. Cochlear ossification does not contraindicate cochlear implantation per se; it does, however, complicate electrode insertion.[49]

There are several theories regarding the pathogenesis of labyrinthine neo-ossification. In 1936 Druss[50] described two types of new bone: metaplastic bone originates from ingrown fibrous scar or connective tissue while osteoplastic bone originates from the adjacent otic capsule after disruption of the endosteum. Postlabyrinthitis ossification is thought to occur via the metaplastic process. During the initial acute stage of infection, bacteria within the perilymphatic spaces induce an acute inflammatory reaction characterized by leukocyte infiltration and fibroblast proliferation.[51] Labyrinthine fibrosis is considered to be the early stage of ossification, and may occur within weeks of initial infection.[28,51,52] Ossification eventually ensues, and this is termed the osseous or late stage of labyrinthitis ossificans. According to Suigiura and Paparella,[51,53] undifferentiated mesenchymal cells originating in the endosteum, modiolar spaces, and basilar membrane likely differentiate into fibroblasts and either subsequently or directly into osteoblasts, and form local or diffuse osseous deposits.

Several investigators have postulated that the pathogenesis of metaplastic bone formation may be related to disruptions of cochlear blood supply, which has been demonstrated experimentally and observed histologically in the temporal bones of patients having undergone a variety of surgical procedures.[25,54–58] This theory has been claimed to be supported by cell culture experiments performed by Gorham and Test,[59] in which low oxygen tension favors bone formation while high oxygen tension favors osteoclastic resorption. Additional investigators have commented on the similar findings between the ossification of vascular occlusion and those of suppurative labyrinthitis.[51,53]

The two types of neo-ossification were further characterized in histologic studies performed by Kotzias and Linthicum[25] on human temporal bones with a variety of pathologic processes including patients who had undergone a variety of neuro-otologic procedures. The metaplastic form is characterized by high cellularity and the relative absence of eosinophilia. There are no osteoblasts on the surface. Although its margins are indistinct, it is confined to the lumen of the cochlea. The osteoplastic form occurs only when there has been disruption of the endosteum, such as occurs during trauma or a surgical defect. It is characterized by less cellularity and increased eosinophilia, and is characteristically lamellar in form, with clear margins and osteoblasts on the surface and not clearly distinct from the endosteal layer.

The postmeningitic neo-ossification is thought to occur via the metaplastic process with the ectopic bone being typically chalky white, whereas the native otic capsule bone is generally ivory in hue.[35] The difference in color and its being confined to the lumen of the cochlea aids in differentiation of the neo-ossified bone and the native otic capsule while drilling the ossified cochlea during the implantation procedure.

Advanced otosclerosis may in rare cases cause luminal obstruction that is usually limited to the round window or first few millimeters of the scala tympani.[12,25,28] It has been suggested by Kotzias and Linthicum[25] that the otosclerotic process may damage the endosteal layer, resulting in the osteoplastic form of neo-ossification. Green and colleagues[28] histologically identified foci of otosclerosis within the areas of neo-ossification. Moreover, all their specimens demonstrated the pathology to be limited to the first 6 mm of the basal turn in the scala tympani. The pattern of ossification induced by trauma is less predictable.[12]

Evaluation of cochlear patency by CT scanning

Multiple investigators have reported discrepancies between the CT interpretation of cochlear patency and the findings at implant surgery, likely due in part to the thicker image slices available at the time these studies were performed, as well as the early stage of experience of the image interpreters. Early fibro-ossific changes are frequently encountered during surgery in postmeningitic patients and are frequently not identified on CT scanning, which would be especially likely when there is little ossification within the fibrous matrix.[30,42,60] The time course for metaplastic ossification is quite variable but is thought to begin with fibrosis as early as 8 days to a few weeks after the initial insult.[25,28,51,52,54] The ultimate time frame and extent of eventual osseous deposition is variable. It has been reported to be detected as early as 2 months postmeningitis in humans by CT scanning.[52] Evidence of ongoing ossification has also been detected to be present histologically in human temporal bones as late as 30 years after the initial insult.[28]

The reported accuracy of high-resolution CT identification of cochlear ossification has ranged from 53% to greater than 90%.[12,35,61–63] A review of these studies is useful because they detail the pattern and likelihood of ossification found among various etiological factors of deafness as well as the potential pitfalls of CT-scan interpretation with regard to particular regions of the cochlea.

Literature reviews for CT assessment of cochlear patency

Jackler In 1987 Jackler and colleagues[62] compared CT interpretations with intraoperative findings on 35 cochlear implant patients (17 adults and 18 children) with a variety of deafness causes. The group included 1 adult and 7 children deafened by meningitis, making up 23% of the study population. CT scans were performed on a GE 8800 system with 1.5-mm contiguous axial sections processed using a bone algorithm. Axial scans were taken parallel to the infraorbital-meatal line, and coronal scans were tilted 105° from this plane. The CT data were reported as either patent or ossified (partial or complete), and detailed the location (round window, basal turn, middle turn, apical turn).

All patients deafened by meningitis had some degree of ossification found at the time of surgery; however, only 5 of 8 had a preoperative CT interpretation suggesting ossification, with the remaining 3 interpreted as normal. This study yielded a 37% false-negative rate among patients deafened by meningitis. However, looking at the specific case data presented, it is apparent that among the 3 instances of postmeningitic false-negative CT interpretation, 2 had partial ossification limited to the round window and the third had soft tissue in the round window region, and that all cases of basal-turn involvement were correctly identified by CT.

When all causes were considered, there were an additional 3 false-negative CT interpretations making a total of 6 out of 13, or a 46% false-negative rate. This total included one patient with Cogan syndrome who had ossification found in the round window and basal turn and one patient with trauma and basal-turn ossification, as well as one patient with prior malignant otitis externa, who had undetected complete cochlear soft tissue obliteration. All the children with congenital deafness (10) or ototoxicity (1) and all of the adults with progressive familial, viral, syphilis, Ménière, and unknown origins had patent readings on CT and no ossification noted at the time of surgery. The effects that these findings had on insertion and outcome are difficult to ascertain, as the 18 children in the study were implanted with a House 3M single-channel device and no performance data were provided; this is especially true in light of the fact that the great majority of patients today are implanted with long multichannel arrays.

Seicshnaydre In 1992 Seicshnaydre and colleagues[63] compared preoperative CT interpretation with intraoperative findings on 31 children who received a Nucleus multichannel cochlear implant, with scanning done using a high-resolution bone algorithm with slice thicknesses of 1 to 1.5 mm in the axial and coronal plane. These investigators analyzed their data differently from the previous study, considering 4 categories with regard to ossification: normal, narrowed basal turn, bony lip at round window, and ossified cochlea. Their cases were also subdivided into postmeningitic and nonmeningitic causes. A look at their specific data reveals the difficulty in interpreting the more subtle findings of narrowed basal turn and abnormalities of the round window. Among patients whose CT scans were interpreted as positive for narrowing or the basal turn, 71% were true positives and 29% were false-positive interpretations after confirmation at surgery. Of note is that all the false-positive cases were in nonmeningitic cases. When looking at abnormalities of the round window, there was an 80% false-positive rate of interpretation in nonmeningitic cases whereas all the meningitic cases were correctly interpreted.

Seidman In 1994 Seidman and colleagues[35] performed a retrospective comparison of preoperative CT radiologic reports and findings during cochlear implant surgery. CT scans were performed on a GE 9800 system with a slice thickness of 1.5 mm nonoverlapping, and used a high-resolution bone algorithm. Their analysis included 32 patients deafened by meningitis. Whereas 22 (69%) patients were found to have intraoperative evidence of ossification, only 7 were properly identified preoperatively. Ten patients were correctly identified as patent while 15 were falsely identified as patent, yielding a 60% (15/25) false-negative rate for preoperative CT interpretation of cochlear ossification among postmeningitic patients in this study. Of interest, these investigators also reported on one false-positive CT interpretation in a patient with osteogenesis imperfecta with a high-resolution CT scan, suggesting cochlear otospongiotic changes and luminal occlusion.

Langman and Quigley In 1996 Langman and Quigley[64] reported a sensitivity of 100% and specificity of 86% for the identification of cochlear obstruction using CT scans taken at 1.5-mm contiguous slices on a GE 9800 scanner; however, as they pointed out, only 14% of the patients in their study were deafened by meningitis. Langman and Quigley did not report data specific to etiology.

Summary of CT findings In summary, it has been the author's observation as well as those reported in the literature that advances in CT technology and radiologist experience have improved the ability to predict luminal obstruction on the basis of CT scanning, as current technology allows for the routine acquisition of 1-mm slice thicknesses.[12,61] A subset of these patients, particularly those deafened by meningitis, may benefit from MR imaging to help distinguish the early fibrous phases of labyrinthitis ossificans from a patent fluid-filled lumen, as both may appear gray on CT scans.[32,65–67] The evaluation of cochlear patency is initially performed by high-resolution CT scanning. Ossified obstruction can reliably be identified, involving the basal segment in isolation or extending distally into the middle and apical turns. Involvement limited to the basal segment on CT may be further evaluated by MR imaging so that a patent fluid-filled distal lumen may be differentiated from soft-tissue obliteration, as this may influence surgical planning (**Figs. 8–11**).

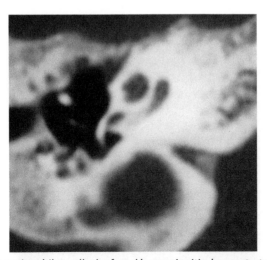

Fig. 8. CT scan of a patient bilaterally deafened by meningitis demonstrates osseous obstruction limited to the proximal basal turn. Although the middle and apical turns appear patent on CT, further evaluation with MR imaging is warranted to further assess the possibility of luminal fibrosis. Note that the relationship between the round window and cochlear aqueduct are nicely demonstrated in this section.

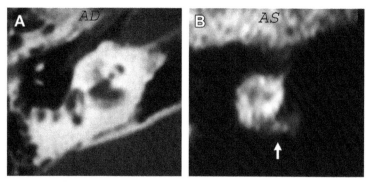

Fig. 9. This patient, bilaterally deafened by meningitis, demonstrated osseous obliteration of the cochlea extending into the middle and apical turns on the right side (*A*). The left cochlea appeared patent by CT scan; however, the coronal MR image (*B*) demonstrates the presence of intermediate signal within the basal turn (*arrow*), suggestive of luminal fibrosis.

Are There Additional Findings that May Complicate the Surgery or Subsequent Patient Management?

The initial objectives of preoperative sectional imaging are the determination of cochlear morphology and luminal patency. Additional useful information may be derived that can optimize safety and facility of surgery, as well as influence subsequent patient management. Proper surgical planning must involve careful review of sectional images so that potential complications may be anticipated and properly managed. Preoperative imaging often provides valuable information that would not preclude implantation, but rather helps assess which would be the technically easier ear to implant.

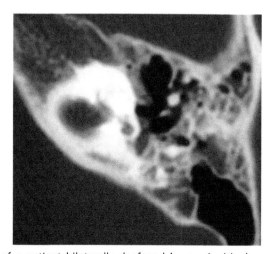

Fig. 10. CT scan of a patient bilaterally deafened by meningitis demonstrates extensive osseous obliteration involving all turns of the cochlea. The opposite side appeared patent. Note the unusual bulbous appearance of the internal auditory canal, which is demonstrated on the T2-weighted MR image in **Fig. 11**.

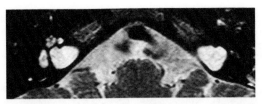

Fig. 11. MR image of the patient depicted in **Fig. 10**. Note the bilaterally abnormal bulbous morphology of the internal auditory canals as demonstrated by the bright signal from cerebrospinal fluid on this T2-weighted image. A bright fluid signal is also present in the lumen of the right cochlea but absent on the left side, which demonstrated extensive osseous obliteration on CT scan.

Vascular anatomy of the ear

Aberrant middle ear vascular anatomy that might complicate mastoidectomy and a facial recess approach to the cochleostomy may be anticipated by the routine acquisition of preoperative CT scanning. An extreme anterior displacement of the sigmoid sinus with approximation against posterior canal wall has been reported in 1.6%, and a high-riding jugular bulb may be present in 6% of the general population.[68] It is rare, though possible, that a jugular bulb or diverticulum may overlie the round window niche or promontory (**Fig. 12**). The distance between the round window and carotid artery may be determined in cases where a drill-out procedure is planned. Abnormal course or dehiscence of the carotid canal may also be detected.

Facial nerve

Preoperative CT scanning is especially useful in identifying the position of the aberrant facial nerve that may be associated with cochlear malformations. It has been well documented in such cases that the course of the facial nerve may be unusual and at increased risk of injury during implantation surgery.[17,69,70] By careful preoperative mapping of the course of the facial nerve canal, such patients may be safely and successfully implanted (**Fig. 13**). Careful review of the position of the facial nerve is

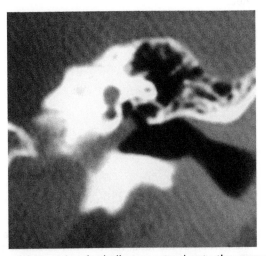

Fig. 12. Note how a dehiscent jugular bulb may extend onto the promontory, potentially interfering with the drilling of a cochleostomy.

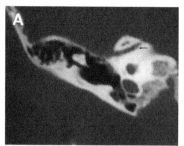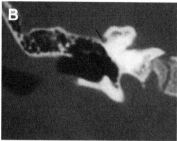

Fig. 13. Coronal CT scan of a patient with a common cavity deformity. (*A*) The facial nerve passes superiorly over the common cochleovestibular chamber (*arrow*). (*B*) A more posterior section, demonstrating that the facial nerve travels along the tegmen (*arrow*). Intraoperatively, the nerve was identified in its descending portion and followed superiorly to the tegmen in the antral region. Here, it formed its second genu with the tympanic portion that coursed along the tegmen tympani, as seen in image *B*. Preoperative knowledge of this anomalous course was felt to enhance the surgical safety of cochlear implantation in this patient.

also warranted in patients without cochlear malformations, as there may be dehiscence of the intratympanic portion that may be encountered during approach to the cochleostomy site.

In some patients with otosclerosis, the presence of spongiotic bone between the apical turn of the cochlea and the pregeniculate facial nerve canal permits unwanted stimulation of the facial nerve during implant use.[71] Careful analysis of the CT study helps to anticipate that certain electrodes will require deprogramming (**Fig. 14**).

Mastoid and tympanic cavity

The mastoid air cell system and tympanic cavity should also be included in the analysis of preoperative CT studies. The degree of mastoid pneumatization is especially useful information when operating on very young children. Though considered fully developed at birth, the depth of the facial recess as well as its degree of pneumatization may be anticipated.

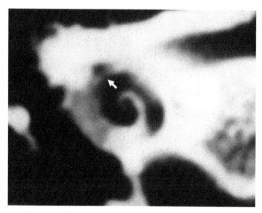

Fig. 14. CT scan of a patient with otosclerosis. Note the otospongiotic changes present adjacent to the labyrinthine portion of the facial nerve in this coronal section (*arrow*). Such pathology could predispose the patient to facial nerve stimulation by the electrodes in this region.

Radiographic findings in conjunction with clinical severity may be considered in side selection as well as determination of the most appropriate course of therapy for patients with associated chronic ear disease. Chronic ear disease need not be an absolute contraindication for cochlear implantation if carefully selected patients are managed with staged procedures. Traditional canal wall surgery or a more extensive exenteration with a blind-sac and oversew type of operation is possible in more severe cases. Subsequent implantation may be performed in a stable, well-protected, and well-healed fat-obliterated mastoid cavity.

The usual landmarks for performing mastoidectomy and facial recess may be distorted or absent in patients with cochlear abnormalities. Careful review of CT images is essential in safely performing surgery on these patients. There are often associated morphologic abnormalities of the vestibular system and ossicular chain.[2] Overall, the lateral semicircular canal is considered the most frequently malformed inner ear structure, which is speculated to be a result of its late embryonic formation.[1,2,72,73]

The cochlear aqueduct

There is a consensus that the cochlear aqueduct plays a role in the pathologic process of labyrinthine ossification. Its role in the pathogenesis of spontaneous and intraoperative CSF fistula is less clear. Gushers during stapedectomy have been traditionally hypothesized to be associated with enlargements of the cochlear aqueduct. Jackler and Hwang[74] doubted that the cochlear aqueduct plays a significant role in the etiology of CSF fistula. Radiographic reports of cochlear aqueduct enlargement are rare.[75] Jackler and Hwang recommended that radiographic enlargement should be reported as a diameter exceeding 2 mm in its narrowest mid otic capsule portion. These investigators pointed out that the lateral otic capsule portion of the cochlear aqueduct is consistently narrow despite variability in the medial opening into the subarachnoid space, and is filled with a complex mesh of loose connective tissue.[74,76]

Traditional arguments implicating the cochlear aqueduct as the source of CSF fistula assert that despite the presence of the tissue mesh, there is a contiguous lumen.[74,77] Jackler and Hwang,[74] however, suggest that there is no correlation between the clinical scenario of perilymphatic gusher and demonstrable radiographic enlargements of the cochlear aqueduct, even casting doubt on the existence in the literature of radiographically demonstrable enlargements of the lateral otic capsule portion of the cochlear aqueduct. Others have argued that even slight increases in the diameter may cause increases in flows, which may be at measurements smaller than can be detected on CT.[78] It has been rebutted, however, that this argument does not take into account the baffling effect of the membranous mesh.[74]

It is plausible, nonetheless, that the cochlear aqueduct may account for the "oozer" but not the "gusher" seen on entering the vestibule during stapes surgery.[79] It is also possible that a similar pathogenesis may exist when easily controllable pulsatile perilymph is encountered during implant surgery at the time of cochleostomy. Its potential management should be anticipated if the presence of an abnormally enlarged cochlear aqueduct is seen on a preoperative CT scan of the implant candidate.

There is at least on case report in the literature, from 1982, of a 15-year-old boy with normal hearing in whom a CSF fistula between the posterior fossa and middle ear via and enlarged cochlear aqueduct was demonstrated by both metrizamide and Pantopaque contrast cisternography performed using conventional polytomography and CT scanning.[80] Middle ear exploration reportedly revealed CSF leaking through a defect in the round window, which was patched. Two years later, during neurosurgical exploration via craniotomy for the treatment of recurrent CSF rhinorrhea and pneumococcal meningitis, it was reported that a tube of arachnoid was passing through a bony defect at the level of the cochlear aqueduct. This tube was believed to be successfully obliterated with muscle, with subsequent resolution of the CSF rhinorrhea and meningitis. The patient was reported as having otherwise normal inner ears and preservation of hearing.

A more likely encounterable and well-documented etiology for CSF leakage is through defective partitioning between the internal auditory canal fundus and the malformed inner ear.[74,80,81] This situation was also documented in the aforementioned article by Park and colleagues[80] in 2 other patients managed for recurrent meningitis and CSF fistula with demonstrable cochlear malformations. Both were children with unilateral deafness and inner ear malformations. One had a unilateral incomplete partition or classic Mondini deformity, and the other had bilateral dilated enlargements of the cochlea and vestibule.

The vestibular aqueduct

The association of enlargement of the vestibular aqueduct and congenital sensorineural hearing loss is well recognized.[6,22,82–86] Radiographically, it may occur in conjunction with other identifiable inner ear anomalies as previously discussed, or as an isolated finding on CT or MR imaging (see **Fig. 3**; **Fig. 15**).[85–91] Radiographic enlargement has been reported using different imaging modalities and criteria, but is generally considered to exist when the aqueduct's diameter is greater than 1.5 to 2.0 mm at its midpoint, measured between the common crus and the external aperture into the posterior fossa.[85,92–94]

The large vestibular aqueduct syndrome is traditionally considered to be a distinct clinical entity in patients with radiographic evidence of enlargement of the vestibular aqueduct.[85,86] Hearing loss is typically bilateral and progressive, with stepwise decrements often associated with episodes of relatively minor head trauma. Moreover, enlargement of the vestibular aqueduct is considered to be a relatively common finding in children with congenital sensorineural hearing loss.[74,85,86] Some investigators regard it as the single most common radiographic finding among patients with congenital sensorineural hearing loss.[74]

The major traditional hypothesis regarding the pathogenesis of this anomaly involves aberrant or arrested development of the endolymphatic duct and sac system, which is based on the observation that in early embryogenesis the duct is shorter,

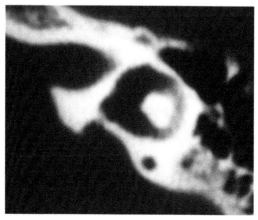

Fig. 15. Axial CT image in a deaf child with an enlarged vestibular aqueduct.

straighter, and proportionally much broader than in later maturity.[85] As more experience has been gained with MR scanning, the defect is currently being described and studied as one involving the entire endolymphatic duct and sac system.[87-91]

There is also some recent evidence supporting a familial component to the disorder.[95] Some recent work is also being done to investigate its genetics basis as well as its association with other known syndromes.[93,96] There are a variety of speculative causes of the hearing loss associated with this disorder based mostly on clinical, radiographic, and surgical observations, as well as some analyses of endolymphatic chemical composition. Among them are: damage secondary to transduction of intracranial CSF pressures; reflux of protein-rich hyperosmolar endolymph from endolymphatic sac into the cochlea through the widely patent duct; and inherent functional abnormalities of endolymphatic sac system leading to abnormal intracochlear fluid composition and dynamics.[85,91,92,94,97] Analyses using high-resolution CT scanning have been able to demonstrate associated modiolar defects in patients with large vestibular aqueducts, further speculating as to the etiology of the associated hearing loss and CSF leaks.[94,98]

The clinical significance of radiographic enlargements of vestibular aqueduct and endolymphatic duct and sac system with regard to the cochlear implant candidate is twofold. It may serve as both a diagnosis and an indicator of the potential for the need to manage an intraoperative CSF leak at the time of cochleostomy. Despite this risk, many such patients have been safely and successfully implanted with the appropriate management.[22,24,99]

Retrocochlear pathology

Appropriate evaluation of retrocochlear pathology with MR imaging must be considered in selected cases, this being especially true in adult patients who have lost hearing in a previously sole hearing ear.

SUMMARY

In summary, preoperative sectional imaging is a vital tool for confirming the presence and nature of an implantable cochlear lumen. Imaging analysis should include the detection of malformations, luminal obstruction, and anatomic variants or middle ear pathology that could complicate the implantation process. Preimplant evaluation of these patients is often complex, taking into account a variety of clinical and electrophysiological data. Appropriate preparedness and experience in handling the potential complications, especially as regards intraoperative CSF leak and facial nerve anomalies, is necessary for safe management. Numerous reports attest to the benefits received by these patients from cochlear implants.[17-24,36]

REFERENCES

1. Jensen J. Malformations of the inner ear in deaf children. Acta Radiol Suppl 1969; 286:1–97.
2. Jackler RK, Luxford WM, House WF. Congenital malformations of the inner ear: a classification based on embryogenesis. Laryngoscope 1987;97(Suppl 40): 2–14.
3. Schuknecht HF, Gulya AJ. Anatomy of the temporal bone with surgical implications. Philadelphia: Lea & Febiger; 1986.
4. Mondini C. Minor works of Carlo Mondini: the anatomical section of a boy born deaf. Am J Otol 1997;18:288–93.

5. Swartz JD, Harnsberger HR. Imaging of the temporal bone. 2nd edition. New York: Thieme Medical Publishers, Inc; 1992.
6. Schuknecht HF. Mondini dysplasia: a clinical and pathological study. Ann Otol Rhinol Laryngol Suppl 1980;89(1 Pt 2):1–23.
7. Phelps PD. Cochlear dysplasias and meningitis. Am J Otol 1994;15(4):551–7.
8. Shelton C, Luxford WM, Tonokawa LL, et al. The narrow internal auditory canal in children: a contraindication to cochlear implants. Otolaryngol Head Neck Surg 1989;100(3):227–31.
9. Phelps PD. Cochlear implants for congenital deformities. J Laryngol Otol 1992; 106(11):967–70.
10. Phelps PD, Lloyd GA, Sheldon PW. Deformity of the labyrinth and internal auditory meatus in congenital deafness. Br J Radiol 1975;48:973–8.
11. Naunton RF, Valvassori GE. Inner ear anomalies: their association with atresia. Laryngoscope 1968;78:1041–9.
12. Lo WM. Imaging of cochlear and auditory brain stem implantation. AJNR Am J Neuroradiol 1998;19:1147–54.
13. Phelps PD, Reardon W, Pembry ME, et al. X-linked deafness, stapes gushers and a distinctive defect of the inner ear. Neuroradiology 1991;33:326–30.
14. Reardon W, Middelton-Price HR, Sandkuijl L, et al. A multipedigree linkage study of X-linked deafness: linkage to Xq13-q12 and evidence for genetic heterogeneity. Genomics 1991;11:885–94.
15. Casselman JW, Kuhweide R, Deimling M, et al. Constructive interference in steady state-3DFT MR imaging of the inner ear and cerebellopontine angle. AJNR Am J Neuroradiol 1993;14(1):47–57.
16. Casselman JW, Kuhweide R, Ampe W, et al. Pathology of the membranous labyrinth: comparison of T1 and T2-weighted and gadolinium-enhanced spin-echo and 3DFT-CISS imaging. AJNR Am J Neuroradiol 1993;14(1):59–69.
17. Molter DW, Pate BR, McElveen JT. Cochlear implantation in the congenitally malformed ear. Otolaryngol Head Neck Surg 1993;108:174–7.
18. Jackler RK, Luxford WM, House WF. Sound detection with the cochlear implant in five ears of four children with congenital malformations of the cochlea. Laryngoscope 1987;97(Suppl 40):2–14.
19. Silverstein H, Smouha E, Morgan N. Multichannel cochlear implantation in a patient with bilateral Mondini deformities. Am J Otol 1988;9:451–5.
20. Tucci DL, Telian SA, Zimmerman-Philips MS, et al. Cochlear implantation in patients with cochlear malformations. Arch Otolaryngol Head Neck Surg 1995; 121:833–8.
21. Slattery WH III, Luxford WM. Cochlear implantation in the congenital malformed cochlea. Laryngoscope 1995;105:1184–7.
22. Woolley AL, Jenison V, Stroer BS, et al. Cochlear implantation in children with inner ear malformations. Ann Otol Rhinol Laryngol 1998;107(6):492–500.
23. Weber BP, Lenarz T, Dillo W, et al. Malformations in cochlear implant patients. Am J Otol 1997;18:S64–5.
24. Hoffman RA, Downey LL, Waltzman SB, et al. Cochlear implantation in children with cochlear malformations. Am J Otol 1997;18(2):184–7.
25. Kotzias SA, Linthicum FH. Labyrinthine ossification: differences between two types of ectopic bone. Am J Otol 1985;6:490–4.
26. Suga F, Lindsay JR. Labyrinthitis ossificans. Ann Otol Rhinol Laryngol 1977;86: 17–29.
27. Rarey KE, Bicknell JM, Davis LE. Intralabyrinthine osteogenesis in Cogan's syndrome. Am J Otolaryngol 1986;7:387–90.

28. Green JD Jr, Marion MS, Hinojosa R. Labyrinthitis ossificans: histopathologic considerations for cochlear implantation. Otolaryngol Head Neck Surg 1991; 104:320–6.

29. Becker TS, Eisenberg LS, Luxford WM, et al. Labyrinthine ossification secondary to childhood bacterial meningitis: implications for cochlear implant surgery. AJNR Am J Neuroradiol 1984;5:539–741.

30. Johnson MH, Hasenstab MS, Seicshnaydre MA, et al. CT of postmeningitic deafness: observations and predictive value for cochlear implants in children. AJNR Am J Neuroradiol 1995;16:103–9.

31. Kaplan SL, Catlin FL, Weaver T, et al. Onset of hearing loss in children with bacterial meningitis. Pediatrics 1984;73:575–8.

32. Silberman B, Garabedian EN, Denoyelle F, et al. Role of modern imaging technology in the implementation of pediatric cochlear implants. Ann Otol Rhinol Laryngol 1995;104:42–6.

33. Dodge PR, Davis H, Feigin RD, et al. Prospective evaluation of hearing impairment as a sequela of acute bacterial meningitis. N Engl J Med 1984;311:869–74.

34. Berlow SJ, Calderelli DD, Matz FJ, et al. Bacterial meningitis and sensorineural hearing loss: a prospective investigation. Laryngoscope 1980;90:1445–52.

35. Seidman DA, Chute PM, Parisier S. Temporal bone imaging for cochlear implantation. Laryngoscope 1994;104:562–5.

36. Balkany T, Gantz B, Nadol JB. Multichannel cochlear implants in partially ossified cochleas. Ann Otol Rhinol Laryngol 1988;97:3–7.

37. Harnsberger HR, Dart DJ, Parkin JL, et al. Cochlear implant candidates: assessment with CT and MR imaging. Radiology 1987;164:53–7.

38. Luxford WM, House WF. House 3M cochlear implant: surgical considerations. International Cochlear Implant Symposium and Workshop—Melbourne, 1985. Clark GM, Busby PA (eds). Ann Otol Rhinol Laryngol Suppl 1987;96(128):12–4.

39. Schuknecht HF. Pathophysiology. In: Schuknecht HF, editor. Pathology of the ear. 2nd edition. Philadelphia: Lea and Febiger; 1993. p. 77–113.

40. Igarashi M, Shuknecht HF. Pneumococcic otitis media, meningitis and labyrinthitis. Arch Otolaryngol 1962;76:126–30.

41. Igarashi M, Saito R, Alford BR, et al. Temporal bone findings in pneumococcal meningitis. Arch Otolaryngol 1974;99:79–83.

42. Balkany T, Dreisbach J, Cohen N, et al. Workshop: surgical anatomy and radiologic imaging of cochlear implant surgery. Am J Otol 1987;8:195–200.

43. Ketten D. The role of temporal bone imaging in cochlear implants. Curr Opin Otolaryngol Head Neck Surg 1994;2:401–8.

44. Otte J, Shucknecht HF, Kerr AG. Ganglion cell populations in normal and pathological human cochlea. Implications for cochlear implantation. Laryngoscope 1978;88:1231–45.

45. Saunders M, Fortnum HM, O'Donaghue GM, et al. Retrospective analysis of children profoundly deafened by bacterial meningitis [abstract no. 34]. In: Lutman ME, Archbold SM, O'Donaghue GM, editors. First European symposium on paediatric cochlear implantation. Nottingham (England): Nottingham Paediatric Implant Programme; 1992.

46. Hinojosa R, Green JD Jr, Marion MS. Ganglion cell populations in labyrinthitis ossificans. Am J Otol 1991;12(Suppl):3–7.

47. Schuknecht HF. Anatomy. In: Schuknecht HF, editor. Pathology of the ear. 2nd edition. Philadelphia: Lea and Febiger; 1993. p. 31–75.

48. Linthicum FH Jr, Fayad J, Otto S, et al. Inner ear morphologic changes resulting from cochlear implantation. Am J Otol 1991;12(Suppl):8–10.

49. Balkany T, Gantz BJ, Steenerson RL, et al. Systematic approach to electrode insertion in the ossified cochlea. Otolaryngol Head Neck Surg 1991;114:4–11.
50. Druss JG. Labyrinthitis secondary to meningococcic meningitis: a clinical and histopathologic study. Arch Otolaryngol 1936;24:19–28.
51. Suigiura S, Paparella MM. The pathology of labyrinthine ossification. Laryngoscope 1967;77:1974–89.
52. Novak MA, Fifer RC, Barkmeier JC, et al. Labyrinthine ossification after meningitis: its implications for cochlear implantation. Otolaryngol Head Neck Surg 1990;103:351–6.
53. Paparella MM, Sugiura S. The pathology of suppurative labyrinthitis. Ann Otol Rhinol Laryngol 1967;76:554–86.
54. Kimura R, Perlman HB. Arterial obstruction of the labyrinth. Part I: Cochlear changes. Part II: Vestibular changes. Ann Otol Rhinol Laryngol 1958;67: 5–40.
55. Belal A. Pathology as it relates to ear surgery. III: surgery of the cerebello-pontine angle tumors. J Laryngol Otol 1983;97:101–15.
56. Belal A, Ylikoski J. Pathology as it relates to ear surgery. II: Labyrinthectomy. J Laryngol Otol 1983;97:1–10.
57. Belal A, Linthicum FH Jr, House WF. Middle fossa vestibular nerve section. A histopathological report. Am J Otol 1979;1:72–9.
58. Belal A. The effects of vascular occlusion on the human inner ear. J Laryngol Otol 1979;93:955–68.
59. Gorham LW, Test WT. Circulatory changes in osteolytic and osteoblastic reaction. Arch Pathol 1964;78:673–80.
60. Jackler RK, Luxford WM, Schindler RA, et al. Cochlear implant candidates: assessment with CT and MR imaging. Radiology 1987;164:53–7.
61. Frau GN, Luxford WM, Lo WM, et al. High resolution computed tomography in evaluation of cochlear patency in implant candidates: a comparison with surgical findings. J Laryngol Otol 1994;108:743–8.
62. Jackler RK, Luxford WM, Schindler RA, et al. Cochlear patency problems in cochlear implantation. Laryngoscope 1987;97:801–5.
63. Seicshnaydre MA, Johnson MH, Hasenstab MS, et al. Cochlear implants in children: reliability of computed tomography. Otolaryngol Head Neck Surg 1992;107: 410–7.
64. Langman AW, Quigley SM. Accuracy of high resolution computed tomography in cochlear implantation. Otolaryngol Head Neck Surg 1996;114(1):38–43.
65. Lasig R, Terwey B, Battmer RD, et al. Magnetic resonance imaging (MRI) and high resolution computer tomography (HRCT) in cochlear implant candidates. Scand Audiol Suppl 1988;30:197–200.
66. Yune HY, Miyamoto RT, Yune ME. Medical imaging in cochlear implant candidates. Am J Otol 1991;12(Suppl):11–7.
67. Phelps PD. Fast spin echo MRI in otology. J Laryngol Otol 1994;108:383–94.
68. Tomura N, Sashi R, Kobayashi M, et al. Normal variations of the temporal bone on high-resolution CT: their incidence and clinical significance. Clin Radiol 1995;50: 144–8.
69. Curtin HD, Vignaud J, Bar D. Anomaly of the facial canal in a Mondini malformation with recurrent meningitis. Radiology 1982;144:335–41.
70. House JR 3rd, Luxford WN. Facial nerve injury in cochlear implantation. Otolaryngol Head Neck Surg 1993;109:1078–82.
71. Kelsall DC, Shallop JK, Brammeier TG, et al. Facial nerve stimulation after Nucleus 22-channel cochlear implantation. Am J Otol 1997;18(3):336–41.

72. Valvassori GE, Naunton RF, Lindsay JR. Inner ear anomalies: clinical and histo-pathological considerations. Ann Otol Rhinol Laryngol 1969;78(5):929–38.
73. Phelps PD. Congenital lesions of the inner ear demonstrated by polytomography. Arch Otolaryngol 1974;100:11–8.
74. Jackler RK, Hwang PH. Enlargement of the cochlear aqueduct: fact of fiction? Otolaryngol Head Neck Surg 1993;109:14–25.
75. Mukherji SK, Baggett HC, Alley J, et al. Enlarged cochlear aqueduct. AJNR Am J Neuroradiol 1998;19(2):330–2.
76. Anson BJ. The endolymphatic and perilymphatic aqueducts of the human ear: development and adult anatomy of their parietes and contents in relation to oto-logical surgery. Acta Otolaryngol 1965;59:140–51.
77. Palva T, Dammert K. Human cochlear aqueduct. Acta Otolaryngol 1969;(Suppl 246): 1. [PMID:4908516].
78. Allen G. Fluid flow in the cochlear aqueduct and cochlear hydrodynamic consid-erations in perilymph fistula, stapes gusher, and secondary endolymphatic hy-drops. Am J Otol 1987;8:319–22.
79. Schuknecht HF, Reisser C. The morphologic basis for perilymphatic gushers and oozers. Adv Otorhinolaryngol 1988;29:1–12.
80. Park TS, Hoffman HJ, Humphreys RP, et al. Spontaneous cerebrospinal fluid otor-rhea in association with a congenital defect of the cochlear aqueduct and Mon-dini dysplasia. Neurosurgery 1982;11(3):356–62.
81. Burton EM, Keith JW, Linden BE, et al. CSF fistula in a patient with Mondini defor-mity: demonstration by CT cisternography. AJNR Am J Neuroradiol 1990;11(1): 205–7.
82. Beal DD, Davey PR, Lindsay JR. Inner ear pathology of congenital deafness. Arch Otolaryngol 1967;85:134–42.
83. Valvassori GE, Clemis JD. The large vestibular aqueduct syndrome. Laryngo-scope 1978;88:723–8.
84. Valvassori GE. The large vestibular aqueduct and associated anomalies of the inner ear. Otolaryngol Clin North Am 1983;16(1):95–101.
85. Jackler RK, de la Cruz A. The large vestibular aqueduct syndrome. Laryngo-scope 1989;99:1238–43.
86. Levinson MJ, Parisier SC, Jacobs M, et al. The large vestibular aqueduct in chil-dren. Arch Otolaryngol 1989;115:54–8.
87. Hirsch BE, Weissman JL, Curtin HD, et al. Magnetic resonance imaging of the large vestibular aqueduct. Arch Otolaryngol Head Neck Surg 1992;118(10):1124–7.
88. Dahlen RT, Harnsberger HR, Gray SD, et al. Overlapping thin-section fast spin-echo MR of the large vestibular aqueduct syndrome. AJNR Am J Neuroradiol 1997;18(1):67–75.
89. Okamoto K, Ito J, Furusawa T, et al. Large vestibular aqueduct syndrome with high CT density and high MR signal intensity. AJNR Am J Neuroradiol 1997; 18(3):482–4.
90. Phelps PD, Mahoney CF, Luxon LM. Large endolymphatic sac. A congenital deformity of the inner ear shown by magnetic resonance imaging. J Laryngol Otol 1997;111(8):754–6.
91. Okamoto K, Ito J, Furusawa T, et al. MRI of enlarged endolymphatic sacs in the large vestibular aqueduct syndrome. Neuroradiology 1998;40(3):167–72.
92. Welling DB, Martyn MD, Miles BA, et al. Endolymphatic sac occlusion for the enlarged vestibular aqueduct syndrome. Am J Otol 1998;19(2):145–51.
93. Tong KA, Harnsberger HR, Dahlen RT, et al. Large vestibular aqueduct syndrome: a genetic disease? AJR Am J Roentgenol 1997;168(4):1097–101.

94. Antonelli PJ, Agnes NV, Lemmerling MM, et al. Hearing loss with cochlear modiolar defects and large vestibular aqueducts. Am J Otol 1998;19:306–12.
95. Abe S, Usami S, Shinkawa H. Three familial cases of hearing loss associated with enlargement of the vestibular aqueduct. Ann Otol Rhinol Laryngol 1997;106(12):1063–9.
96. Phelps PD, Coffey RA, Trembath RC, et al. Radiological malformations of the ear in Pendred syndrome. Clin Radiol 1998;53(4):268–73.
97. Wilson DF, Hodgson RS, Talbot JM. Endolymphatic sac obliteration for large vestibular aqueduct syndrome. Am J Otol 1997;18(1):101–6 [discussion: 106–7].
98. Lemmerling MM, Mancuso AA, Antonelli PJ, et al. Normal modiolus: CT appearance in patients with a large vestibular aqueduct. Radiology 1997;204:213–9.
99. Aschendorff A, Marangos N, Laszig R. Large vestibular aqueduct syndrome and its implication for cochlear implant surgery. Am J Otol 1997;18(Suppl 6):S57.

Genetic Approach to Evaluation of Hearing Loss

Melinda Cohen, MS, John A. Phillips III, MD*

KEYWORDS

- Genetics • Hearing loss • Inheritance • Syndromic
- Non syndromic • OMIM • Gene reviews

Key Points: GENETIC APPROACH TO EVALUATION OF HEARING LOSS

1. Information on the genetic basis of and testing for disorders with hearing loss is increasing rapidly.

2. Otologists, genetics professionals, and specialized laboratory testing are needed for the diagnosis, education, counseling, and management of patients and families with familial hearing loss.

3. A variety of electronic databases can provide rapid access to information needed on genetic causes of hearing loss.

4. The genetic approach to the evaluation of hearing loss requires otologic, audiologic, and physical examinations; the use of family history; and ancillary and molecular genetic testing.

THE GENETICS REVOLUTION

The Human Genome Project has provided a wealth of information on the sequence and organization of the human genome, which is the genetic equivalent of the Rosetta stone. This data has enabled scientists to decipher the code of the estimated 20,000 genes contained in the approximately 3.3 billion bases of the human genome. In addition, comparisons of the genomes of different normal individuals have shown that about 1 out of 1300 bases differ at a frequency of 1% or more. These frequent variations are referred to as polymorphisms. Thus, every gene is likely to contain polymorphisms, which may be functionally important. In addition, rarer variations that occur in

---

Disclosure statement: none.

Division of Medical Genetics and Genomic Medicine, Vanderbilt University School of Medicine, DD-2205 Medical Center North, Nashville, TN 37232-2578, USA

* Corresponding author.

E-mail address: john.a.phillips@Vanderbilt.Edu

Otolaryngol Clin N Am 45 (2012) 25–39

doi:10.1016/j.otc.2011.08.015

0030-6665/12/$ – see front matter © 2012 Elsevier Inc. All rights reserved.

less than 1% of people can be identified, which, either alone or in combination with environmental factors, can cause human genetic diseases.

New findings on the genetic basis of hearing loss are reported at an ever-increasing rate in a growing variety of books, journals, and databases. Unfortunately, up-to-date information on clinical and laboratory findings of disorders causing hearing loss and the accuracy and availability of genetic tests cannot be found in a single source. Electronic databases can provide medical professionals rapid access to current clinical and genetic information. These electronic databases can be searched interactively for specific symptoms and signs to produce a list of differential diagnoses and access corresponding genetic tests. The use of these databases should improve the ability of otologists to identify rare or recently discovered genetic causes of hearing loss and the subtleties that differentiate the various alternative diagnoses.

Identifying the genetic basis of hearing loss is becoming more useful. For example, newborn screening and molecular testing for hearing loss have enhanced detection and improved the outcome of infants with congenital hearing loss. In this article, the authors review the principles of inheritance, genetic terminology, types of mutations, outline a genetic approach to the diagnosis of hearing loss, show how information on genetic disorders and testing can be obtained, and outline how otologists and geneticists can work together to strengthen the clinical applications of genetics to hearing loss.

GENETIC TERMINOLOGY, GENETIC VARIATIONS, EFFECTS OF VARIATIONS ON GENE FUNCTION, AND FORMS OF INHERITANCE
Selected Genetic Terms

Alleles are versions of a gene that occur at a single locus. When a person has a pair of identical alleles, they are homozygous (a homozygote) and when the alleles are different, they are heterozygous (a heterozygote or carrier).[1] A compound heterozygote is a genotype in which two different mutant alleles of the same gene are present. The terms homozygous, heterozygous, and compound heterozygous can refer to either a person or a genotype.

Expressivity is the severity of expression of the phenotype or the extent to which a genetic defect is expressed. When the severity of disease differs in those who have the same genotype, the phenotype has variable expressivity.

Genotype is the set of different versions of the gene (alleles) that occur at a given locus.

Heterogeneity is explained as follows: Genetic disorders often include several phenotypes that are similar but are actually determined by different genotypes. Genetic *heterogeneity* can result from different mutations at the same locus (allelic heterogeneity), mutations at different loci (locus heterogeneity), or both. Recognition of genetic heterogeneity is important in clinical diagnosis, prognosis, and genetic counseling regarding recurrence risks. Phenotypic heterogeneity occurs when clinically different phenotypes are caused by different mutations in the same gene.

Imprinting is the process by which certain genes or chromosomal regions are modified during meiosis so that gene expression varies depending on parental origin.

Locus is the position occupied by a gene on a chromosome. Different forms of the gene (alleles) can occupy a locus.

Mutation is used in medical genetics in two ways:

1. To indicate a new genetic change that has not been previously known in a kindred
2. To indicate a disease-causing allele

Penetrance is the fraction of individuals with a disease-causing genotype that has any signs or symptoms of the disease. When the frequency of expression of a phenotype is less than 100% (eg, some of those who have the appropriate genotype completely fail to express it), the gene is said to show reduced penetrance. Penetrance is an all-or-none concept.

Phenotype is the observed morphologic, clinical, cellular, or biochemical characteristics determined by genotype and environment (ie, phenotype = genotype + environment).

Pleiotropy means there are multiple phenotypic effects of a single gene or gene pair. Pleiotropy is most often used when the effects are not obviously related.

Uniparental disomy (UPD) occurs when both members of a chromosome pair are inherited from one parent and neither chromosome is inherited from the other parent.

Genetic Variations

Frameshift mutations are insertions or deletions of several codon bases that are not multiples of 3.[1] Such changes disrupt the codon reading frame and usually cause the creation of a premature termination (or stop) codon that ends translation of the encoded protein.

Missense mutations are single base pair substitutions that result in the translation of a different amino acid for the altered codon (unit of 3 bases).

Nonsense mutations introduce a premature termination (or stop) codon that encodes a truncated protein product.

Polymorphism is the occurrence in a population of two or more alleles, each at a frequency of at least 1%. Alleles with a lower frequency than 1% are often referred to as rare variants.

Effects of Variations on Gene Function

In autosomal dominant (AD) disorders, disease occurs despite the presence of a normal gene or allele. There are at least four mechanisms that allow the mutant AD allele to overpower the remaining normal allele and cause AD disorders[1]:

Dominant negative is explained as follows: Instead of a simple deficiency or dysfunction of the protein product, an abnormal protein is synthesized that causes an abnormal phenotype by interfering with the function of the product of the normal allele (dominant negative effect) as is seen in DFNA2A (Online Mendelian Inheritance in Man [OMIM] # 600101) and DFNA9 (OMIM # 601369).[1–3]

Gain of function occurs when the mutant protein can gain properties through mutation (simple gain of function) or become toxic to the cell through acquisition of a novel property as in some forms of DFNA5 (OMIM # 600994).[1–3]

Haploinsufficiency occurs when the contribution of a normal allele is insufficient to prevent disease, because of a loss-of-function mutation of the other allele. A phenotype occurs in heterozygotes despite one of the pair of alleles being fully functional because loss of half of the normal activity of two genes causes disease. Haploinsufficiency often occurs with mutations in genes encoding transcription factors, structural proteins, or cell surface receptors. An example is DFNA2A (OMIM # 600101).[1–3]

Two-hit mutation is an inherited mutation of one copy of some autosomal genes (first hit or mutation). For example, mutations in the neurofibromatosis type 2 (NF2) gene can result in pedigrees with dominantly inherited tumors, such as acoustic neuromas in NF2 (OMIM # 101000). Random loss of the other normal allele caused by a rare event occurring in a somatic cell (second hit or mutation) eliminates both copies of the gene in such cells and renders them cancerous. Thus, although the predisposition to tumors in NF2 is inherited as an AD trait, the mutations that lead to cancer are recessive at the cellular level because both copies of the gene must be dysfunctional for this type of cancer to develop.[1–3]

Forms of Inheritance

Mendelian inheritance

AD inheritance describes a trait or disorder in which the phenotype is expressed in those who have inherited only one copy or allele of a particular gene mutation along with a normal allele.[1] These individuals are referred to as heterozygotes. The term autosomal indicates that the gene resides on one of the 22 pairs of autosomes, which are the non-sex chromosomes. AD disorders are inherited equally by males and females. Offspring of a heterozygous parent have a 50% chance of inheriting the mutation. De novo mutations are those mutations that occur for the first time in the index case. Factors, such as de novo mutations, mosaicism, penetrance, and variable expressivity, can contribute to differences in the recurrence risk or clinical severity of AD disorders.

Autosomal recessive (AR) inheritance describes a trait or disorder in which the phenotype is only expressed in those who have two copies (alleles) of a gene that is mutated at a particular autosomal locus. These individuals are referred to as homozygotes if the mutations in their two alleles are identical and as "compound heterozygotes" if their alleles differ. Carriers are persons who have one mutant allele and one normal allele and who typically do not express the disease phenotype. Unaffected parents of a child with an AR disorder are obligate carriers who have a 25% recurrence risk as a couple. The term consanguinity is used to describe couples who are genetically related and, therefore, more likely to share alleles that cause autosomal recessive disorders.

X-linked dominant (XLD) inheritance describes a dominant trait or disorder in which the phenotype is caused by a mutation in a gene on the X chromosome. Although the phenotype is seen in both females (who are heterozygous) and males (who have only one X chromosome and are, thus, hemizygous), males tend to be more severely affected. Offspring of affected heterozygous females have a 50% risk to inherit the mutation. All of the daughters and none of the sons of affected males inherit the mutation.

X-linked recessive inheritance also describes a trait or disorder in which the phenotype is caused by a mutation in a gene on the X chromosome. It differs from XLD in that the phenotype is seen only in hemizygous males and homozygous females. Although carrier females who have only one copy of the mutation do not usually express the phenotype, some may be affected because of non-random X-chromosome inactivation or, rarely, X-chromosome inactivation as a result of chromosomal translocation involving the healthy allele. Offspring of carrier females have a 50% risk to inherit the mutation and all daughters of affected males are obligate carriers.

Causes of Nonmendelian Inheritance

Imprinting is the process whereby certain genes or chromosomal regions are modified during meiosis so that gene expression varies depending on parental origin. For example, some genes are only expressed if paternally inherited, such as familial paragangliomas with sensorineural hearing loss (OMIM # 168000), whereas others must be maternally inherited to be expressed. Nonmendelian inheritance of a disease can occur if an individual inherits imprinted gene alleles from only one parent such that both copies are silenced.[1,3]

UPD occurs when both members of a chromosome pair are inherited from one parent and neither is inherited from the other parent. An abnormal phenotype and nonmendelian disease expression can occur if the chromosomal region involved includes imprinted genes. For example, one form of retinitis pigmentosa can be caused by uniparental paternal disomy of the USH2A gene (OMIM # 608400).[1,3]

Mitochondrial (MT) inheritance describes a trait or disease that is transmitted through the separate genome of the mitochondria, which are cytoplasmic organelles. Mutations in genes, such as MTRNR1, that cause aminoglycoside-induced deafness (OMIM # 580000) are always maternally inherited because ova contain mitochondria, whereas sperm do not. Related terms include homoplasmy (all mitochondria in a cell have the mutation) or heteroplasmy (some mitochondria have the mutation and some do not).[1-3]

OVERVIEW OF GENETIC DISORDERS CAUSING HEARING LOSS

Genetic disorders that cause hearing loss can be grouped into disorders that are syndromic or nonsyndromic. Disorders that cause syndromic hearing loss are associated with congenital malformations or with medical problems involving other organ systems. In contrast, disorders that cause nonsyndromic hearing loss can have anomalies of the middle or inner ear but do not have congenital anomalies of the external ear or medical problems of other organ systems.[2-6]

Syndromic Hearing Loss

More than 400 genetic syndromes that include hearing loss have been reported, and there are approximately 800 OMIM entries, when accessed in December 2010, that include deafness.[3] Although syndromic hearing loss can account for up to 30% of prelingual deafness, its contribution to all deafness is much smaller. The following syndromic causes of hearing loss will be grouped by their mode of inheritance.[2,3]

Syndromic hearing loss disorders with AD modes of inheritance

Waardenburg syndrome (WS) is the most common AD syndrome causing hearing loss. WS has variable expressivity of sensorineural hearing loss and pigmentary abnormalities of the hair including a white forelock, and the eyes with heterochromic irides. WS1 (OMIM # 193500) has dystopia canthorum or lateral displacement of the inner canthus of the eye, whereas WS2 (OMIM # 193510, 600193, 606662, 608890, 611584) does not. WS3 (OMIM # 148820) has upper-limb anomalies and WS4 (OMIM # 277580, 613265, 613266) has Hirschsprung disease. Because WS1 and WS3 are both caused by PAX3 mutations, they are examples of phenotypic heterogeneity. WS2, caused in some but not all cases by MITF or SNA12 mutations, and WS4, caused by EDNRB, EDN3, or SOX10 mutations, are both examples of locus heterogeneity.[2,3]

Branchio-oto-renal syndrome (BOR) (OMIM # 113650, 610896) is the second most common AD syndrome causing hearing loss. BOR causes conductive, sensorineural, or mixed hearing loss associated with branchial cleft cysts or fistulae; ear anomalies, including preauricular pits; and renal anomalies with high penetrance, but variable expressivity. EYA1 gene mutations are reported to cause BOR1 (OMIM # 113650), whereas SIX5 mutations cause BOR2 (OMIM # 610896).[2,3]

Stickler syndrome is an AD disorder characterized by progressive sensorineural hearing loss, cleft palate, spondyloepiphyseal dysplasia, and osteoarthritis. Stickler syndrome types 1 and 2 (STL1 and STL2, OMIM # 108300, 604841) have severe myopia, and a predisposition to retinal detachment. STL1 and 2 are caused by COL2A1 or COL11A1 mutations, respectively. STL3 (OMIM # 184840), which lacks retinal detachment, is caused by COL11A2 mutations.[2,3]

NF2 (OMIM # 101000) is characterized by hearing loss caused by bilateral acoustic neuromas or vestibular schwannomas. Hearing loss usually begins with unilateral slowly progressing hearing loss in the third decade from a vestibular schwannoma but onset can be bilateral and rapidly progressing. A definitive diagnosis requires magnetic resonance imaging with gadolinium contrast. Individuals with NF2 are at increased risk for meningiomas, astrocytomas and ependymomas. These different tumors represent pleiotropic effects of two-hit NF2 mutations explained previously. Molecular testing of presymptomatic at-risk family members for the NF2 mutant allele segregating in the family can facilitate early diagnosis and treatment.[2,3]

Syndromic hearing loss disorders with AR modes of inheritance

Usher syndrome is the most common AR syndromic cause of hearing loss, accounting for more than 50% of the individuals who are deaf-blind in the United States. Affected individuals are born with sensorineural hearing loss and usually develop visual impairment from retinitis pigmentosa (RP) after the first decade. Night blindness and progressive loss of peripheral vision occur in the second decade. The multiple genocopies of Usher syndrome are differentiated by the degree of hearing impairment and vestibular function testing. *Usher syndrome type I* (OMIM # 276900, 276904, 601067, 612632, 602083, 602097, 606943) has congenital severe to profound sensorineural hearing loss and abnormal vestibular dysfunction. Traditional amplification is ineffective and communication is usually manual. *Usher syndrome type II* (OMIM # 605472, 276901, 611383) usually has congenital mild to severe sensorineural hearing loss and normal vestibular function. Hearing aids frequently provide effective amplification and communication is usually oral. *Usher syndrome type III* (OMIM # 276902) has progressive hearing loss and deterioration of vestibular function.[2,3]

Pendred syndrome (OMIM # 274600) is the second most common AR cause of syndromic hearing loss. It is characterized by congenital sensorineural hearing loss that is usually severe to profound and a euthyroid goiter that develops in early puberty (40%) or adulthood (60%). Hearing loss is associated with Mondini dysplasia or dilated vestibular aqueduct that can be detected by computed tomography (CT) examination of the temporal bones (**Fig. 1**). Vestibular function is usually abnormal. SLC26A4 (OMIM # 605646) mutations are detected in approximately 50% of multiplex kindreds

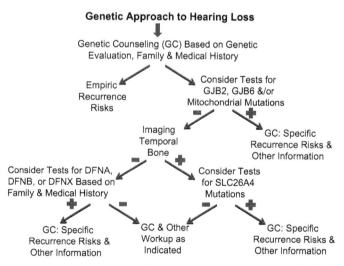

Fig. 1. Genetic approach to hearing loss. DFN refers to nonsyndromic deafness loci which can be autosomal dominant (DFNA), autosomal recessive (DFNB), or X linked (DFNX). See sections on DNFA, DFNB, Claire's Case History and Pendred syndrome for explanations of GJB2, GJB6 and SLC26A4 mutations.

and are also a cause of nonsyndromic hearing loss (see **Fig. 1** and DFNB4 discussed later).[2,3]

Jervell and Lange-Nielsen syndrome (OMIM # 220400, 612347) is the third most common AR cause of syndromic hearing loss. It has congenital hearing loss and a prolonged QT interval (abnormal QTc [c = corrected] greater than 440 msec). Affected individuals can have syncopal episodes and sudden death. Because screening electrocardiogram (ECG) is not highly sensitive, children with hearing loss and a positive family history for sudden death, sudden infant death syndrome, syncope, or long QT syndrome should have a thorough cardiac evaluation. Molecular testing can also be used but allelic and locus heterogeneity caused by mutations in the KCNQ1 (OMIM # 607542) and KCNE1 (OMIM # 176261) genes can complicate testing.[2,3]

Biotinidase deficiency (OMIM # 253260) is an AR disorder that causes a deficiency of biotin, which is a cofactor for carboxylases essential for gluconeogenesis (pyruvate carboxylase), fatty acid synthesis (acetyl CoA carboxylase), and catabolism of several branched-chain amino acids (propionyl-CoA carboxylase and beta methylcrotonoyl-CoA carboxylase). If biotinidase deficiency is not detected by newborn screening and treated by daily oral biotin, affected individuals can develop alopecia, ataxia, conjunctivitis, dermatitis, seizures, hypotonia, developmental delay, and visual problems. Sensorineural hearing loss occurs in at least 75% of symptomatic children and it is usually irreversible.[2,3]

Refsum disease (OMIM # 266500, 26510) is characterized by severe progressive sensorineural hearing loss and retinitis pigmentosa. It is caused by faulty phytanic acid metabolism.[2,3]

Syndromic hearing loss disorders with an X-linked mode of inheritance

Alport syndrome (OMIM # 104200, 203780, 301050) has progressive sensorineural hearing loss and glomerulonephritis that leads to end-stage renal disease and variable ophthalmologic findings. Hearing loss usually does not occur before 10 years of age. AD, AR, and X-linked (XL) forms (see OMIM # mentioned earlier) are described. AD, AR and XL forms account for rare, ~15% and ~85% of syndromic hearing loss disorders, respectively.[2,3]

Mohr-Tranebjaerg syndrome (OMIM # 304700) has progressive, postlingual hearing loss associated with visual disability, dystonia, fractures, and intellectual disability. TIMM8A mutations disrupt translocation of proteins from the cytosol across the inner MT membrane.[2,3]

Syndromic hearing loss with MT inheritance

A 3243 A to G transition in the MT gene MTTL1 is reported in 2% to 6% of individuals with diabetes mellitus in Japan (OMIM # 590050). Approximately 60% of those with diabetes mellitus and this mutation develop sensorineural hearing loss. Heteroplasmy is thought to affect the penetrance and variable expressivity of this disorder.[2,3]

Nonsyndromic Hearing Loss

Nonsyndromic hearing loss has no associated medical problems or congenital anomalies of the external ear but it can be associated with abnormalities of the middle ear or inner ear. Importantly, more than 70% of hereditary hearing loss is nonsyndromic.[2–5]

Nonsyndromic hearing loss grouping by mode of inheritance

The different genetic loci for nonsyndromic deafness are designated as DFN (for deafness loci) and they are designated as A, B, or X based on their mode of inheritance. Thus, DFNA has an AD, DFNB has an AR, and DFNX has an XL mode of inheritance. Nonsyndromic deafness can also be caused by MT inheritance.[2]

Contributions of DFNA, DNFB, and DNFX to prelingual and postlingual onset of nonsyndromic hearing loss

In the prelingual nonsyndromic hearing loss group, inheritance is 75% to 80% AR (DFNB, see OMIM # 220290, 600974, 603678, 605646, 603681, 612645), 20% to 25% AD (DFNA, see OMIM # 601544, 606346, 607453), and 1.0% to 1.5% XL (DFNX, see OMIM # 304400, 304500, 300030, 300066, 30614).[2–5] Most reported post-lingual nonsyndromic hearing loss families have an AD mode of inheritance and are DFNA, whereas most prelingual severe to profound hearing loss is AR and DFNB. Most XL (DFNX) forms cause nonsyndromic hearing loss and can be either prelingual or postlingual.[2–5]

Genetic heterogeneity of DFNA and DNFB forms of nonsyndromic hearing loss

DFNA and DFNB nonsyndromic forms of hearing loss have high genetic heterogeneity. Most cases of DFNB nonsyndromic hearing loss (OMIM # 220290) are caused by mutations in a single gene (GJB2); however, most cases of DFNA nonsyndromic hearing loss do not have mutations at a single locus.[2–5]

Contributions of MT inheritance to nonsyndromic hearing loss

Nonsyndromic MT hearing loss presents with moderate to profound hearing loss caused by a mutation in either the MT-RNR1 or MT-TS1 gene. MT-RNR1 mutations can be associated with aminoglycoside ototoxicity or late-onset sensorineural hearing loss. Bilateral and severe to profound hearing loss occurs within a few days to weeks after receiving an aminoglycoside antibiotic, such as gentamycin, tobramycin, amika-cin, kanamycin, or streptomycin. MT-TS1 mutations typically present as childhood onset of sensorineural hearing loss, which can be associated with palmoplantar ker-atoderma in some families.[2,3,6]

GENETIC INFORMATION AND TESTING RESOURCES

Information on the large number and variety of human genetic disorders causing hearing loss may seem impenetrable to many physicians and their patients. However, learning to access this complex data is critical to applying newly discov-ered genetic information to patient care. Taking a careful family history (including a 3-generation pedigree) and using centralized databases on the Internet, such as GeneReviews and OMIM, are powerful and straightforward ways to identify hearing loss disorders that are genetic (see **Fig. 1**).[2–6] As these databases grow, they will also provide more comprehensive access to current treatments, specialized laboratory tests, opportunities for research participation, and educational materials for patients and their families. Every physician should develop his or her medical bioinformatics skills and use these resources to obtain current information. Physicians also need to be able to help patients and their families use this information to become more aware of their risks for the genetic disorders that affect hearing. We should also make fami-lies aware of the opportunities to participate in research to discover better ways to treat and prevent these diseases.

The OMIM database can be searched interactively to generate a list of differential diagnoses associated with symptoms and signs and the mode of inheritance observed in patients and their relatives.[3] Such differential diagnoses may include rare or recently discovered disorders. Accessing and using different databases can improve an otologist's diagnostic skills, revealing the subtle differences among alternative diagnoses. The following sections introduce the reader to using the World Wide Web to obtain information about the genetic disorders that cause hearing loss.

Claire's Case History

Claire was the 2.64-kg product of a 36-week, uncomplicated pregnancy to a 38-year-old woman with G2P1. Labor and delivery were unremarkable. Claire was in the regular nursery for three days and required two days of phototherapy for hyperbilirubinemia. Newborn hearing screening (NBHS) was not mandatory and was not done. At two weeks, when her bilirubin was checked, NBHS was attempted without success.

Claire smiled by two weeks of age. Her parents became concerned about her lack of response to sounds by one month of age but were reassured by her pediatrician. When she was two months old, her parents requested a hearing evaluation. At 4.5 month old, she was diagnosed by audiology as having profound sensorineural hearing loss (SNHL). Claire was fitted with hearing aids at 5.5 months of age and began weekly speech and language therapy at 6 months of age. She had cochlear implants done at 12 and 18 months of age. She was evaluated by a geneticist at 7.5 months of age and was found to have a normal physical examination, normal ECG, and no family history of deafness, sudden infant death, white forelock, or conditions associated with familial deafness or parental consanguinity. Genetic testing confirmed that she had DFNB1 caused by compound heterozygosity for a GJB2 1 BP deletion (35delG) and a GJB6 partial deletion (ΔGJB6-D13S1830). Her parents were told they have a 25% recurrence risk and they were given the GeneReviews for this disorder.[5] Claire continues to receive weekly speech and language therapy and is doing well at 4.5 years old. Her parents' goal is to have Claire mainstreamed into regular school with minimal accommodations by kindergarten.

GENETIC APPROACH TO EVALUATING AND TESTING FOR HEARING LOSS

Hearing loss is a common birth defect.[8] One of every 500 newborns has bilateral permanent sensorineural hearing loss 40 dB or greater and by adolescence the prevalence increases to 3.5 out of 1000.[9] More than 50% of prelingual deafness is genetic and most of these cases are nonsyndromic and have an AR mode of inheritance (see **Fig. 1**). About 50% of nonsyndromic AR hearing loss type 1 (referred to as DFNB1) is caused by mutations of the GJB2 or GJB6 genes, which encode the connexin 26 and 30 proteins, respectively. In the general population, the carrier rate is 1 out of 33 for a GJB2 allele that causes DFNB1, and the frequency of DFNB1 caused by GJB2 mutations alone is approximately 1 out of 4400 births.[2,3,5]

Newborn Hearing Screening

Congenital hearing loss can be detected by NBHS, which has been advocated by the American College of Medical Genetics, the March of Dimes, and the National Institutes

---

Key Points: CLAIRE'S CASE

1. More than 50% of babies born with hearing loss have no known risk factors for hearing loss and 90% are born to normal-hearing parents.

2. Claire was born in a state that did not have mandatory NBHS. Her suspected hearing loss was not confirmed until she was 4.5 months old. NBHS could have led to an earlier diagnosis of SNHL, earlier intervention, and less parental anxiety. To remedy this gap in NBHS, Claire's parents' successfully advocated legislation entitled Claire's Law that now mandates NBHS in Tennessee.[7]

3. The goal of NBHS is early detection and intervention for all hearing-impaired infants at an early age to prevent psychosocial, educational, and language problems. Infants not identified with hearing loss by 6 months of age or younger frequently have delays in speech and language development.

of Health. NBHS is required in 35 states plus the District of Columbia. In most of the remaining states, it is offered to all newborns but is not required. The states of California and Texas remain exceptions in that they offer NBHS to select populations or by request.[10-12]

Confirmation of Hearing Loss

An evaluation for genetic causes is needed for newborns identified by NBHS, for those who are found to be at risk for hearing loss by NBHS, and for those who are confirmed as having hearing loss (see **Fig. 1**). Genetic forms of hearing loss must be distinguished from acquired (nongenetic) causes of hearing loss. The genetic forms of hearing loss are diagnosed by otologic, audiologic, and physical examination; family history; ancillary testing (eg, CT examination of the temporal bone); and molecular genetic testing.[2-6]

Genetic Evaluation and Counseling for Hearing Loss

This process leads to the accurate diagnosis of hereditary conditions and the communication of information to families. The process includes the following:

1. Collection of family and medical histories
2. Physical examination by an experienced clinical geneticist
3. Testing for mutations if needed to clarify cause, prognosis, recurrence, or to guide treatment
4. Sharing of information with the family with follow-up and support services

A genetic approach to hearing loss is shown in **Fig. 1**, which incorporates genetic evaluation; genetic counseling; family history; and temporal bone imaging and genetic testing, if needed. The issues that arise in genetic evaluations and genetic counseling can differ for every family and are often dependent on the number and relationships of affected family members, the age of onset and severity of deafness present in affected relatives, linguistic and cultural orientation, and the results of temporal bone imaging and genetic tests that may be required.

The success of genetic counseling in relaying information to families and the determination of types of hereditary deafness through clinical evaluations and laboratory tests depends on appropriate referrals by medical professionals, including otolaryngologists. A working relationship between otolaryngologists and clinical geneticists for the referral and evaluation of patients with hereditary deafness or deafness of unknown cause is important.

ETHICAL CONSIDERATIONS REGARDING GENETIC TESTING FOR HEARING LOSS
Ethical Considerations Regarding Genetic Testing in Children

Genetic testing in children presents ethical issues because they are legally unable to provide informed consent. Children aged younger than 7 years are rarely developmentally ready to make an informed decision, so informed-consent issues arise because genetic testing can have a profound effect on their future. For example, the results of genetic testing can alter the child's self-image and future aspirations. It can also affect the relationship between the child and his or her parents. Although it is strongly recommended that genetic testing in childhood be avoided, it should be stressed that results of a genetic evaluation for hearing loss, including the genetic testing of infants and children aged younger than 7 years, can alter the patients' management regarding the choice of hearing augmentation and cochlear implantation (see **Fig. 1**).[2-6] Both the

American Academy of Pediatrics and the American Society of Human Genetics have published statements regarding the ethical issues involved.[13,14]

In general, testing children for diagnostic purposes or predictive testing is considered acceptable as long as results can have a significant impact on clinical management. Patients' parents should give informed consent after they have been educated about the disorder and given an explanation of the possible outcomes of the genetic testing, including any potential pitfalls (false positives, false negatives, failure to detect a mutation) that may arise. Where feasible, assent should also be obtained from the child. Some laboratories require documentation of informed assent if the child is older than 7 years.

Responsibility to Relatives at Risk

The standard of care is to inform patients of the risks to family members for genetic disorders and to encourage patients to inform their family members of the condition. This discussion should be documented in patients' medical records. Health care providers should be available to assist patients in informing family members. Genetic counselors can help with issues, such as providing verbal and written information regarding the condition and facilitating genetic testing for family members at risk.[15,16]

HOW TO FIND THE INFORMATION YOU NEED: GENETICS ON THE WORLD WIDE WEB
Online Mendelian Inheritance in Man

OMIM is maintained by the National Center for Biotechnology Information (NCBI). It is available without charge on the Internet at http://www.ncbi.nlm.nih.gov/omim.[3] It is updated regularly and contained more than 20,000 entries in December 2010. Each entry contains a wealth of information about the history, signs, symptoms, diagnosis, management, and research findings of a given condition or gene as well as detailed gene- and disease-focused genomic maps. Access through hyperlinks to a variety of other Web sites is another important strength. These hyperlinks include genes and disease from NCBI, the Cardiff Human Gene Mutation Database (HGMD), Mito-Map (a human MT genome database), and PubMed.

Gene Tests-GeneReviews

Gene Tests-GeneReviews is a comprehensive Web site that contains a medical genetics laboratory directory, genetics clinic directory, and disease information that is available at http://www.ncbi.nlm.nih.gov/sites/GeneTests.[2,4–6] The teaching materials at the home Web site of GeneReviews (http://www.ncbi.nlm.nih.gov/projects/GeneTests/static/concepts/conceptsindex.shtml) include an excellent glossary, which has interactive access to in-depth knowledge as well as downloadable slides. This Web site also includes GeneReviews, which provides excellent reviews of hereditary hearing loss and deafness, DFNA2, DFNA3, DFNB1, and nonsyndromic hearing loss and deafness, and MT (see **Fig. 1**). This Web site also provides the geographic location and contact information for medical genetics evaluation and counseling services that are updated every 6 to 12 months.

Internet resources for health professionals can be found at the Web sites listed in **Table 1**. These resources include the American Academy of Pediatrics, the National Newborn Screening and Genetics Resource Center, the NCBI databases, and the National Organization for Rare Disorders.

For information resources for patients and families, a selection of Web sites that may be useful are provided in **Table 2**. A referral to genetic counseling professionals may

Table 1
Internet resources for health professionals

Web Site and URL	Description
American Academy of Pediatrics http://aappolicy.aappublications.org/cgi/content/full/pediatrics;118/3/e934	Newborn screening fact sheets discussing detection, evaluation, and treatment
Clinical Trials http://clinicaltrials.gov	Registry of clinical trials in the United States and the world
GeneReviews-Gene Tests-GeneClinics http://www.ncbi.nlm.nih.gov/sites/GeneTests/	International directory of genetics clinics and genetic testing laboratories Expert-authored, peer-reviewed disease descriptions and educational material
Hereditary Hearing Loss Homepage www.hereditaryhearingloss.org	Provides current overview of hereditary hearing loss for researchers and clinicians; lists data and links for all known gene localizations and identifications for monogenic, nonsyndromic hearing impairment
National Newborn Screening and Genetics Resource Center http://genes-r-us.uthscsa.edu/NCBI	Resources regarding newborn screening and genetics for health professionals, parents, and families
NCBI databases http://www.ncbi.nlm.nih.gov	Develops, distributes, supports, and coordinates access to databases and software for the scientific and medical communities
National Organization for Rare Disorders http://www.rarediseases.org	Information about rare genetic conditions, support services, and research
OMIM http://www.ncbi.nlm.nih.gov	Extensive compilation of human genes and genetic phenotypes. Focuses on the relationship between phenotype and genotype

also be helpful to families, especially when there are concerns about recurrence risks or reproductive decision making (see later discussion).

HOW GENETICISTS AND OTOLOGISTS CAN WORK TOGETHER
When to Consider Referral to a Geneticist or Genetic Counselor

Otologists have long been aware of the genetic cause of many types of hearing loss and the need to inform their patients and their families about recurrence risks. However, in many situations, it is helpful to refer the family to a genetics clinic for information related to more accurate recurrence risks for members of the immediate and extended family. The purpose of the referral may also include assistance in diagnosis, patient education and management, assuring informed consent, and assisting families in reproductive and other decision making or the facilitation of testing. Genetics professionals for a specific geographic region can be located through the Gene Tests or National Society of Genetic Counselors Web sites.[2,4–6,17]

Diagnostic Assistance

If a patients has multiple anomalies, atypical medical problems, or dysmorphic features in addition to his or her hearing loss, a diagnostic genetic evaluation is warranted. Because of the complexity of possible causes, cost, and the variable

Table 2
Resources for patients and families

Web Site and URL	Description
Alexander Graham Bell Association for the Deaf and Hard of Hearing http://nc.agbell.org	Advocacy, education, research, and financial aid for individuals with hearing loss
American Society for Deaf Children http://www.deafchildren.org	Supports, educates, advocates families of hearing impaired children
Boys Town National Research Hospital http://www.boystownhospital.org	Provides clinical care, research opportunities, and educational outreach programs
Connexins and Deafness http://davinci.crg.es/deafness	Detailed information about connexins and deafness
Genetic Alliance http://www.geneticalliance.org	Network of more than 1000 disease-specific advocacy organizations
Harvard Medical School Center for Hereditary Deafness www.hearing.harvard.edu	Family friendly information about hereditary hearing loss and deafness
Medical Genetics, University of Kansas Medical Center http://www.kumc.edu/gec/support	Information on inherited conditions, birth defects, and support groups for families, educators, and health care providers
National Association of the Deaf www.nad.org	Civil rights organization of, by and for deaf and hard of hearing individuals in the United States

sensitivity of genetic tests, a genetics clinic referral is almost always more cost-effective than ordering a series of tests, such as mutation analyses (see **Fig. 1**). A referral may also be helpful if features of the examination or family history are suggestive of a genetic condition, which may or may not be related to the hearing loss.

Education and Management

A genetics referral may provide assistance with up-to-date disease education and management, including arranging appropriate medical, psychosocial, and educational referrals. If DNA testing is not available, the options of DNA banking or participation in a research study may be offered. Because there are multiple forms of syndromic and nonsyndromic hearing loss that can have different modes of inheritance, a genetic evaluation, pedigree analysis, and possibly genetic testing are needed to provide genetic counseling regarding the probability and characteristics of associated problems for specific families.

Informed Consent/Decision Making and Facilitation of Testing

The genetics team can be helpful in providing sufficient information to ensure informed consent, an essential component of genetic testing, and in facilitating specimen handling. A referral to a genetic counselor (a master's level professional who is trained to obtain family histories, evaluate risks, and counsel patients and families about available options) may be especially helpful for the discussion of reproductive options and the pros and cons of genetic testing for patients and other family members. The counselor can help families inform extended family members of possible risks and facilitate the referral of relatives to genetics clinics near their homes.

Hereditary hearing loss can be inherited in an AD, AR, or XL mode, as well as by MT inheritance. Informed consent and genetic counseling before molecular testing can clarify the sensitivity and the pros and cons of molecular testing. Importantly, the family can be engaged in deciding what they might do differently if a specific molecular test is positive. If they decide that no changes in management, risk assessment, or determination of the specific genetic diagnosis will arise from a given test, they usually choose not to pursue such tests. When informative tests are not available or the required affected relatives are unwilling to be tested to prove the validity of the test, empiric recurrence risk figures, coupled with current genetic and molecular information on the disorder, can be provided by genetic counseling.

SUMMARY

As new genes are discovered and molecular genetic diagnostic testing becomes more available, clinicians will need to have an understanding of how these tests can best be used to guide patient management. Staying current with such information will require familiarity with online resources. Genetics professionals are able to assist with the management of such patients and serve as a valuable resource.

ACKNOWLEDGMENTS

The authors thank Jackie Cundall RN, BSN, Newborn Hearing Screening Coordinator, Tennessee Department of Health for her long-term and dedicated efforts in expanding the NBHS program in Tennessee. The authors also thank Claire's parents for reviewing this article and providing the motivation for Claire's Law, which has subsequently helped all newborns with hearing loss in Tennessee.

REFERENCES

1. Nussbaum RL, McInnes RR, Willard HF. Thompson & Thompson Genetics in Medicine. 7th edition. Philadelphia (PA): Saunders; 2007. p. 115–46, 175–84, 323–5, 531–50.
2. Smith RJ, Hildebrand MS, Van Camp G. Deafness and hereditary hearing loss overview. Genereviews [Internet]. In: Pagon RA, Bird TC, Dolan CR, et al, editors. Seattle (WA): University of Washington; 1993. Available at: http://www.ncbi.nlm. nih.gov/books/NBK1434. Accessed November 24, 2010.
3. OMIM (Online Mendelian Inheritance in Man). McKusick-Nathans Institute of Genetic Medicine, Johns Hopkins University (Baltimore, MD) and National Center for Biotechnology Information, National Library of Medicine (Bethesda, MD). Available at: http://www.ncbi.nlm.nih.gov/omim. Accessed November 24, 2010.
4. Smith RJ, Sheffield AM, Van Camp G. Nonsyndromic hearing loss and deafness, DFNA3. GeneReviews [Internet]. In: Pagon RA, Bird TC, Dolan CR, et al, editors. Seattle (WA): University of Washington; 1993. Available at: http://www.ncbi.nlm. nih.gov/books/NBK1536. Accessed November 24, 2010.
5. Smith RJ, Van Camp G. Nonsyndromic Hearing Loss and Deafness, DFNB1. GeneReviews [Internet]. In: Pagon RA, Bird TC, Dolan CR, et al, editors. Seattle (WA): University of Washington; 1993. Available at: http://www.ncbi.nlm.nih.gov/ books/NBK1272. Accessed November 24, 2010.
6. Pandya A. Nonsyndromic hearing loss and deafness, mitochondrial. GeneReviews [Internet]. In: Pagon RA, Bird TC, Dolan CR, et al, editors. Seattle (WA): University of Washington; 1993. Available at: http://www.ncbi.nlm.nih.gov/books/NBK1422. Accessed November 24, 2010.

7. Public Chapter No. 768 (Senate Bill No. 3191) enacted by the general assembly of the state of Tennessee, July 1, 2008 entitled "Claire's Law".

8. Hilgert N, Smith RJ, Van Camp G. Forty-six genes causing nonsyndromic hearing impairment: which ones should be analyzed in DNA diagnostics? Mutat Res 2009;681:189–96.

9. Morton CC, Nance WE. Newborn hearing screening – a silent revolution. N Engl J Med 2006;354:2151–64.

10. American College of Medical Genetics. Genetics evaluation guidelines for the etiologic diagnosis of congenital hearing loss. Genetic evaluation of congenital hearing loss expert panel. (pdf) Available at: www.acmg.net. 2002. Accessed September 21, 2010.

11. American College of Medical Genetics. Statement on universal newborn hearing screening. Available at: www.genetics.faseb.org. 2000. Accessed September 21, 2010.

12. National Newborn Screening & Genetics Resource Center. Available at: http://genes-r-us.uthscsa.edu/resources/newborn/newborn_menu.htm. Accessed December 28, 2010.

13. ASHG/ACMG policy statement. Ethical, legal, and psychosocial implications of genetic testing in children and adolescents. Am J Hum Genet 1995;57:1233–41.

14. American Academy of Pediatrics Committee on Bioethics. Policy statement: ethical issues with genetic testing in pediatrics. Pediatrics 2001;107:1451–5.

15. Clayton EW. Ethical, legal, and social implications of genomic medicine. N Engl J Med 2003;349:562–9.

16. American Society of Human Genetics Policy Statement. Professional disclosure of familial genetic information. Am J Hum Genet 1998;62:474–83.

17. National Society of Genetic Counselors Web site. Available at: http://www.nsgc.org. Accessed December 28, 2010.

Pediatric Cochlear Implantation: Candidacy Evaluation, Medical and Surgical Considerations, and Expanding Criteria

Selena E. Heman-Ackah, MD, MBA[a], J. Thomas Roland Jr, MD[a],
David S. Haynes, MD[b], Susan B. Waltzman, PhD[a],*

KEYWORDS

- Pediatric cochlear implantation • Candidacy evaluation
- Medical considerations • Surgical considerations

PEDIATRIC CANDIDACY EVALUATION

Patient selection is one of the most important determinants of cochlear implant success within the pediatric population.[1] Therefore, comprehensive candidacy evaluation is critical to the patient success. The purpose of the candidacy evaluation is to determine the medical and audiometric suitability of the patient for cochlear implantation. Within the pediatric population, the candidacy evaluation varies slightly by age, but maintains a core of essential components. The pediatric cochlear implantation candidacy evaluation should comprise a battery of testing, including a medical evaluation, imaging evaluation, audiologic evaluation, speech and language evaluation, and patient/family counseling. **Table 1** provides a synopsis of the components of the cochlear implantation evaluation.

Dr Roland is a member of the Advanced bionics, Cochlear Americas and Med El Advisory Boards.
a Department of Otolaryngology, New York University Cochlear Implant Center, New York University School of Medicine, 660 First Avenue, 7th Floor, New York, NY 10016, USA
b Otology Group of Vanderbilt, Department of Otolaryngology–Head and Neck Surgery, Vanderbilt Bill Wilkerson Center, Vanderbilt University, 1215 21st Avenue South, 7209 Medical Center East, South Tower, Nashville, TN 37232, USA
* Corresponding author.
E-mail address: susan.waltzman@nyumc.org

Otolaryngol Clin N Am 45 (2012) 41–67
doi:10.1016/j.otc.2011.08.016
0030-6665/12/$ – see front matter © 2012 Elsevier Inc. All rights reserved.

Table 1
Components of the cochlear implant evaluation

Evaluation	Components
Medical	History
	Prenatal exposures (TORCH infections, teratogens)
	Perinatal concerns (prematurity, low birth weight, neonatal intensive care unit low Apgar score, hyperbilirubinemia, sepsis, intubation)
	Postnatal concerns (ototoxins, meningitis, mumps)
	Family history
	Physical examination
	Syndromes
	Otitis media
	Pneumococcal vaccination
Imaging	High-resolution computed tomography of temporal bones
	Magnetic resonance imaging of the internal auditory canal
Audiologic	Pure tone audiometry
	Speech discrimination
	Hearing aid evaluation
	Speech perception assessment
Speech and language	Assess language development
	Screen for articulation disorders
Physiologic	Auditory brainstem response test
	Electrically evoked auditory brainstem response test
Cognitive and development	Assess for cognitive and developmental delays
Patient and family counseling	Establish patient and family expectation
	Assess family commitment to aural rehabilitation protocol
	Selection of cochlear implant device
	Informed consent

Medical Evaluation

Various medical considerations must be factored when considering cochlear implantation in the pediatric population to facilitate patient selection, create realistic expectations, and design optimal rehabilitation protocol. The cochlear implantation team should be aware of the source of hearing loss. During the medical evaluation, a complete history and physical examination should be performed with the goals of identifying cause of hearing loss and evaluating birth history, family history, and history of otologic disease. In addition, immunization history should be confirmed because appropriate immunization is critical in pediatric cochlear implant candidates.

Sensorineural hearing loss within the pediatric population may be secondary to unknown cause, acquired cause, or hereditary cause. Unknown cause accounts for 15% to 44% of pediatric patients with sensorineural hearing loss[2]; successful implantation and rehabilitation have been documented in pediatric patients with sensorineural hearing loss of unknown cause.[3]

In most reports[2] approximately 15% to 40% of sensorineural hearing loss in pediatric patients is of acquired cause. Prenatal exposure to certain infections and teratogens has been associated with congenital sensorineural hearing loss. Thus, while obtaining the medical history, history of intrauterine exposure to cytomegalovirus, herpes virus, rubella, syphilis, toxoplasmosis, and varicella should be deciphered. In addition, history of intrauterine exposure to teratogens including alcohol, drug abuse, methyl mercury, and thalidomide should be obtained. During the perinatal period, low birth weight, anoxia, low Apgar score, hyperbilirubinemia, or sepsis have been associated with sensorineural hearing loss. A complete perinatal history should be obtained highlighting these factors as well as history of prematurity, intubation, and neonatal intensive care unit admission because all of these factors may contribute to sensorineural hearing loss. Gentamicin is commonly used in the management of neonatal sepsis.[4] History of aminoglycoside administration, including gentamicin, furosemide and other ototoxin administration, mumps, and meningitis should be noted.

Sensorineural hearing loss has a hereditary cause in most pediatric patients, accounting for approximately 40% to 50% in most reports[2]; therefore, a complete family history should be obtained, with a focus on relatives with congenital or early-onset hearing loss. Hereditary sensorineural hearing loss may be categorized as nonsyndromic sensorineural hearing loss or syndromic sensorineural hearing loss; nonsyndromic sensorineural hearing loss accounts for most hereditary congenital hearing loss.[2] Mutations within the connexin 26 genes, namely the *GJB 2* and *GJB 6* genes, are responsible in most cases.[5–7] Patients with deafness associated with mutations in the connexin 26 genes have been found to be excellent candidates for cochlear implantation because they perform equal to or better than other cochlear implant patients in reading comprehension, nonverbal cognition, speech performance, language perception, speech perception, and speech intelligibility.[5,8,9]

Patients should be evaluated for signs and symptoms consistent with syndromic forms of sensorineural hearing loss. Patients with various forms of syndromic sensorineural hearing loss have been implanted with successful aural rehabilitation including Usher syndrome, Pendred syndrome, Refsum disease, Jervell Lange-Nielsen syndrome, Waardenburg syndrome, branchio-oto-renal syndrome, and CHARGE syndrome.[10–19] Of concern amongst this group are patients with syndromes that have characteristic findings that complicate implantation or aural rehabilitation. Both Usher syndrome and Refsum disease include retinitis pigmentosa and progressive blindness; thus, early cochlear implantation should be performed before onset of severe visual deficiency to optimize outcome.[10] The first sign of vestibular dysfunction in patients with Usher syndrome is delayed walking.[10] If it is age appropriate, age at onset of walking should be obtained during the medical interview. Patients with CHARGE syndrome have variable benefit from cochlear implantation secondary to difficulties in aural rehabilitation associated with developmental delay and mental retardation.[19] Although Jervell Lange-Nielsen syndrome is a rare syndrome, patients with congenital sensorineural hearing loss should undergo electrocardiography because of the potential associated prolonged QT interval and propensity of arrhythmia, and cardiac syncope. Patients presenting with a history of a seizure disorder, on anticonvulsants, and with an associated hearing loss should be considered to have Jervell Lange-Nielsen syndrome. Patients with the confirmed diagnosis of Jervell Lange-Nielsen syndrome, preoperative cardiology consultation should be performed, and evaluation of the patient's immediate family suggested. Because of the significant risk of cardiac event with the administration of general anesthesia, a pacemaker or defibrillator should be considered before cochlear implantation and β-blockers should be administered within the perioperative period.[20–22] A complete otolaryngology physical examination should be performed with a focus on identifying craniofacial anomalies or physical findings that may elucidate any of the associated syndromes outlined earlier.

In addition, the patient should be screened for chronic otitis media. A history of episodes and frequency of otitis media should be performed. A pressure equalization tube may be required at the time of, before, or after cochlear implantation for management of chronic otitis media with effusion.[23]

A history of immunization is a critical component of the medical cochlear implantation evaluation. The rate of meningitis amongst children with hearing loss has been shown to be higher than in those children without hearing loss. Further, children with cochlear implants are at a higher risk for meningitis than children with hearing loss who have not received cochlear implants. Several risk factors have been associated with these findings, including lack of appropriate immunization.[24–26] Approximately 90% of cases of meningitis after pediatric cochlear implantation are caused by infections with *Streptococcus pneumonia*.[24] In October 2003, the United States Centers for Disease Control and Prevention (CDC) published recommendations that all cochlear implant recipients receive age-appropriate vaccination against *Streptococcus* pneumonia. These recommendations were updated in 2010.[27,28] **Table 2** provides a summary of the current immunization guidelines. All children younger than 24 months should receive the 7-valent pneumococcal conjugate vaccine (PCV7). Children aged 24 months to 59 months who have not previously been vaccinated should undergo a modified vaccination protocol as depicted in **Table 2**. All patients older than 5 years should receive the 23-valent pneumococcal polysaccharide vaccine (PPV23). All patients receiving cochlear implantation should be up to date on age-appropriate pneumococcal vaccination at least 2 weeks before cochlear implantation if possible according to the CDC recommendations. Within the medical evaluation, the immunization record should be reviewed to assess compliance with CDC recommendations for pneumococcal vaccination. If discrepancies exist, vaccinations should be administered to maintain compliance with pneumococcal vaccination recommendations.

Imaging Evaluation

Cochleovestibular anomalies are common amongst pediatric cochlear implant candidates because they often correlate with sensorineural hearing loss. Therefore, preoperative evaluation of cochleovestibular anatomy is an important component of the pediatric cochlear implant evaluation. The goals of the preoperative imaging evaluation are to determine whether there are cochleovestibular anomalies that preclude implantation, to evaluate for evidence of luminal obstruction, to identify findings that may complicate the surgery or subsequent patient management, and to determine which ear may be the most appropriate to implant.

In evaluating patients for cochleovestibular anomalies, the patient is assessed for an implantable cavity in proximity to stimulable neural elements with projections that

Table 2
CDC recommendations for pneumococcal vaccination

Age at First PCV$_{13}$ Dose	PCV$_{13}$ Primary Series	PCV$_{13}$ Booster Dose	PPSV Dose
2–6 months	3 doses, 2 months apart	1 dose at 12–15 months of age	Indicated at $\geq$24 months of age
7–11 months	2 doses, 2 months apart	1 dose at 12–15 months of age	Indicated at $\geq$24 months of age
12–23 months	2 doses, 2 months apart	—	Indicated at $\geq$24 months of age
2–6 years	2 doses, 2 months apart	—	After PCV$_{13}$ series
6–18 years	1 dose	—	After PCV$_{13}$ dose
$\geq$18 years	—	—	Prior to implant

PCV$_{13}$: 13-valent pneumococcalconjugate; PPSV: 23-valent pneumococcalpolysaccharide (Pneumovax®).

contact the auditory cortex. Up to 35% of pediatric cochlear implant candidates have cochleovestibular anomalies.[29] When present, cochleovestibular anomalies occur bilaterally in 65% of patients and are similar in 93% of patients.[30] The most commonly used classification system for cochleovestibular malformations, by Jackler and colleagues,[30] is presented in **Table 3**. Although complete labyrinthine aplasia and cochlear aplasia represent the least commonly encountered deformities, their presence precludes the option of cochlear implantation. Alternative methods of language rehabilitation must be explored within this patient population. During the imaging evaluation, cochlear aplasia must be differentiated from common cavity deformity because the propensity for cochlear implantation differs in these 2 conditions. Patients with common cavity deformity, cochlear hypoplasia, incomplete partition deformity, lateral semicircular canal dysplasia, and enlarged vestibular aqueduct may successfully undergo cochlear implantation.[29] However, knowledge of these deformities preoperatively is critical to success in implantation because the presence of the deformities governs electrode array choice and necessitates alterations in operative technique.

During the imaging evaluations, evidence of luminal obstruction is assessed. Luminal obstruction may result from inner ear inflammation, abnormal bone metabolism, or trauma. The most common cause of luminal obstruction within the pediatric population is postmeningitis labyrinthitis ossificans. Luminal obstruction may also result from hematogenous infections including septicemia, mumps, rubella, and viral infections or from suppurative labyrinthitis secondary to otitis media or cholesteatoma. Early-onset Paget disease may cause luminal obstruction. In addition, luminal obstruction may result from temporal bone fractures. The findings of luminal obstruction may interfere with complete insertion of cochlear implant electrode. Thus, identification of luminal obstruction must be determined preoperatively to assist in preoperative planning regarding side of implantation and intraoperative technique for cochleostomy and drill-out.

Findings that may complicate cochlear implant surgery or subsequent patient management are appraised during the imaging evaluation. Amongst pediatric patients with vestibulocochlear anomalies, approximately 15% of patients have an aberrant facial nerve course.[29,31] An aberrant facial nerve may preclude the traditional facial recess approach for cochleostomy and electrode insertion. Vascular anomalies may complicate cochlear implant surgery as well. Extreme anterior position of the sigmoid sinus may contract exposure to the facial recess. This situation has been reported in approximately 1.6% of patients.[32] High-riding jugular bulbs are present in up to 6% of patients.[32] Jugular diverticuli are exceedingly rare. In addition, the presence of high-riding jugular bulbs or jugular diverticuli overlying the round window niche or promontory may complicate cochlear implantation surgery. Aberrant carotid artery and dehiscent carotid artery may complicate drill-out procedure in patients with ossified

Table 3	
Classification of cochleovestibular anomalies (Jackler and colleagues[30])	
Cochlear Status	**Malformation (%)**
Absent or malformed cochlea	Complete labyrinthine aplasia (1)
	Cochlear aplasia (2)
	Cochlear hypoplasia (11.2)
	Common cavity (19.4)
	Incomplete partition (42)
Normal cochlea	Lateral semicircular canal dysplasia (7.1)
	Enlarged vestibular aqueduct (17.3)

cochlea. During the imaging evaluation, mastoid and tympanic pneumatization is evaluated. The imaging is screened for evidence of enlarged vestibular or cochlear aqueduct. Enlargement of either the vestibular aqueduct or the cochlear aqueducts may be associated with an increased risk of cerebrospinal fluid (CSF) gusher.[33–35] However, this assertion remains controversial.[36,37]

High-resolution computed tomography (HRCT) of the temporal bones and high-resolution magnetic resonance imaging (MRI) of the otic capsule and internal auditory canal are the most commonly used imaging modalities in the pediatric cochlear implant imaging evaluation. However, the protocol by which these 2 imaging modalities are used remains variable. HRCT of the temporal bones is beneficial in identifying cochlear dysplasia, labyrinthine ossification, position of the facial nerve, aeration of the temporal bone, position of the sigmoid sinus, high-riding jugular bulb, carotid artery dehiscence, jugular diverticuli, size of the vestibular aqueduct, narrowing of the cochlear nerve canal, modiolar deficiency, and lateral semicircular canal dysplasia. There is considerable overlap in the imaging ability of HRCT of the temporal bone and MRI of the internal auditory canal. MRI of the internal auditory canal may be used to identify cochlear dysplasia, labyrinthine ossification, the position of the sigmoid sinus, the size of the vestibular aqueduct, narrowing of the cochlear nerve canal, modiolar deficiency, lateral semicircular canal dysplasia, evaluation of the internal auditory canal neural contents, and the caliber of the cochlear nerve. On comparison of the 2 modalities, MRI has been found to be superior in identifying early ossification of the labyrinth and soft tissue anomalies in the inner ear, the most important of which is presence or absence of the cochlear nerve.[38] HRCT of the temporal bones is superior at identifying the bony labyrinth, including enlarged vestibular aqueduct and caliber of the cochlear nerve canal.[39] No benefit has been shown in using dual-modality (HRCT and MRI) screening in the pediatric population before cochlear implantation.[40] Specificity and negative predictive value for MRI alone and HRCT alone are both high; there is no significant difference between the ability of MRI and HRCT to predict abnormal inner ear anatomy at the time of surgery.[40] For this reason, the choice of primary screening modality in imaging before cochlear implantation is left to the discretion of the cochlear implant team and center. If the patient has any symptoms that may warrant an MRI, this imaging modality should be used preoperatively given the current US Food and Drug Administration (FDA) guidelines precluding MRI in patients with existing cochlear implants.

Audiologic Evaluation

The audiologic evaluation is used to identify current aural performance and to guide aural rehabilitation after cochlear implantation. The main components of the audiologic evaluation include pure tone average assessment, hearing aid evaluation, speech perception testing, and electrophysiologic evaluation.

Current pediatric guidelines for cochlear implantation stipulate parameters for pure tone audiometry, speech perception, and aided performance required for cochlear implant candidacy. **Table 4** details the current FDA guidelines for the most recently approved devices in pediatric cochlear implantation. In general, unaided pure tone audiometry is performed to ensure sensorineural hearing loss with threshold of greater than or equal to 90 dB hearing level (HL). In addition, otoacoustic emissions should be performed. Presence of normal otoacoustic emissions in the presence of sensorineural hearing loss should increase the suspicion for auditory neuropathy/auditory dyssynchrony (AN/AD), the diagnosis of which greatly impacts aural rehabilitation methodology and expected outcomes.

Before consideration for cochlear implantation, pediatric candidates usually undergo a trial period with a hearing aid. The length of the hearing aid trial is determined by the implant center based on the characteristics of the candidate, including level of hearing loss, previous hearing aid experience, and other disabilities. Pediatric patients must undergo binaural hearing aid trials for a minimum of 3 to 6 months to document lack of or minimal improvement in auditory development. With children aged 24 months and younger, lack of auditory skills development is assessed by lack of meeting auditory milestones and poor performance on speech perception tests, including the Infant-Toddler Meaningful Auditory Integration Scale, Meaningful Auditory Integration Scale, or Early Speech Perception Test. In children approximately aged 2 years and older, lack of auditory skills development is assessed by open-set word recognition and open-set sentence recognition testing, including the Lexical Neighborhood Test and the Multisyllabic Lexical Neighborhood Test. Additional speech perception tests used in the pediatric cochlear implant candidacy evaluation include the Bamford-Kowal-Bench (BKB) Sentences, Early Speech Perception Test (Low Verbal Version or Standard Version), Glendonald Auditory Screening Procedure, Ling Sound Test, Minimal Pairs, Monosyllable-Trochee-Spondee Test, Northwestern University Children's Perception of Speech Test, Phonetically Balanced Kindergarten Word List, and Word Intelligibility by Picture Identification.

Electrophysiologic Evaluation

Electrophysiologic testing is of particular importance in evaluating younger pediatric patients ($\leq$24 months of age) and patients with development delay. Electrophysiologic testing serves as an objective measure of audiologic function. The electrophysiologic evaluation may include auditory brainstem response testing or electrically evoked auditory brainstem response testing. Auditory brainstem response testing serves as an objective measure of degree of sensorineural hearing loss in the pediatric cochlear implant evaluation in prelingually deaf and developmentally delayed patients. In addition, auditory brainstem response testing assists in the screening and diagnosis of AN/AD. Patients with AN/AD present with normal otoacoustic emissions and evidence of sensorineural hearing loss on auditory brainstem response testing. Patients with AN/AD have a more variable outcome in cochlear implantation.

Electrically evoked auditory brainstem response testing is most commonly used in pediatric patients less than the age of 24 months, patients with significant developmental delay, patients with observed vestibulocochlear anomalies identified during the imaging evaluation, and patients in whom no residual hearing has been detected on routine audiometry or traditional auditory brainstem response testing. This test confirms electrical stimulability of the auditory system via auditory brainstem response testing in these pediatric patient groups. The presence of stimulability and auditory brainstem response has been correlated with postoperative stimulability after cochlear implantation.[41,42] Electrically evoked auditory brainstem response testing assists in the selection of the ear for implantation in patients without any residual hearing, in patients with longstanding history of sensorineural hearing loss, and patients with inner ear malformations.[43–45]

Electrophysiologic testing is of great assistance in evaluating patients with AN/AD. Amongst pediatric patients with AN/AD, approximately 50% show some degree of open-set speech perception abilities.[46] Failure to achieve open-set speech perception after cochlear implantation in pediatric patients is believed to be secondary to cochlear nerve deficiency, lack of electrical-induced neural synchronization, and coexisting developmental delays.[46] Electrically elicited compound action potential testing may be beneficial in assessing which patients with AN/AD perform successfully

Table 4
Guidelines for most recently FDA-approved devices for pediatric cochlear implantation

Device Name	Device Manufacturer	Most Recent Approval	Pediatric Approval	Indications
Clarion HiResolution TM Bionic Ear System: HiRes 90KTM receiver HiFocus electrode array HiFocus Helix electrode array	Advanced Bionics Corporation (Advanced Bionics, Sylmar, CA, USA)	2003	12 mo–17 y	Profound, bilateral sensorineural hearing loss (>90 dB HL) Use of appropriately fit hearing aids for at least: 6 mo for children aged 2–17 y 3 mo for children aged 12–23 mo Minimum use of hearing aids is waived with evidence of cochlear ossification Little or no benefit from appropriately fit hearing aids In children <4 y defined as failure to reach developmentally appropriate auditory milestones measured by: Infant-Toddler Meaningful Auditory Integration Scale Meaningful Auditory Integration Scale <20% correction simple open-set word recognition test at 70 dB SPL In children >4 years defined as: scoring <12% on a difficult open-set word recognition test at 70 dB SPL scoring <30% on an open-set sentence test at 70 dB SPL
Nucleus Freedom implant with Contour AdvanceTM Electrode CI512 and CI513	Cochlear Corporation (Cochlear Americas, Centennial, CO, USA)	2009	12 mo–17 y	Children 12–24 mo Bilateral, profound sensorineural hearing loss (>90 dB HL) Limited benefit from appropriate binaural hearing aids Lack of progress in development of simple auditory skills Participation in intensive aural rehabilitation over 3–6 mo Quantified by Meaningful Auditory Integration Scale or Early Speech Perception Test Children 25 mo to 17 y and 11 mo Severe to profound sensorineural hearing loss (>65 dB HL) Limited benefit from appropriate binaural hearing aids 3–6 mo hearing aid trial Scoring <30% on open-set Multisyllabic Lexical Neighborhood Test or Lexical Neighborhood Test depending on the child's cognitive and linguistic skills

Med-El Pulsar CI100	Med-El (MED-EL, Durham, NC, USA)	2005	12 mo–17 y	Bilateral, profound sensorineural hearing loss (>90 dB at 1000 Hz)
				Little or no benefit from appropriately fit binaural hearing aids
				Younger children
				Lack of progress in development of simple auditory skills
				Participation in intensive aural rehabilitation over 3–6 mo
				Older children
				Scoring <20% on Multisyllabic Lexical Neighborhood Test or Lexical
				Neighborhood Test depending on child's cognitive ability and
				linguistic skills
				3–6 mo hearing aid trial

after cochlear implantation, because robust response has been correlated with improved performance.[46]

Speech and Language Evaluation

The speech and language evaluation should be performed in all pediatric patients before cochlear implantation. This strategy allows for the determination as to whether factors in addition to hearing impairment are contributing to hindrance in auditory development. Numerous children with developmental, cognitive, and language delay have been implanted with successful aural rehabilitation after modified aural rehabilitation protocols to optimized speech perception and production.[47,48] Children with cognitive and developmental delays have been found to develop speech perception skills at a slower rate compared with children without.[49] Despite this finding, cochlear implantation in patients with cognitive and developmental delay has been shown to improve quality of life, increase listening and communication skills, enhance self-sufficiency, and enhance their ability to interact with others.[47,48]

During the speech and language evaluation, the pediatric patients are screened for developmental language and articulation disorders. In addition, a description of the patient's communication status with respect to normative data by age is performed. This strategy assists in the development of appropriate goals and expectations of cochlear implantation and in the design of rehabilitation program for use postoperatively.

Patient and Family Counseling

After completion of the medical, imaging, audiologic, physiologic, speech and language, and cognitive and development evaluation, patient and family counseling is performed. The goal of the patient and family counseling is to summarize the findings of the cochlear implant evaluation and provide the family with recommendations from the cochlear implant team. At this time, expectations for cochlear implantation outcome are established. Explanation and assurance of understanding regarding the components and extent of postoperative aural rehabilitation are explained to the family. The level of commitment of the patient and family to the requirements of aural rehabilitation is assessed. Any questions asked by the family are answered. The family should be provided with literature regarding the available devices for implantation, and with the assistance of the cochlear implantation team, a decision regarding desired device for implantation are made. The patient's family is provided with a detailed description of the cochlear implantation procedure, informed consent is obtained, and the procedure and all options to the procedure are discussed.

SURGICAL CONSIDERATIONS

Various surgical considerations must be factored when performing cochlear implantation within the pediatric population. The cochlear implant surgeon must be aware of the potential need for alterations in the cochlear implantation procedure to accommodate cochleovestibular anomalies within the pediatric population and the considerations in electrode array choice to optimize postoperative aural rehabilitation. The surgeon should be abreast of techniques for simultaneous, bilateral cochlear implantation in children. In addition, the cochlear implant surgeon should be aware of complications that may accompany cochlear implantation in the pediatric population to minimize associated morbidity. The surgical section presented here is an overview of important considerations in pediatric cochlear implantation.

The Traditional Pediatric Cochlear Implantation Procedure

The traditional approach for cochlear implantation in the pediatric population uses the transmastoid, facial recess approach similar to that used in the adult population. Because the cochlear and the facial recess are adult size at birth, there is no additional risk related to cochleostomy and electrode insertion. The main components of the traditional pediatric implant procedure include incision and receiver placement design, simple mastoidectomy with facial recess, drill-out for receiver placement, securing of the receiver, cochleostomy, electrode placement, device telemetry, and closure. Mild variations are performed based on surgeon preference, but there are general principles that govern each stage:

- The procedure is performed with the patient under general anesthesia.
- Minimal or no shaving is performed in the postauricular region to facilitate exposure.
- The incision is designed and marked with a marking pen.
- A superior extension may be incorporated to facilitate implant receiver placement.
- The placement of the receiver is designed 2 cm posterior to the postauricular incision and superior to the imaginary line extending from the lateral canthus and superior aspect of the external auditory canal.
- The proposed position of the receiver is marked.
- Facial nerve monitoring is used through the duration of the procedure.
- The patient is prepared and draped in the normal sterile fashion.
- The skin incision is infiltrated in 1:100,000 epinephrine (or 2% lidocaine 1:100,000 epinephrine) in older children or 1:200,000 epinephrine in younger children.
- The skin incision is created as designed and skin flaps are elevated to the level of the posterior external auditory canal.
- Periosteal incisions are created and the Palva flap is elevated.
- Fascia for occlusion of the cochleostomy may be obtained from the most posterior portion of the Palva flap.
- The periosteum is then elevated posteriorly and superiorly for placement of the electrode receiver.
- The angulation of the receiver has evolved over time without impact on patient satisfaction, cosmesis, or clinical and functional outcomes.[50] A recent survey revealed that the average placement of cochlear implant receiver is currently 56.8° relative to the skull base.[50]
- The implant template may be used to facilitate assessing adequacy of periosteal elevation and to mark positioning of receiver.
- The cortex may be drilled out to facilitate stability of the receiver, prevent cutaneous complication (including implant exposure), and to improve cosmetic appearance via a lower profile.
- The bone in the periphery of the drill-out may be completed to the level of the dura, creating a central island of bone if necessary to facilitate deeper inset of the receiver.
- Simple mastoidectomy is performed with identification of the facial nerve and thinning of the posterior canal wall, facilitating exposure and light penetrance into the facial recess.
- The facial recess should be funnel shaped, not a tunnel, to allow thorough visualization of and access to the posterior mesotympanic structures.
- Maximum exposure is of utmost importance to allow proper cochleostomy placement and this can be accomplished by skeletonizing the facial nerve and

the chorda tympani nerve without injury to the nerves and removing the bone anterior to the facial nerve over the stapedius muscle.

- The round window niche is visualized and drilled for complete visualization of the round window membrane.
- Copious irrigation and attention to drill shaft position are used to minimize the risk of heat transmission and trauma to the facial nerve.
- The cochleostomy is then performed.
- The positioning of the cochleostomy varies by institution and by surgeon preference. However, placement of the cochleostomy inferior or anteroinferior to the round window membrane has been found to facilitate atraumatic insertion of cochlear implant electrodes within the central scala tympani.[51,52]
- The size of electrode varies slightly by device. The smallest cochleostomy should be performed for safe and easy advancement of the cochlear implant electrode without resistance.
- Using a 1-mm diamond burr, the cochlea is drilled to expose endosteum.
- Using a Barbara needle, straight pick, or McGee oval window rasp, with care not to displace bone fragments into the cochlea, the cochleostomy is widened.
- In addition, suctioning over the cochleostomy should not be performed to decrease risk of trauma.
- Many surgeons choose to use the round window for insertion depending on the electrode being used and the anatomic visualization of the round window.
- Round window insertion is facilitated by removal of the superior and posterior bony overhanging round window niche.
- The device is next placed into position.
- The receiver is secured. Various techniques are used for securing the device without significant impact on outcome.
- Once the device is secured, the electrode is atraumatically advanced through to cochleostomy with a goal of complete insertion.
- The cochleostomy is packed with fascia, muscle, periosteum or fat to prevent perilymph fistula and to seal the cochlea to prevent bacterial penetration into the cochlea in the event of otitis media.
- At this time, neural response telemetry may be performed. Intraoperative neural response telemetry has been shown to provide valuable information regarding electrical output, the response of the auditory system to electrical stimulation, and preliminary device programming data.[53]
- On completion of the neural response telemetry, the periosteum is closed and the incision is closed.
- Intraoperative radiograph of the skull may be taken to confirm electrode positioning.
- The patient is awakened from general anesthesia and transferred to the postanesthesia recovery unit.
- Patients may be monitored overnight; however, cochlear implantation in the pediatric population may safely be performed on an outpatient basis without increased incidence of morbidity or complications.[54]

Cochlear Implantation in Pediatric Patients with Vestibulocochlear Anomalies

Approximately one-third of pediatric patients undergoing cochlear implantation have some degree of vestibulocochlear abnormality. However, these patients have successfully undergone a cochlear implantation procedure. Knowledge of the presence of the malformation and minor alterations of the cochlear implantation procedure facilitates successful implantation and aural rehabilitation.

Incomplete partitioning

Incomplete partitioning is the most commonly encountered vestibulocochlear anomaly.[29] With incomplete partitioning, the cochlea completes 1 to 1.5 turns instead of the 2.5 associated with normal cochlear development around the modiolus. The 1.5 turns typically comprise the basal turn with the apparent confluence of the middle and apical turn. In patients with true Mondini-type cochleas (incomplete partitioning) regular full electrodes can be used successfully and the cochlear implantation procedure may be performed as described earlier. The main concern within these patients is partial insertion of the electrode because of the lack of 2.5 complete turns to the cochlea. Despite this concern, patients with incomplete partitioning and cochlear hypoplasia have undergone successful aural rehabilitation and function well after cochlear implantation. The main issue in these patients is optimizing the number of electrodes implanted and the functionality of these electrodes.

Common cavity deformity

Common cavity deformity is the second most common vestibulocochlear anomaly in the pediatric population. Common cavity deformity represents a confluence of the cochlea and vestibule into a common rudimentary cavity lacking internal architecture. Neural components within the common cavity have been histologically shown to lie within the periphery of the common cavity. Ideal electrode placement in the common cavity therefore requires placement of the electrode along the periphery of the common cavity with a circumferential vector of stimulation. For these reasons, straight-banded, circumferentially stimulating electrode array may be of benefit in patients with common cavity deformity. With common cavity deformity, a transmastoid antral approach most often can be used without need for facial recess to perform cochleostomy. An attempt should be made to avoid positioning the cochleostomy directly opposite the internal auditory canal. The electrode is inserted along the lateral wall to prevent kinking and bending. Intraoperative fluoroscopy has been shown to facilitate successful implantation in patients with common cavity deformity.[55,56] Newer portable intraoperative computed tomography scanners can also be used.

Intraoperative fluoroscopy

Intraoperative fluoroscopy has been proposed for cochlear implantation in pediatric patients with vestibulocochlear anomalies. Intraoperative fluoroscopy allows real-time assessment of cochlear implant electrode positioning during insertion. Intraoperative fluoroscopy has been found to be safe for patients and pose minimal risk to operative staff.[56] Radiation exposure to the patient should not exceed 200 rad for the duration of the procedure. Most contemporary fluoroscopy units produce radiation doses less than 10 rad per minute. The average exposure during cochlear implantation is for less than 3 minutes' total fluoroscopy time. In cochlear implantation with intraoperative fluoroscopy, the C-arm is positioned and target image acquisition confirmed after induction of general anesthesia, before initiation of the procedure. The C-arm is placed with the beam director beneath the operative table in an anti-Stenvers view. The beam is narrowed, centered, and magnified to facilitate visualization of the cochlea. The implantation procedure then proceeds as described earlier.

Intraoperative fluoroscopy has been shown to facilitate cochlear implant placement in patients with vestibulocochlear anomalies. It allows for real-time visualization of the electrode during the insertion process and the insertional stop point is delineated, which can minimize kinking and bending of the electrode and prevent internal auditory canal insertions. It has also been described for use in cases in which the intracochlear behavior of the electrode array cannot be predicted, in use with new electrode designs, and in patients with intraluminal obstruction of the cochlea (ie, labyrinthitis ossificans).[57]

Cochlear Implantation in Pediatric Patients with Ossified Cochleae

Since the introduction of the 7-valent pneumococcal conjugate vaccine and the *Haemophilus influenza* type B vaccine, the incidence of postmeningitic sensorineural hearing loss has declined.[58,59] However, in cases of pediatric meningitis, 5% of patients present with profound sensorineural hearing loss.[60] Early bilateral cochlear implantation, before complete cochlear obstruction from labyrinthitis ossificans, has been associated with improved outcomes in terms of completeness of insertion, speech intelligibility, and sound localization.[59,61] Cochlear ossification associated with postmeningitic deafness in the pediatric population requires additional surgical consideration to drill out the area of obstruction, allowing for implant electrode advancement.

Ossification in postmeningitic patients can be classified in 3 categories:

1. obliteration of the round window niche
2. obstruction limited to the inferior segment
3. upper segment obstruction.

Slight variations in operative technique are associated with implantation in each of these scenarios.

Obliteration of the round window niche

With obliteration of the round window niche from a fibrous tissue obliteration to dense calcific bony occlusion, drill-out must be performed within the region of the round window niche for exposure of the scala tympani. No evidence of the round window niche can be identified in the most severe cases. With obliteration of the round window niche, drill-out should be performed approximately 1.5 mm inferior to the pyramidal process, allowing for exposure to the region of the round window.[62] If not visible, the niche can be identified by encountering less dense and more lightly colored bone within this region. Following this bone anteriorly reveals the scala tympani, allowing for cochleostomy performance and electrode insertion.

Obstruction limited to the inferior segment

In most cases, limited obstruction of the basal turn of the cochlea is identified. The character of the obstruction may vary from a fibrous tissue band to dense calcified bony plate. The length of obstruction within the inferior segment greatly impacts the surgical approach to implantation. Involvement limited to the inferior 8 to 10 mm of the basal turn may be subjugated by drilling out over the round window niche as described earlier with extension along the basal turn of the cochlea. The open lumen may be encountered beyond the drill-out by tunneling through with a fine pick, delicate drill, or hand-held laser.[62] Once luminal patency is observed, cochlear implant electrode may be inserted.

Upper segment obstruction

In the final scenario of involvement within the ascending segment of the cochlea, the initial drill-out is performed as described earlier. Once the inferior 8 to 10 mm of the cochlea are opened, various options for implantation have been described. Partial insertion may be performed. With ossified cochleae and partial insertions, the use of double-array electrodes via a basal and middle turn cochleostomy has been found to result in more usable electrode contacts than single-stranded arrays. The use of a depth gauge or test electrode may be useful in determining which electrode to insert.

In general, if the test electrode cannot be inserted beyond the proximal basal segment into the pars ascendens and superior, a double array is considered.[63] A double array necessitates creation of an additional, second cochleostomy in the second turn of the cochlea. To prepare for the second cochleostomy, the incus, incus bar, and stapes superstructure are removed to maximize access anterior to the oval window. Using a 1-mm diamond burr and copious irrigation, this superior cochleostomy is created immediately anterior to the oval window, adjacent to the annular ligament of the stapes footplate. The cochleariform process serves as the superior limit of dissection and a landmark for facial nerve location. Drilling below the cochleariform process parallel to the tensor tympani muscle is critical to avoid damage to the facial nerve. One array is placed in the basal turn tunnel (described earlier) and the other array is inserted either retrograde or anterograde through the superior cochleostomy, based on patient anatomy and manufacturer recommendations. (Cochlear [Cochlear Americas, Centennial, CO, USA] prefers anterograde and MED-EL [MED-EL, Durham, NC, USA] encourages retrograde.) If no lumen is found in the upper cochlea, an apical tunnel can be created through the new bone using a rasp or 0.5-mm to 1-mm diamond bur. This tunnel should be directed toward the tensor tympani, away from the probable location of neural elements. The second array can then be placed in this superior tunnel. In general, the electrodes should not overlap and forceful insertion or overinsertion, leading to kinking or tip roll-over, should be avoided. Each cochleostomy should be effectively packed with periosteum or fascia to firmly secure the electrode position.

Pediatric patients with incomplete insertion with at least 10 electrodes have been shown to obtain open-set speech recognition.[64] If the ossification is limited to the scala tympani, the cochleostomy may be extended superiorly 1 to 2 mm, allowing for insertion of the electrode within the scala vestibule.[62,65] If both the scala tympani and scala vestibule are involved beyond the inferior segment, a perimodiolar trough may be drilled out.[66] This technique requires a radical mastoidectomy. The tympanic membrane (TM), malleus, and incus are removed, and the external auditory canal is obliterated. The carotid artery is skeletonized. The inferior segment is drilled out as described earlier, and the drill-out is continued to create an open trough around the modiolus. The electrode is then placed through the inferior segment tunnel into the trough and secured in place with fascia and tissue glue.

Complications in Pediatric Cochlear Implantation

Cochlear implantation within the pediatric population is safe and effective. Although major complications are rare, the cochlear implant surgeon should be well versed of the potential associated complications and potential means for their prevention. The rate of complications in pediatric cochlear implantation is on average approximately 10%.[67–70] Most complications reported represent minor complications, with major complications accounting for only 20% to 30% of all complications on average.[67–70] The presence of inner ear malformation has been correlated with an increased rate of complication in pediatric cochlear implantation.[69] Complications after cochlear implantation may be classified as early (within the first 2 weeks of implantation) and late (greater than 2 weeks after cochlear implantation).

Infection

Amongst the early complications of cochlear implantation, infection is the most commonly reported, presenting as wound infections or otitis media.[67–69] Infection comprises approximately half of all complications, early and late, after cochlear implantation. For this reason, perioperative antibiotics are commonly administered, including a brief postoperative course of oral antibiotics after discharge. Additional early complications of hematoma and seroma, which occur in approximately 2% of patients, may contribute to the development of postoperative wound infection. For this reason, care should be taken to ensure a completely dry field before closure of incision. In addition compressive dressing is applied postoperatively to prevent the accumulation of blood or serous fluid. When large seromas and hematomas occur, evacuation should be performed; whereas small stable collections may be monitored closely.

Facial nerve paresis

Despite the fact that facial nerve sheath exposure is commonly reported in pediatric cochlear implantation, facial nerve paresis is an uncommon complication of cochlear implantation surgery.[67–70] In up to 9% of patients, facial nerve sheath and nerve exposure has been reported.[67] Intraoperative facial nerve monitoring should be used in all cochlear implant procedures to minimize injury. In addition, during posterior tympanotomy and cochleostomy, copious irrigation should be used and care should be taken to prevent inadvertent contact of the drill shaft with the facial nerve. Injury to the chorda tympani nerve is a more common. Rates of chorda tympani injury have been reported in up to 20% of pediatric patients.[67] With the increase in bilateral cochlear implantation, care should be taken to maintain the integrity of the chorda tympani nerve while opening the facial recess.

CSF fistulas

CSF fistulas may present early or late after cochlear implantation in the pediatric population. CSF fistulas have been reported to present in up to 1% of pediatric patients after cochlear implantation.[68,71] Secondary meningitis has been reported in only a small percentage of pediatric patients after cochlear implantation.[69] CSF fistulas may be prevented by securely packing the cochleostomy around the electrode after implantation with fascia or muscle to prevent leakage.

Device failures

In addition, device failures may present early or late after cochlear implantation. Device failure has been reported to occur at a rate of up to 2%.[67–71] There are no methods available to prevent late device failures; however, early device failures may be circumvented. Intraoperative telemetry may be helpful in ensuring the function of the cochlear implant device at the time of implantation, decreasing the risk of early failure.

Cholesteatomas

Cholesteatomas have been reported after cochlear implantation as late complications.[67] Iatrogenic, undiagnosed TM perforation or preexisting chronic ear disease may be the inciting factors in cholesteatoma formation. TM perforation and cholesteatoma place the patient at risk for electrode exposure.[67] Multiple surgical options exist for the management of TM perforation, chronic ear disease, or cholesteatoma in the setting of planned cochlear implantation. Ideally, risk factors for the development of cholesteatoma or chronic otitis media (such as chronic, purulent otorrhea, large TM perforation, or significant TM retraction pockets) are identified at the initial cochlear implantation evaluation. Surgical strategy should be individualized and incorporate a range of factors, including the extent of middle ear disease and mastoid disease, the size of the TM perforation or retraction pocket, and the presence of ongoing or active infection.

Evidence exists to support both single-stage and multistage procedures to address chronic ear disease and cholesteatoma before cochlear implantation.[72,73] Multistage procedures require postponement or delay of implantation until creation of a safe, dry ear is confirmed, whereas single-stage procedures can be combined with and performed at the same time as cochlear implantation.[72] In cases of TM perforations or small retraction pockets, cartilage tympanoplasty techniques can be used to prevent the development of secondary, acquired cholesteatoma. If cholesteatoma is found, a radical mastoidectomy with removal of all squamous epithelium and closure of the external auditory canal (ie, creation of a blind sac) is an option. This procedure can be single-stage or multistage and attempts to create a safe cavity for the cochlear implantation device by removing all potentially infected tissue and squamous epithelium. Although rates of cholesteatoma recurrence are low with this technique, the inability to visually monitor the surgical cavity (because of closure of the canal) is a frequently cited drawback of this approach.[72,73]

EXPANDING CRITERIA

With the advancement of cochlear implant technology and investigation of the impact of cochlear implantation in various populations, the criteria for cochlear implantation continues to evolve. Cochlear implantation is currently being performed bilaterally within the pediatric population. In addition, children less than the age of 12 months have been implanted with great degrees of success. Cochlear implantation has also been performed in adolescent children with congenital sensorineural hearing loss and pediatric patients with residual hearing.

Cochlear Implantation in Children Younger than 12 Months

The foundation for advanced use and acquisition of language is laid by early hearing experience in childhood. With the newborn hearing screening programs, profound sensorineural hearing loss is more commonly being diagnosed within the first month of life. Auditory rehabilitation, including conventional amplification, beginning before age 6 months has been shown to significantly improve vocabulary, speech intelligibility, general language ability, social-emotional development, parental bonding, and parental grief resolution when compared with later aural rehabilitation.[74,75] Early cochlear implantation has been shown to improve phonological processing skills.[76] These improvements in receptive and expressive language have been shown to increase with age in children with cochlear implants as well.[77] For these reasons, the lower age limitation for cochlear implantation has continued to evolve.

Outcomes of implantation in patients younger than 12 months

Cochlear implantation is currently approved by the FDA for pediatric patients aged 12 months and older. Recently, implantation has been reported in children younger than 12 months. The current body of literature has revealed a trend toward benefit in terms of auditory rehabilitation and linguistic ability.[78–83] When compared with patients implanted between age 1 and 2 years, patients implanted before the age of 12 months have been shown to have superior speech understanding.[84] Patients implanted younger than 12 months have been found to have a receptive and expressive language skills growth rate similar to normal-hearing peers.[78–83] These advances in expressive language appear early in the development of speech acquisition.[85] Colletti and colleagues[86] evaluated the long-term (4-year to 9-year) outcomes of pediatric patients implanted within 3 cohorts: (1) patients implanted before age 12 months, (2) patients implanted at age 12 months to 23 months, and (3) patients implanted at age 24 months to 36 months. Compared with the patients implanted at or after 12 months of age, the patients implanted before the age of 12 months were found to have receptive language growth exceeding patients within the other 2 groups and overlapping that of normal-hearing children. At 9-year follow-up, 100% of the patients implanted before age 12 months, 38% of the patients implanted at age 12 to 23 months, and 20% of the patients implanted at age 24 to 36 months performed within the 76 to 100 percentile on speech receptive testing.

Operative considerations in cochlear implantation in patients younger than 12 months

Certain additional operative considerations are associated with cochlear implantation in pediatric patients younger than 12 months. As stated earlier, the blood volume within the pediatric patient is significantly less than that of the adult population. Within children younger than 12 months, the total systemic blood volume is approximately 80 mL per kg. Blood losses of less than 10% within the pediatric population can induce hypovolemia and its associated effects.[87] Therefore, small degrees of blood loss in the pediatric population can have catastrophic effects. The main sources of blood loss during pediatric cochlear implantation include bleeding from emissary veins and slow losses from bone marrow.[77] Care should be taken to maintain meticulous hemostasis throughout the duration of cochlear implantation in children younger than 12 months to prevent potential complications.

Although the size of the cochlear and the facial recess reaches adult size by birth, changes occur in the position of the facial nerve and pneumatization of the mastoid during childhood. Within children younger than 12 months, lateral and superficial displacement of the facial nerve and semicircular canals has been described as well as underdevelopment of the mastoid tip.[78,79,88] To prevent injury during cochlear implantation in children less than 12 months, minimal inferior extension of the skin incision and careful identification of the facial nerve should be performed. Facial nerve monitoring should be used in all cochlear implantation procedures regardless of age.

Additional operative considerations within patients younger than 12 months include soft tissue manipulation, receiver placement, and electrode migration. The skin of children younger than 12 months typically is significantly thinner than the adult population, making trauma to the skin flap and soft tissue a concern.[78,79,88] The skull thickness of younger pediatric patients can be less than a few millimeters. Dura exposure during receiver drill-out has been advocated to decrease device profile, improve cosmesis, and reduce risk of external damage from trauma.[78,89] With thinner receiver/stimulators now available, dural exposure and extensive drilling of a well or seat may not be so important for reducing device profile on the scalp and securing the device. Alternatively, others advocate that tight soft tissue closure is important in achieving device stability.[89] With younger children, significant changes in skull circumference may occur, potentially altering the distance between receiver placement and electrode insertion. Despite this, to date, there has been no evidence of device migration in the younger pediatric population[78]; however, further long-term studies are necessary.

Bilateral Cochlear Implantation

Binaural hearing in normal-hearing individuals allows listeners to hear more effectively in ambient noise and to localize the source of sound. Individuals with normal hearing in only 1 ear show deficiency in both tasks. Even mild to moderate unilateral hearing loss has been found to be associated with poorer academic performance and poorer speech development.[90,91] Binaural hearing allows the listener to take advantage of signals from the head shadow, binaural summation, and binaural squelch effects, improving speech recognition in noise and sound localization performance.[92] Similarly, children with unilateral cochlear implants have been shown to have difficulty with speech recognition in noisy environments, trouble with sound localization, and problems with the head shadow effect.[93] Because of these findings, binaural cochlear implantation has been introduced in children with bilateral profound sensorineural hearing loss.

Benefits in audition and vocalization

The proven benefits of bilateral cochlear implantation are multiplicitous. Pediatric patients with bilateral cochlear implantation have been shown to use significantly more audition and vocalization in communication 1 year after cochlear implantation than pediatric patients with unilateral cochlear implantation.[94] These findings were reported to be independent of age at time of implantation or duration of deafness.[94] Similar findings were reported by Wie and colleagues.[95] Bilateral cochlear implantation was shown to improve the ability to develop complex expressive and receptive spoken language early in the postimplantation period. After 12 to 48 months of cochlear implant use, pediatric patients have been found to develop expressive and receptive language skills within the normative range for their age.[95]

Benefits in speech perception

Bilateral cochlear implantation has been found to improve speech understanding in noise. Benefits in speech perception in noise from bilateral cochlear implantation have been shown early after cochlear implantation and have been found to continually improve up to 24 months after second implant placement.[96] Bilateral cochlear implantation has been shown to improve sound localization in addition to speech understanding both in quiet and in noise compared with patients with unilateral implantation alone or unilateral implantation plus contralateral hearing aid.[97–100] On right versus left discrimination, patients using both bilateral cochlear implants were found to outperform patients using 1 ear alone and patients with unilateral cochlear implants.[101,102] Similarly, in a review of pediatric patients after sequential bilateral cochlear implantation, sound localization was evaluated before sequential and after sequential bilateral implantation.[96] With unilateral implantation, none of the pediatric patients was able to successfully lateralize sound. After sequential bilateral implantation, 57% of children were able to lateralize at 6 months of bilateral cochlear implant use and 83% were able to lateralize at 24 months of bilateral cochlear implant use.[96] When assessing minimum audible angle, patients with bilateral cochlear implants are able to discern a smaller minimum audible angle than unilateral cochlear implant use.[96,103] Similarly, children with bilateral cochlear implants have been found to perform better on sound localization tasks than children with unilateral cochlear implants with contralateral hearing aids.[103]

Simultaneous and sequential cochlear implantation

Bilateral cochlear implantation may be performed in a simultaneous or sequential manner. Both simultaneous and sequential bilateral cochlear implants have been shown to have benefit over unilateral cochlear implantation; however, there seems to be a critical period after which the benefit of sequential bilateral cochlear implantation diminishes. Wolfe and colleagues[104] evaluated the postactivation speech recognition results in noise and in quiet from sequentially implanted children comparing the early and late implanted ear. No statistically significant difference was noted for speech recognition in quiet between early and late implanted ears when the second implant was performed before 4 years of age.[104] Alternatively, patients who underwent sequential implantation at greater than 4 years of age have statistically significant differences in speech recognition in quiet between ears.[104] No statistically significant difference in bilateral benefit in noise was noted in patients receiving the second implant before 4 years of age and those receiving the second implant after 4 years of age.[104] In comparing patients with simultaneous cochlear implantation, short interval (6–12 months) implantation, and long interval (more than 2 years) implantation, Gordon and Papsin reported a noticeable advantage to simultaneous or short interval implantation when compared with long interval implantation.[105]

In addition, the age of first-side implantation was found to be a contributing factor in the outcome of sequential cochlear implantation within the pediatric population.[97] Despite this finding, patients receiving sequential implantation greater than 2 years after implantation up to 10 years after initial implantation have been noted to benefit from bilateral cochlear implantation compared with unilateral implantation.[96,103,104,106] In addition, these benefits have been found to increase with time after bilateral implantation regardless of interval.[96,103,104,106] These data suggest that sequential bilateral or early bilateral cochlear implantation may be of greater benefit in the pediatric population. Despite this finding, if sequential or early implantation cannot be accomplished, patients receiving late sequential bilateral implantation obtain significant benefit from bilateral implantation, warranting the procedure.

Simultaneous bilateral cochlear implantation is a safe and effective method for bilateral cochlear implantation. In a review of 50 patients with simultaneous bilateral cochlear implantation compared with sequential bilateral cochlear implantation, total operative time was found to be significantly shorter amongst the simultaneous bilateral patients.[107] Total hospital stay was decreased in the simultaneous bilateral group compared with the sequential bilateral group.[107] The reported rates of complication with simultaneous bilateral cochlear implantation parallel that reported in the literature for unilateral cochlear implantation.[107]

Cochlear Implantation in Adolescents with Congenital Long-term Deafness

Cochlear implantation in prelingually deaf children and postlingually deaf adults has extensively been explored within the literature. Recently, the issues revolving cochlear implantation within prelingually deaf adolescents have been explored. Outcomes within this population show a high degree of variability.

Various factors have been found to affect success in cochlear implantation within prelingually deafened adolescents. Pure tone thresholds of 40 dB or less have been reported in prelingually deaf individuals implanted during adolescence.[108] In addition, this study provides data regarding mode of communication after cochlear implantation in the adolescent population.[108] Although more common with cued speech users than sign language user, some adolescent patients, after delayed cochlear implantation, were able to convert to oral communication.[108] In a review of congenitally deaf children implanted at a mean age of 12 years (range 8–17 years), congenitally deaf individuals implanted later in childhood were found to be able to obtain open-set speech understanding.[109] The length of deafness, length of device use, and mode of communication have all been found to contribute to outcomes.[109] These patients were noted to have mean preoperative sentence recognition scores on common phrases tests of 31% and BKB test of 29%.[109] Postoperative mean sentence recognition scores on common phrases and BKB tests improved to 73% and 65%, respectively.[109] Schramm and colleagues[110] reported similar findings with regard to open-set word and sentence test scores. Preimplantation open-set word test score (range 0%–24%) improved significantly (range 0%–74%) in 60% of prelingually deaf adolescent patients 6 months after implantation.[110] Similarly, open-set sentence test scores ranged from 0% to 98% within this cohort.[110] Patients continued to show improvement throughout the study period of 12 months.[110] Arisi and colleagues[111] presented a prospective study of 45 individuals implanted at age 11 years or greater. One-third of patients were found to be good performers after cochlear implantation.[111] Improved performance was correlated with daily use of implant. In addition, degree of hearing loss at time of deafness diagnosis affects success of cochlear implant use in adolescent patients; patients with hearing loss of 100 dB HL or less were more likely to be good performers than individuals with a greater degrees of hearing loss.[111] Additional factors that have been found to influence cochlear implant outcomes in congenitally deaf patients implanted during adolescence include the cause of hearing loss, use of speech therapy, education, device used, and therapeutic strategy.[111]

Cochlear Implantation in Pediatric Patients with Residual Hearing

Recently, pediatric patients with residual hearing have been undergoing cochlear implantation. As stated earlier regarding late implantation in adolescent patients with congenital hearing loss, patients with residual hearing are more likely to be good performers after cochlear implantation.[111] Similar reports have been reported in pediatric patients with congenital hearing loss who have received implants.[112] Increased auditory experience in children with residual hearing has been found to positively influence postoperative perception skills.[113] In a review of pediatric patients with pure tone thresholds of greater than 70 dB HL in whom all patients received good aided benefit in the frequencies ranging from 500 to 2000 Hz, mean speech perception scores were found to significantly improve after cochlear implantation.[114] The mean open-set speech recognition scores of 21.4% were reported before implantation. One year after implantation, the mean open-set speech recognition scores improved to 83.6%.[114]

Using minimal trauma techniques for cochleostomy and insertion, residual hearing may be preserved in the pediatric population after cochlear implantation. In a review by Skarzynski and colleagues,[115] residual hearing after cochlear implantation was maintained within 5 dB in 62% of pediatric and adult patients. In addition, only 19% of patients within this study lost all measurable residual hearing after cochlear implantation.[115] Hybrid technology, which provides electroacoustic stimulation, has been investigated for second-side implantation within the pediatric population.[116] Pediatric patients implanted on 1 side with the standard 24-mm electrode array and in the contralateral ear with the hybrid 10-mm electrode array were found to have equivalent performance in both ears.[116]

These data suggest that pediatric patients with residual hearing may have an advantage in performance over patients with no residual hearing. With minimally invasive techniques, cochlear implantation within the pediatric population can be performed without significant deleterious impact on residual hearing. With further investigation of electroacoustic stimulation, pediatric patients with residual hearing may benefit from the hybrid technology. However, further investigation is necessary to delineate the full impact of implantation within children with residual hearing and expand the criteria for cochlear implantation within this population.

SUMMARY

Since the introduction of cochlear implantation in clinical practice, its preoperative evaluation, implementation, and criteria for use continue to evolve. Patient selection is essential to success in cochlear implantation. The preoperative evaluation is designed to identify appropriate candidates for implantation and should include medical evaluation, cochlear imaging, audiologic and hearing aid evaluation, speech and language evaluation, electrophysiologic testing, psychological testing, and speech perception testing. Within the evaluation of pediatric patients, the cause of sensorineural hearing loss should be identified because it may affect perioperative care, surgical techniques during implantation, and postoperative rehabilitation. Within the pediatric population, the criteria for implantation continue to evolve. Most recently, implantation is being undertaken in patients who are younger than 12 months. Bilateral cochlear implantation is often used in the pediatric population to improve directional hearing and hearing in noise.

REFERENCES

1. Daya H, Figueirdo JC, Gordon KA, et al. The role of graded profile analysis in determining candidacy and outcome for cochlear implantation in children. Int J Pediatr Otorhinolaryngol 1999;49:135–42.
2. Riga M, Psarommatis I, Lyra C, et al. Etiological diagnosis of bilateral, sensorineural hearing impairment in a pediatric Greek population. Int J Pediatr Otorhinolaryngol 2005;69:449–55.
3. Rajput K, Brown T, Bamiou DE. Aetiology of hearing loss and other related factors versus language outcome after cochlear implantation in children. Int J Pediatr Otorhinolaryngol 2003;67:497–504.
4. Rao SC, Ahmed M, Hagan R. One dose per day compared to multiple doses per day of gentamicin for treatment of suspected or proven sepsis in neonates, 2006 for treatment of suspected or proven sepsis in neonates. Cochrane Database Syst Rev 2006;25:CD005091.
5. Siem G, Fagerheim T, Jonsrud C, et al. Causes of hearing impairment in the Norwegian paediatric cochlear implant program. Int J Audiol 2010;49:596–605.
6. Kenneson A, Van Naarden Braun K, Boyle C. GJB2 (connexin 26) variants and nonsyndromic sensorineural hearing loss: a HuGE review. Genet Med 2002;4: 258–74.
7. Dahl HH, Sauders K, Kelly TM, et al. Prevalence and nature of connexin 26 mutations in children with non-syndromic deafness. Med J Aust 2001;175: 191–4.
8. Dahl HH, Wake M, Sarant J, et al. Language and speech perception outcomes in hearing-impaired children with and without connexin 26 mutation. Audiol Neurootol 2003;8:263–8.
9. Sinnathuray AR, Toner JG, Clarke-Lyttle J, et al. Connexin 26 (GJB2) gene-related deafness and speech intelligibility after cochlear implantation. Otol Neurotol 2004;25:935–42.
10. Loundon N, Marlin S, Busquet D, et al. Usher syndrome and cochlear implantation. Otol Neurotol 2003;24:216–21.
11. Vescan A, Parnes LS, Cucci RA, et al. Cochlear implantation and Pendred's syndrome mutation in monozygotic twins with large vestibular aqueduct syndrome. J Otolaryngol 2002;31:54–7.
12. Siem G, Fruh A, Leren TP, et al. Jervell and Lange-Nielsen syndrome in Norwegian children: aspects around cochlear implantation, hearing and balance. Ear Hear 2008;29:261–9.
13. Chorbachi R, Graham JM, Ford J, et al. Cochlear implantation in Jervell and Lange-Nielsen syndrome. Int J Pediatr Otorhinolaryngol 2002;66:213–21.
14. Green JD, Schuh MJ, Maddern BR, et al. Cochlear implantation in Jervell and Lange-Neilsen syndrome. Ann Otol Rhinol Laryngol Suppl 2000;185:27–8.
15. Raine CH, Kurukulasuriva MF, Bajaj Y, et al. Cochlear implantation in Refsum's disease. Cochlear Implants Int 2008;9:97–102.
16. Cullen RD, Zdanski C, Roush P, et al. Cochlear implants in Waardenburg syndrome. Laryngoscope 2006;116:1273–5.

17. Sugii A, Iwaki T, Doi K, et al. Cochlear implant in a young child with Waardenburg syndrome. Adv Otorhinolaryngol 2000;57:215–9.
18. MacArdie BM, Bailey C, Phelps PD, et al. Cochlear implants in children with craniofacial syndromes: assessment and outcomes. Int J Audiol 2002;41:347–56.
19. Lanson BG, Green JE, Roland JT Jr, et al. Cochlear implantation in children with CHARGE syndrome: therapeutic decisions and outcomes. Laryngoscope 2007; 117:1260–6.
20. Moss AJ, Schwartz PJ, Crampton RS, et al. The long QT syndrome. Prospective longitudinal study of 328 families. Circulation 1991;84:1136–44.
21. Yanmei F, Yaqin W, Haibo S, et al. Cochlear implantation in patients with Jervell and Lange-Nielsen syndrome, and a review of literature. Int J Pediatr Otorhinolaryngol 2008;72:1723–9.
22. Wilson WR, Geer GE, Grubb BP. Implantable cardioverter-defibrillators in children: a single-institutional experience. Ann Thorac Surg 1998;65:775–8.
23. Barañano CF, Sweitzer RS, Mahalak ML, et al. The management of myringotomy tubes in pediatric cochlear implant recipients. Arch Otolaryngol Head Neck Surg 2010;136:557–60.
24. Biernath KR, Reefhuis J, Whitney CG, et al. Bacterial meningitis among children with cochlear implants beyond 24 months after implantation. Pediatrics 2006; 117:284–9.
25. Parner ET, Reefhuis J, Schendel D, et al. Hearing loss diagnosis followed by meningitis in Danish children, 1995-2004. Otolaryngol Head Neck Surg 2007; 136:428–33.
26. Cohen NL, Hirsch BE. Current status of bacterial meningitis after cochlear implantation. Otol Neurotol 2010;31:1325–8.
27. CDC. Pneumococcal vaccination for cochlear implant candidates and recipients: updated recommendation of the Advisory Committee on Immunization Practices. MMWR Morb Mortal Wkly Rep 2010;59:258–61.
28. Reefhuis J, Whitney C, Mann E. A public health perspective on cochlear implants and meningitis in children. Otol Neurotol 2010;31:1329–30.
29. Papsin BC. Cochlear implantation in children with anomalous cochleovestibular anatomy. Laryngoscope 2005;115(1 Pt 2 Suppl 106):1–26.
30. Jackler RK, Luxford WM, House WF. Congenital malformations of the inner ear: a classification based on embryogenesis. Laryngoscope 1987;97:2–14.
31. Sennaroglu L, Sarac S, Ergin T. Surgical results of cochlear implantation in malformed cochlea. Otol Neurotol 2006;27:615–23.
32. Tomura N, Sahi R, Kobayashi M, et al. Normal variations of the temporal bone on high-resolution CT: their incidence and clinical significance. Clin Radiol 1995;50: 144–8.
33. Chadha NK, James AL, Gordon KA, et al. Bilateral cochlear implantation in children with anomalous cochleovestibular anatomy. Arch Otolaryngol Head Neck Surg 2009;135:903–9.
34. Kim CS, JuKwon B, Chang SO, et al. CSF gusher in cochlear implantation. Cochlear Implants Int 2004;5:67–9.
35. Kim LS, Jeong SW, Huh MJ, et al. Cochlear implantation in children with inner ear malformations. Ann Otol Rhinol Laryngol 2006;115:205–14.
36. Dettman S, Sadeghi-Baralighi A, Ambett R, et al. Cochlear implants in forty-eight children with cochlear and/or vestibular abnormality. Audiol Neurootol 2010;16: 222–32.
37. Jackler RK, Hwang PH. Enlargement of the cochlear aqueduct: fact or fiction? Otolaryngol Head Neck Surg 1993;109:14–25.

38. Parry DA, Booth T, Roland PS. Advantages of magnetic resonance imaging over computed tomography in preoperative evaluation of pediatric cochlear implant candidates. Otol Neurotol 2005;26:976–82.
39. Trimble K, Blaser S, James AL, et al. Computed tomography and/or magnetic resonance imaging before pediatric cochlear implantation? Developing an investigative strategy. Otol Neurotol 2007;28:317–24.
40. Gleeson TG, Lacy PD, Bresnihan M, et al. High resolution computed tomography and magnetic resonance imaging in the pre-operative assessment of cochlear implant patients. J Laryngol Otol 2003;117:692–5.
41. Kileny PR, Zwolan TA, Zimmerman-Philips S, et al. Electrically evoked auditory brainstem response in pediatric patients with cochlear implants. Arch Otolaryngol Head Neck Surg 1994;120:1083–90.
42. Kileny PR, Zwolan TA. Perioperative transtympanic electric ABR in paediatric cochlear implant candidates. Cochlear Implants Int 2004;5(Suppl 1):23–5.
43. Kileny PR, Zwolan TA, Boerst A, et al. Electrically evoked auditory potential: current clinical applications in children with cochlear implants. Am J Otol 1997;18:S90–2.
44. Kim AH, Kileny PR, Arts HA, et al. Role of electrically evoked auditory brainstem response in cochlear implantation of children with inner ear malformations. Otol Neurotol 2008;29:626–34.
45. Nikolopoulos TP, Mason SM, Gibbin KP, et al. The prognostic value of promontory electric auditory brain stem response pediatric cochlear implantation. Ear Hear 2000;21:236–41.
46. Teagle HF, Roush PA, Woodard JS, et al. Cochlear implantation in children with auditory neuropathy spectrum disorder. Ear Hear 2010;31:325–35.
47. Donaldson AI, Heavner KS, Zwolan TA. Measuring progress in children with autism spectrum disorder who have cochlear implants. Arch Otolaryngol Head Neck Surg 2004;130:666–71.
48. Filipo R, Bosco E, Mancini P, et al. Cochlear implants in special cases: deafness in the presence of disabilities and/or associated problems. Acta Otolaryngol Suppl 2004;552:74–80.
49. Pyman B, Blamey P, Lacy P, et al. The development of speech perception in children using cochlear implants: effects of etiologic factors and delayed milestones. Am J Otol 2000;21:57–61.
50. Campisi P, James A, Hayward L, et al. Cochlear implant positioning in children: a survey of patient satisfaction. Int J Pediatr Otorhinolaryngol 2004;68:1289–93.
51. Meshik X, Holden TA, Chole RA, et al. Optimal cochlear implant insertion vectors. Otol Neurotol 2010;31:58–63.
52. Briggs RJS, Tykocinski M, Stidham K. Cochleostomy site: implications for electrode placement and hearing preservation. Acta Otolaryngol 2005;125:870–6.
53. Cosetti MK, Shapiro WH, Green JE, et al. Intraoperative neural response telemetry as a predictor of performance. Otol Neurotol 2010;31:1095–9.
54. Lui JH, Roland PS, Waller MA. Outpatient cochlear implantation in the pediatric population. Otolaryngol Head Neck Surg 2000;122:19–22.
55. Roland JT Jr, Coelho DH, Pantelides H, et al. Partial and double-array implantation of the ossified cochlea. Otol Neurotol 2008;29:1068–75.
56. Coelho DH, Waltzman SB, Roland JT Jr. Implanting common cavity malformations using intraoperative fluoroscopy. Otol Neurotol 2008;29:914–9.
57. Fishman AJ, Roland JT Jr, Alexiades G, et al. Fluoroscopically assisted cochlear implantation. Otol Neurotol 2003;24:882–6.

58. Poehling KA, Talbot TR, Griffin MR, et al. Invasive pneumococcal disease among infants before and after introduction of pneumococcal conjugate vaccine. JAMA 2006;295:1668–74.
59. Philippon D, Bergeron F, Ferron P, et al. Cochlear implantation in postmeningitic deafness. Otol Neurotol 2009;31:83–7.
60. Baraff LJ, Schriger DL. Outcomes of bacterial meningitis in children: a meta-analysis. Pediatr Infect Dis J 1993;12:389–94.
61. Tsuji RK, Goffi-Gomez MV, Peralta CO, et al. Neural response thresholds in the Nucleus Contour cochlear implant before and after stylet removal. Acta Otolaryngol 2009;129:1330–6.
62. Young NM, Tan TQ. Current techniques in management of postmeningitic deafness in children. Arch Otolaryngol Head Neck Surg 2010;136:993–8.
63. Balkany T, Gantz BJ, Steenerson RL, et al. Systematic approach to electrode insertion in ossified cochlea. Otolaryngol Head Neck Surg 1996;114:4–11.
64. Cohen NC, Waltzman SB. Partial insertion of Nucleus multichannel cochlear implant: technique and results. Am J Otol 1993;14:357–61.
65. Steenerson RL, Gray LB, Wynens MS. Scala vestibule cochlear implantation for labyrinthine ossification. Am J Otol 1990;11:360–3.
66. Gantz BJ, McCabe BF, Tyler RS. Use of multi-channel cochlear implants in obstructed and obliterated cochleas. Otolaryngol Head Neck Surg 1988;98:72–81.
67. Bhatia K, Gibbin KP, Nikolopoulos TP, et al. Surgical complications and their management in a series of 300 consecutive pediatric cochlear implantations. Otol Neurotol 2004;25:730–9.
68. Francis HW, Buchman CA, Visaya JM, et al. Surgical factors in pediatric cochlear implantation and their early effects on electrode activation and functional outcomes. Otol Neurotol 2008;29:502–8.
69. Loundon N, Blanchard M, Roger G, et al. Medical and surgical complications in pediatric cochlear implantation. Arch Otolaryngol Head Neck Surg 2010;136:12–5.
70. McJunkin J, Jeyakumar A. Complications in pediatric cochlear implants. Am J Otolaryngol 2010;31:110–3.
71. Hou JH, Zhao SP, Ning F, et al. Postoperative complications in patients with cochlear implants and impacts of nursing intervention. Acta Otolaryngol 2010; 130:687–95.
72. Hellingman CA, Dunnebier EA. Cochlear implantation in patients with acute or chronic middle ear infectious disease: a review of the literature. Eur Arch Otorhinolaryngol 2009;266:171–6.
73. El-Kashlan HK, Arts H, Telian SA. External auditory canal closure in cochlear implant surgery. Otol Neurotol 2003;24:404–8.
74. Moeller MP. Early intervention and language development in children who are deaf and hard of hearing. Pediatrics 2000;106:605–27.
75. Yoshinaga-Itano C. Early intervention after universal neonatal hearing screening: impact on outcomes. Ment Retard Dev Disabil Res Rev 2003;9:252–66.
76. Spencer LJ, Oleson JJ. Early listening and speaking skills predict later reading proficiency in pediatric cochlear implant user. Ear hear 2008;29:270–80.
77. Hay-McCutcheon MJ, Kirk KI, Henning SC, et al. Using early language outcomes to predict later language ability in children with cochlear implants. Audiol Neurootol 2008;13:370–8.
78. Roland JT Jr, Cosetti M, Wang KH, et al. Cochlear implantation in very young children: long-term safety and efficacy. Laryngoscope 2009;119:2205–10.
79. Waltzman SB, Roland JT Jr. Cochlear implantation in children younger than 12 months. Pediatrics 2005;116:e487–93.

80. Dettman SJ, Pinder D, Briggs RJ, et al. Communication development in children who receive the cochlear implant younger than 12 months: risks versus benefit. Ear Hear 2007;28:11S–8S.

81. Colletti V, Carner M, Miorelli V, et al. Cochlear implantation at under 12 months: report on 10 patients. Laryngoscope 2005;115:445–9.

82. Valencia DM, Rimell FL, Friedman BJ, et al. Cochlear implantation in infants less than 12 months of age. Int J Pediatr Otorhinolaryngol 2008;72:767–73.

83. Tait M, DeRaeve L, Nikolopoulos TP. Deaf children with cochlear implants before the age of 1 year: comparison of preverbal communication with normally hearing children. Int J Pediatr Otorhinolaryngol 2007;71:1605–11.

84. Lesinski-Schiedat A, Illg A, Heermann R, et al. Paediatric cochlear implantation in the first and in the second year of life: a comparative study. Cochlear Implants Int 2004;5:146–59.

85. Schauwers K, Gillis S, Govaerts PJ. The characteristics of prelexical babbling after cochlear implantation between 5 and 20 months of age. Ear Hear 2008; 29:627–37.

86. Colletti L. Long-term follow-up of infants (4–11 months) fitted with cochlear implants. Acta Otolaryngol 2009;129:361–6.

87. Johr M, Ho A, Wagner CS, et al. Ear surgery in infants under one year of age: its risks and implications for cochlear implant surgery. Otol Neurotol 2008;29: 310–3.

88. Birman C. Cochlear implant surgical issues in the very young child. Cochlear Implants Int 2009;10:19–22.

89. Balkany TJ, Whitley M, Shapira Y, et al. The temporalis pocket technique for cochlear implantation: anatomic and clinical study. Otol Neurotol 2009;30: 903–7.

90. Khairi MD, Daud M, Noor RM, et al. The effect of mild hearing loss on academic performance in primary school children. Int J Pediatr Otorhinolaryngol 2010;74: 67–70.

91. Lieu JE, Tye-Murray N, Karzon RK, et al. Unilateral hearing loss is associated with worse speech-language scores in children. Pediatrics 2010;125:e1348–55.

92. Brown KD, Balkany TJ. Benefits of bilateral cochlear implantation: a review. Otolaryngol Head Neck Surg 2007;15:315–8.

93. Ruscetta MN, Arjmand EM, Pratt SR. Speech recognition abilities in noise for children with severe-to-profound unilateral hearing impairment. Int J Pediatr Otorhinolaryngol 2005;69:771–9.

94. Tait M, Nikolopoulos TP, DeRaeve I, et al. Bilateral versus unilateral cochlear implantation in young children. Int J Pediatr Otorhinolaryngol 2010;74:206–11.

95. Wie OB. Language development in children after receiving bilateral cochlear implants between 5 and 18 months. Int J Pediatr Otorhinolaryngol 2010;74: 1258–66.

96. Sparreboom M, Snik AF, Mylanus EA. Sequential bilateral cochlear implantation in children: development of the primary auditory ability of bilateral stimulation. Audiol Neurootol 2011;16:203–13.

97. Zeitler DM, Kessler MA, Terushkin V, et al. Speech perception benefits of sequential bilateral cochlear implantation in children and adults: a retrospective analysis. Otol Neurotol 2008;29:314–25.

98. Dunn CC, Noble W, Tyler RS, et al. Bilateral and unilateral cochlear implant users compared on speech perception in noise. Ear Hear 2010;31:296–8.

99. Dunn CC, Tyler RS, Oakley S, et al. Comparison of speech recognition and localization performance in bilateral and unilateral cochlear implant users

matched on duration of deafness and age at implantation. Ear Hear 2008;29: 352–9.

100. Eapen RJ, Buss E, Adunka MC, et al. Hearing-in-noise benefits after bilateral simultaneous cochlear implantation continue to improve 4 years after implantation. Otol Neurotol 2009;30:153–9.

101. Galvin KL, Mok M, Dowell RC, et al. Speech detection and localization results and clinical outcomes for children receiving sequential cochlear implants before four years of age. Int J Audiol 2008;47:636–46.

102. Lovett RE, Kitterick PT, Hewitt CE, et al. Bilateral or unilateral cochlear implantation for deaf children: an observational study. Arch Dis Child 2010;95:107–12.

103. Litovsky RY, Johnstone PM, Godar S, et al. Bilateral cochlear implants in children: localization acuity measured with minimum audible angle. Ear Hear 2006;27:43–59.

104. Wolfe J, Baker S, Caraway T, et al. 1-year postactivation results for sequentially implanted bilateral cochlear implant users. Otol Neurotol 2007;28:589–96.

105. Gordon KA, Papsin BC. Benefits of short interimplant delay in children receiving bilateral cochlear implants. Otol Neurotol 2009;30:319–31.

106. Scherf F, Van Deun DL, Van Wieringen A, et al. Three-year postimplantation auditory outcomes in children with sequential bilateral cochlear implantation. Ann Otol Rhinol Laryngol 2009;118:336–44.

107. Ramsden JD, Papsin BC, Leung R, et al. Bilateral simultaneous cochlear implantation in children: our first 50 cases. Laryngoscope 2009;119:2444–8.

108. Kos MI, Deriaz M, Guyot JP, et al. What can be expected from a late cochlear implantation? Int J Pediatr Otorhinolaryngol 2009;73:189–93.

109. Waltzman SB, Roland JT Jr, Cohen NL. Delayed implantation in congenitally deaf children and adults. Otol Neurotol 2002;23:333–40.

110. Schramm D, Fitzpatrick E, Seguin C. Cochlear implantation for adolescents and adults with prelinguistic deafness. Otol Neurotol 2002;23:698–703.

111. Arisi E, Forti S, Pagani D, et al. Cochlear implantation in adolescents with prelinguistic deafness. Otolaryngol Head Neck Surg 2010;142:804–8.

112. Gantz BJ, Rubinstein J, Tyler R, et al. Long term results of cochlear implants in children with residual hearing. Ann Otol Rhinol Laryngol 2000;185:S33–6.

113. Zwolan TA, Zimmerman-Phillips S, Ashbaugh CJ, et al. Cochlear implantation of children with minimal open-set speech recognitions skills. Ear Hear 1997;18: 240–51.

114. Mondain M, Sillon M, Vieu A, et al. Cochlear implantation in prelingually deafened children with residual hearing. Int J Pediatr Otorhinolaryngol 2002;63: 91–7.

115. Skarzynski H, Lorens A, D'Haese P, et al. Preservation of residual hearing in children and post-lingually deafened adults after cochlear implantation: an initial study. ORL J Otorhinolaryngol Relat Spec 2002;64:247–53.

116. Gantz BJ, Dunn CC, Walker EA, et al. Bilateral cochlear implants in infants: a new approach - Nucleus Hybrid S12 project. Otol Neurotol 2010;31:1300–9.

Surgical Techniques in Cochlear Implants

Brannon Mangus, MD[a],*, Alejandro Rivas, MD[a], Betty S. Tsai, MD[a],
David S. Haynes, MD[a], J. Thomas Roland Jr, MD[b]

KEYWORDS

- Cochlear implants • Round window insertion • Cochleostomy

OVERVIEW OF SURGICAL TECHNIQUES FOR COCHLEAR IMPLANTS

The first report of auditory perception from an electrical stimulation occurred in 1790 when Alessandro Volta passed current across his own head using batteries. He experienced a "boom within his head" and the perceived a sound similar to "boiling, thick soup."[1] The first cochlear implantation was performed by Djourno and Eyriès in Paris in 1957. With this implant, the patient was able to discriminate between large changes in frequencies and appreciate environmental noises and some words but had no speech understanding. Dr William F. House collaborated with Dr James Doyle, a neurosurgeon, and Jack Urban, an engineer, to develop a practical and reliable means to restore hearing through electrical stimulation and implanted two deaf volunteers in 1961 with some success of auditory stimulation, but both devices had to be removed due to infections.[2] By 1984, the cochlear implant had gained Food and Drug Administration approval and multichannel implants were being developed. In 1988, the National Institutes of Health released a statement that suggested multichannel implants would be more effective than single-channel implants.[3] At the same time, new processing strategies were being developed, which ultimately led the National Institutes of Health to conclude at their 1995 meeting that "a majority of those individuals with the latest speech processors for their implants will score above 80% correct on high-context sentences even without visual cues."[4] The success of the cochlear implant has progressed so much that in 2008, Gifford and colleagues[5] reported the need for more difficult material to assess patient performance because more than 25% of cochlear implant patients achieve 100% scores on standard sentence material. As of 2008, more than 120,000 cochlear implants have been implanted worldwide.[2]

No disclosures.
David S Haynes is Consultant for Cochlear America, Zeiss.
[a] Otology Group of Vanderbilt, Department of Otolaryngology–Head and Neck Surgery, Vanderbilt Bill Wilkerson Center, Vanderbilt University, 1215 21st Avenue South, 7209 Medical Center East, South Tower, Nashville, TN 37232, USA
[b] Department of Otolaryngology, New York University Cochlear Implant Center, New York University School of Medicine, 660 First Avenue, 7th Floor, New York, NY 10016, USA
* Corresponding author.
E-mail address: brannon.mangus@vanderbilt.edu

Otolaryngol Clin N Am 45 (2012) 69–80
doi:10.1016/j.otc.2011.08.017
0030-6665/12/$ – see front matter © 2012 Elsevier Inc. All rights reserved.

oto.theclinics.com

EVOLUTION OF INCISIONS

As the cochlear implant has evolved since its inception, so has the cochlear implant incision.[6] The original incisions were based on the concept that wide exposure of the internal receiver stimulator (R/S) was necessary for placement and fixation. It was also generally believed that the incision should not cross the implant or electrode array. Because of these concepts, as well as the early practice of "thinning" the flap over the magnet, initially the majority of cochlear implant complications were flap related, sometimes necessitating implant removal.[7–9] Despite the evolution in incision design, the underlying principles of the incision have remained the same and include the following:

1. Planned incision should not be near the internal R/S to prevent potential extrusion or pain.
2. Blood supply must not be compromised.
3. Linea temporalis, mastoid tip, and spine of Henle should be accessible without undue retraction.

The original, anteriorly based C-shaped postauricular incision worked well with single-channel implants but had to be modified to a larger C-shaped incision when multichannel devices came into use due to the increased size of the R/Ss. The larger C-shaped incisions were associated with a high rate of device extrusion. The C-shaped incisions preserved blood supply from branches of the superficial temporal artery but transected occipital artery branches. Also, this incision was thought to be incompatible with patients who had a pre-existing postauricular incision due to compromised blood supply.[10] In response to the complications associated with the C-shaped incision, an extended endaural incision was developed and widely used in Europe due to its small incision and lower risk. The endaural incision was abandoned, however, due to a high incidence of skin breakdown at the external auditory meatus and scalp numbness. In Australia, an inferiorly based inverted U-shaped incision was developed to replace the C-shaped incision. The inverted U-shaped incision, which was later modified into an inverted J-shaped incision, maximized the blood supply from both the superficial temporal and occipital arteries but still had similar complications to the C-shaped incision, including scalp numbness. A benefit of the inverted J-shaped incision was that it could incorporate a pre-existing postauricular incision.[6,8,9,11–14] The inverted J-shaped incision has been modified and shortened over time into the standard postauricular incision, which is the most commonly used incision at this time (**Fig. 1**). Many centers

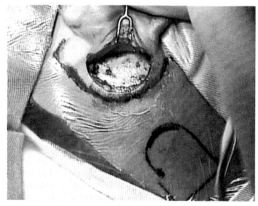

Fig. 1. Skin incision and flap elevation. Left ear.

(including New York University [NYU] and Vanderbilt University) now use a minimal access incision, which is a 2-cm to 4-cm, oblique, straight postauricular incision. The advantages of this incision are that there is minimal hair shaving, less tissue elevation/manipulation, shorter operative times, faster healing, less swelling, and the potential for earlier activation. Disadvantages include decreased visibility, need for more skin retraction, and limited access for drilling the bony well for the implant.[6,14] (For an illustration of the evolution of the skin incision, see **Fig. 2.**)

SECURING THE COCHLEAR IMPLANT

Because device migration can lead to infection, extrusion, and the need for revision surgery, different methods of securing the internal R/S and the cochlear implant electrode have been proposed.[15,16]

Traditionally, the R/S has been secured using tie-down sutures that were passed through monocortically drilled holes on each side of the R/S.[17] Other techniques for securing the R/S include

- Drilling two 4-mm titanium screws on either side of the well and connecting them with a 3-0 nylon suture[18]
- Applying polypropylene mesh over the R/S and securing the mesh with titanium screws[19]
- Cementing the R/S with ionomeric bone cement[20]
- Securing the proximal portion of the electrode by placing it in a drilled-out groove connecting the well and mastoid, thus eliminating the need for fixation of any type[21]
- Sewing the periosteum together over the implant.[22]

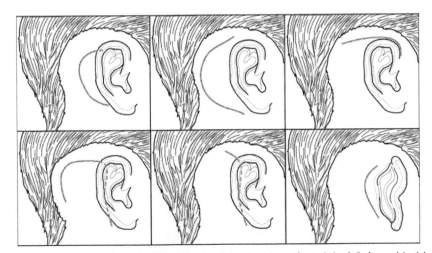

Fig. 2. The evolution of the cochlear implantation incision. The original C-shaped incision evolved into the large C-shaped incision to accommodate the larger multichannel implant. Due to the high complication rate of the C-shaped incision, the endaural incision was adopted in Europe and widely used. The U-shaped incision, however, which evolved into the J-shaped incision, was widely used in Australia and the United States. The J-shaped incision was able to accommodate a pre-existing postauricular incision and eventually was modified to become the standard postauricular incision most commonly used today. (*From* Flint P, editor. Cummings otolaryngology—head and neck surgery. 5th edition. Philadelphia: Mosby: Elsevier; 2010; with permission of Elsevier.)

In 2009, Balkany and colleagues[23] described the temporalis pocket technique obviating drilling a well or fixation of any type. The theory behind this technique is based on the anatomic limitations of the temporalis pocket, which is bounded "anteriorly by dense condensations of pericranium anteriorly at the temporal-parietal suture, posteroinferiorly at the lamboid suture, and anteroinferiorly by the bony ridge of the squamous suture."

Electrode migration is reported to be second only to device failure as a cause of reimplantation.[24,25] To prevent electrode migration, Balkany and Telischi[26] described the split bridge technique. This technique uses the incus buttress as a fixation point for the electrode changing the force vector of extrusion by 90°. Cohen and Kuzma also took advantage of the incus buttress by securing the electrode to the buttress with a titanium clip.[27] Several other techniques have been developed to minimize electrode migration, including tightly packing the cochleostomy with tissue, placing a coil of electrode against the tegmen mastoideum, and using precurved electrode arrays.[25]

At Vanderbilt University and NYU, no effort is made to fix the electrode at the fantail or at the facial recess. Attempts are made to coil the redundant electrode array in the mastoid cavity, usually securing the coil in against the tegmen (**Fig. 3**). A tight pocket technique for securing the R/S, snugged up with or without periosteal sutures, is currently preferred (**Fig. 4**). This technique has shortened operative times, eliminating the need for (potentially biofilm-forming) additional foreign material. No significant R/S migrations have occurred at either center.

MINIMALLY INVASIVE TECHNIQUES
Mastoidectomy with Posterior Tympanotomy Approach

In 1961, Dr House introduced the mastoidectomy with posterior tympanotomy approach (MPTA) for cochlear implantation.[28] Since then, the MPTA has stood the test of time and become the most commonly used approach. As the name implies, a mastoidectomy is performed followed by a posterior tympanotomy, which opens the facial recess exposing the round window. Several techniques have been developed and explored to try to minimize the extent of surgery needed to place the implant and the risk to the facial nerve and chorda tympani associated with the MPTA.

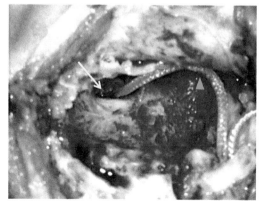

Fig. 3. Electrode in cochleostomy (*arrow*) with excess electrode coiled in mastoid cavity (*arrow head*). Left ear.

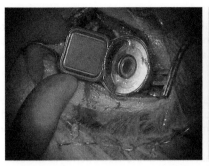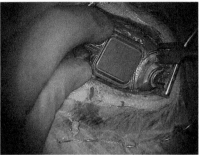

Fig. 4. Placing the R/S into the periosteal pocket. Left ear.

Suprameatal Route

In 1999, Kronenberg and colleagues[29,30] developed a technique that avoids a mastoid-ectomy altogether and introduces the electrode into the middle ear via a suprameatal route. This suprameatal approach is based on a retroauricular tympanotomy approach to the middle ear in which the facial nerve is protected by the body of the incus. Draw-backs to the suprameatal approach include the following[31]:

- The electrode is stretched during insertion into the cochleostomy.
- Low-lying dura is a relative contraindication.
- A round window insertion and inferior cochleostomy is difficult.
- Additionally, the revision surgery rate is much higher with this technique (J. Thomas Roland Jr, MD, personal communication, 2011).

Endaural Approach

Another nonmastoidectomy technique uses an endaural approach for access to the cochleostomy and a superoposterior transcanal wall approach for the electrode. This endaural approach, also known as the Veria operation, requires a special perfo-rator for drilling a direct tunnel and a safety electrode forceps for inserting the electrode.[32,33]

Minimal Access Incision Techniques

Minimal access incision techniques[14,34,35] have also been described. A percutaneous cochlear implant technique that involves a single, image-guided drill passed from the mastoid cortex through the facial recess to access the cochlea has been developed. The percutaneous cochlear implant technique uses an intraoperative CT scan and three fiducial markers in the bone surrounding the mastoid to plan a safe trajectory for the drill and has been validated in vitro[36–38] and in vivo.[39,40] Access to correct cochleostomy or round window insertion may also be limited and the 3-D approach to scala tympani insertion is limited.

COCHLEOSTOMY VERSUS ROUND WINDOW INSERTION

Because the human brain has the capability to integrate both acoustic and high-frequency electrically processed information,[41] much attention has been paid to the possibility and benefit of electroacoustic stimulation (EAS). The goal of EAS is to use the cochlear implant for high-frequency loss and use a hearing aid to improve the residual low-frequency hearing. Benefits of EAS when compared with electrical stimulation only or acoustic stimulation only include improved listening to speech in quiet, in noise, or in competition with another speaker.[2,41–53] Other benefits of EAS include improvement in identification of melodies and reception of musical sounds[47,49,54] With the benefits of EAS in mind, many investigators have sought the least traumatic way to insert the electrode array in hopes of preserving residual low-frequency hearing.

Traditional Cochleostomy Technique

- The traditional way to drill the cochleostomy is through the promontory anterior and inferior to the round window membrane using a 1-mm to 1.5-mm diamond burr (**Fig. 5**).
- The round window membrane is usually 1-mm to 1.5-mm inferior to the stapes tendon.[6]
- If necessary, the round window niche is removed to identify the round window.
- Meticulous drilling with a 1-mm diamond burr is then used and continued until the "blue" lining of the endosteum is visible, taking care to avoid inadvertent penetration of the endosteum because this may expose the inner ear to significant acoustic trauma, up to 130 dB.[55] The endosteum is at the same level and is continuous with the round window membrane.
- The size of the cochleostomy is determined by the size of the electrode array, which ranges from 1.0 mm to 1.4 mm.
- Once the endosteum is exposed, great care is taken to prevent bone dust or blood from entering into the cochleostomy. Some centers encourage the use of hyaluronic acid or dilute surgical-grade glycerin at this point to prevent entrance of blood and bone dust.[56] These substances have a buoyant density greater than bone dust and blood, thus preventing ingress to the scala tympani.
- At this point, a straight pick is used to open the endosteum and the electrode is inserted (**Fig. 6**).
- Suction is prohibited at this stage to avoid loss of perilymphatic fluid. Systemic and/or topical intratympanic steroids may be used in hearing preservation cases.

The use of the traditional cochleostomy approach in combination with a short/hybrid electrode in patients with residual low-frequency hearing has resulted in improved hearing in noise and music perception.[48,54] Although temporal bone studies have shown that the basal turn structures can be damaged with the traditional

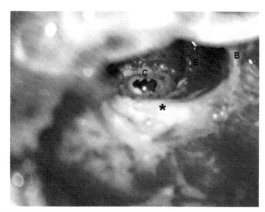

Fig. 5. Opened facial recess. (B, incus buttress; C, cochleostomy; E, stapes; *, facial nerve). Left ear.

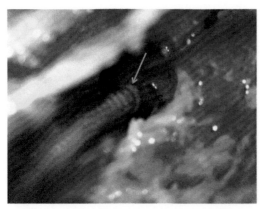

Fig. 6. Cochleostomy with electrode (*arrow*) in place (C, cochleostomy). Left ear.

cochleostomy approach,[57,58] this approach is preferred by many surgeons to avoid the complicated negotiation of the hook region of the cochlea and initiate insertion at an appropriate angle up the scala tympani in the proximal basal turn of the cochlea (pars inferior).

Round Window Approach

The round window approach to electrode insertion has gained much attention due to the potential for reduced damage to intracochlear structures, as demonstrated in by several temporal bone studies.[59–61]

- To avoid insertion into the wall of the scala tympani, the electrode is inserted into the round window at an oblique/anterior angle to the surface. The electrode itself seals the insertion incision, and further sealing is accomplished with muscle and/ or periosteum.
- Good visualization of the round window may be achieved in most cases by removing the bony round window niche with a 1-mm diamond as well as per-forming an adequate facial recess with drilling away of the bone anterior to the descending facial nerve over the stapedius muscle (**Figs. 7** and **8**).

Use of the round window approach with a standard electrode has resulted in pres-ervation in residual low-frequency hearing and the benefit of EAS in children.[62] In addi-tion to avoiding the potential trauma that the inner ear experiences from the 130 dB produced from drilling the traditional cochleostomy,[55] the round window approach may reduce postoperative vertigo.[62,63]

Concerning the cochleostomy versus round window debate, James and colleagues[50] concluded, "it appears that the correct approach to opening the cochlea, whether via the round window or... via an anterior-inferior cochleostomy, is vital to avoid basal trauma, whether a long or short electrode is used." Even if hearing is not preserved, it is expected that minimally invasive techniques and preservation of fine structures will optimize postoperative performance.

POSTOPERATIVE RADIOGRAPH/TELEMETRY...NEED OR NO NEED

Previously, intraoperative radiographs of the skull have been routinely used to confirm electrode placement into the cochlea and detect possible electrode kinking. The initial

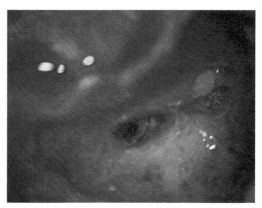

Fig. 7. Round window niche lip removed exposing the round window membrane. Left ear.

MED-EL surgical manual stated, "A postoperative x-ray is not required, but is recommended for verification of electrode insertion and as a baseline reference for electrode placement."[64] Intraoperative plain radiographs were also purported to play a role in the initial programming of patients.[65] Intraoperative plain radiographs, however, have not been found useful for uncomplicated cochlear implantations because their usefulness in patient management is negligible[66] and subsequent versions of MED-EL's surgical manual have not mentioned plain radiographs.[67] The authors' technique is to only obtain intraoperative plain radiographs in unique or suspect cases. Many centers, including the NYU group, routinely perform intraoperative radiographs to verify the absence of tip rollover, verify intracochlear insertion, and act as a baseline for postoperative analysis should electrode extrusion be suspected. Intraoperative CT scanning has recently been available at the authors' center. The authors have found the scanner useful for complex cases of severe malformations or in cases of significant osteoneogenesis. Scanning in the operating room allows making intraoperative decisions regarding electrode placement in difficult cases, eliminates the need for postoperative scanning, and potentially reduces revision surgical cases. Intraoperative fluoroscopy is commonly used by the NYU team in cases of cochlear anomalies and obstructed cochleas. This technique has been shown to prevent intrameatal

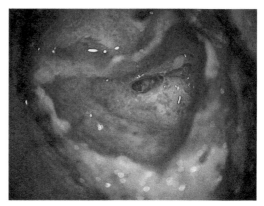

Fig. 8. Round window membrane where electrode will be placed. Left ear.

internal auditory canal (IAC) electrode insertions and verify an insertional stop point in common cavities and hypoplastic cochlea cases.[68,69]

Neural-response telemetry and impedence testing obtained intraoperatively can also help confirm proper functioning of the device and correct placement. Spread of excitation testing can also detect electrode tip rollover. Intraoperative measurements, fluoroscopy, and intraoperative radiographs may alert surgeons to a malfunctioning or misplaced device allowing a surgeon to replace the implant at that time, saving a patient from a future operation.

SUMMARY

Advanced technology, new surgical techniques, and refining established techniques are hallmarks of cochlear implant surgery. Minimally invasive techniques, shorter operative times, and near-zero complication rates are the current benchmarks. Further advancements, including image-guided surgery, hearing preservation even with full insertion, and telemetry-based advanced programming, are expected to be standard in the future.

REFERENCES

1. Stevens SS. On hearing by electrical stimulation. J Acoust Soc Am 1937;8:191–5.
2. Wilson BS, Dorman MF. Cochlear implants: a remarkable past and a brilliant future. Hear Res 2008;242:3–21.
3. National Institutes of Health. Cochlear implants. NIH Consensus Statement 1988; 7:1–9.
4. National Institutes of Health. Cochlear implants in adults and children. NIH Consensus Statement 1995;13:1–30.
5. Gifford RH, Shallop JK, Peterson AM. Speech recognition materials and ceiling effects: considerations for cochlear implant programs. Audiol Neurootol 2008; 13:193–205.
6. Flint P, editor. Cummings otolaryngology—head and neck surgery. 5th edition. Philadelphia: Mosby: Elsevier; 2010. p. 2237.
7. Cohen NL, Hoffman RA. Complications of cochlear implant surgery in adults and children. Ann Otol Rhinol Laryngol 1991;100:708–11.
8. Cohen NL, Hoffman RA, Stroschein M. Medical or surgical complications related to the Nucleus multichannel cochlear implant. Ann Otol Rhinol Laryngol Suppl 1988;135:8–13.
9. Gibson Wpr HH, Prowse C. A new incision for placements of cochlear implants. J Laryngol Otol 1995;109:821–5.
10. Hoffman RA, Cohen NL. Surgical pitfalls in cochlear implantation. Laryngoscope 1993;103:741–4.
11. Harris JP, Cueva RA. Flap design for cochlear implantation: avoidance of a potential complication. Laryngoscope 1987;97:755–7.
12. Haberkamp TJ, Schwaber MK. Management of flap necrosis in cochlear implantation. Ann Otol Rhinol Laryngol 1992;101:38–41.
13. el-Naggar M, Hawthorne M. Delayed extrusion of a cochlear implant: a case report of an implant extruding 21 months after the original operation. J Laryngol Otol 1995;109:56–7.
14. O'Donoghue GM, Nikolopoulos TP. Minimal access surgery for pediatric cochlear implantation. Otol Neurotol 2002;23:891–4.

15. Webb RL, Lehnhardt E, Clark GM, et al. Surgical complications with the cochlear multiple-channel intracochlear implant: experience at Hannover and Melbourne. Ann Otol Rhinol Laryngol 1991;100:131–6.

16. Hoffman RA, Cohen NL. Complications of cochlear implant surgery. Ann Otol Rhinol Laryngol Suppl 1995;166:420–2.

17. Cohen NL, Roland JT Jr, Fishman A. Surgical technique for the nucleus contour cochlear implant. Ear Hear 2002;23:59S–66S.

18. Lee DJ, Driver M. Cochlear implant fixation using titanium screws. Laryngoscope 2005;115:910–1.

19. Davis BM, Labadie RF, McMenomey SO, et al. Cochlear implant fixation using polypropylene mesh and titanium screws. Laryngoscope 2004;114:2116–8.

20. Rudel C, Zollner W. Ionomeric cement—a bone glue for device fixation. Ear Nose Throat J 1994;73:189–91.

21. Loh C, Jiang D, Dezso A, et al. Non-sutured fixation of cochlear implants using a minimally-invasive approach. Clin Otolaryngol 2008;33:259–61.

22. Molony TB, Giles JE, Thompson TL, et al. Device fixation in cochlear implantation: is bone anchoring necessary? Laryngoscope 2010;120:1837–9.

23. Balkany TJ, Whitley M, Shapira Y, et al. The temporalis pocket technique for cochlear implantation: an anatomic and clinical study. Otol Neurotol 2009;30: 903–7.

24. Rivas A, Marlowe A, Chinnici J. Replacement of the cochlear prosthesis: indications and results in adults. San Diego (CA): Published abstract for Combined Otolaryngology Spring Meeting; 2007.

25. Connell SS, Balkany TJ, Hodges AV, et al. Electrode migration after cochlear implantation. Otol Neurotol 2008;29:156–9.

26. Balkany T, Telischi FF. Fixation of the electrode cable during cochlear implantation: the split bridge technique. Laryngoscope 1995;105:217–8.

27. Cohen NL, Kuzma J. Titanium clip for cochlear implant electrode fixation. Ann Otol Rhinol Laryngol Suppl 1995;166:402–3.

28. House WF. Cochlear implants. Ann Otol Rhinol Laryngol 1976;85(Suppl 27):1–93.

29. Kronenberg J, Migirov L, Dagan T. Suprameatal approach: new surgical approach for cochlear implantation. J Laryngol Otol 2001;115:283–5.

30. Kronenberg J, Baumgartner W, Migirov L, et al. The suprameatal approach: an alternative surgical approach to cochlear implantation. Otol Neurotol 2004;25: 41–4 [discussion: 4–5].

31. Postelmans JT, Tange RA, Stokroos RJ, et al. The suprameatal approach: a safe alternative surgical technique for cochlear implantation. Otol Neurotol 2010;31: 196–203.

32. Kiratzidis T, Iliades T, Arnold W. Veria Operation. II. Surgical results from 101 cases. ORL J Otorhinolaryngol Relat Spec 2002;64:413–6.

33. Kiratzidis T, Arnold W, Iliades T. Veria operation updated. I. The trans-canal wall cochlear implantation. ORL J Otorhinolaryngol Relat Spec 2002;64: 406–12.

34. Mann WJ, Gosepath J. Technical Note: minimal access surgery for cochlear implantation with MED-EL devices. ORL J Otorhinolaryngol Relat Spec 2006; 68:270–2.

35. Stratigouleas ED, Perry BP, King SM, et al. Complication rate of minimally invasive cochlear implantation. Otolaryngol Head Neck Surg 2006;135:383–6.

36. Labadie RF, Mitchell J, Balachandran R, et al. Customized, rapid-production microstereotactic table for surgical targeting: description of concept and in vitro validation. Int J Comput Assist Radiol Surg 2009;4:273–80.

37. Balachandran R, Mitchell JE, Blachon G, et al. Percutaneous cochlear implant drilling via customized frames: an in vitro study. Otolaryngol Head Neck Surg 2010;142:421–6.
38. Warren FM, Balachandran R, Fitzpatrick JM, et al. Percutaneous cochlear access using bone-mounted, customized drill guides: demonstration of concept in vitro. Otol Neurotol 2007;28:325–9.
39. Labadie RF, Noble JH, Dawant BM, et al. Clinical validation of percutaneous cochlear implant surgery: initial report. Laryngoscope 2008;118:1031–9.
40. Labadie RF, Balachandran R, Mitchell JE, et al. Clinical validation study of percutaneous cochlear access using patient-customized microstereotactic frames. Otol Neurotol 2010;31:94–9.
41. von Ilberg C, Kiefer J, Tillein J, et al. Electric-acoustic stimulation of the auditory system. New technology for severe hearing loss. ORL J Otorhinolaryngol Relat Spec 1999;61:334–40.
42. Kiefer J, Pok M, Adunka O, et al. Combined electric and acoustic stimulation of the auditory system: results of a clinical study. Audiol Neurootol 2005;10:134–44.
43. Gantz BJ, Turner CW. Combining acoustic and electrical hearing. Laryngoscope 2003;113:1726–30.
44. Wilson BS, Lawson DT, Muller JM, et al. Cochlear implants: some likely next steps. Annu Rev Biomed Eng 2003;5:207–49.
45. Gstoettner W, Kiefer J, Baumgartner WD, et al. Hearing preservation in cochlear implantation for electric acoustic stimulation. Acta Otolaryngol 2004;124: 348–52.
46. Gstoettner WK, Helbig S, Maier N, et al. Ipsilateral electric acoustic stimulation of the auditory system: results of long-term hearing preservation. Audiol Neurootol 2006;11(Suppl 1):49–56.
47. Gantz BJ, Turner C, Gfeller KE, et al. Preservation of hearing in cochlear implant surgery: advantages of combined electrical and acoustical speech processing. Laryngoscope 2005;115:796–802.
48. Gantz BJ, Turner C, Gfeller KE. Acoustic plus electric speech processing: preliminary results of a multicenter clinical trial of the Iowa/Nucleus Hybrid implant. Audiol Neurootol 2006;11(Suppl 1):63–8.
49. Kong YY, Stickney GS, Zeng FG. Speech and melody recognition in binaurally combined acoustic and electric hearing. J Acoust Soc Am 2005;117:1351–61.
50. James CJ, Fraysse B, Deguine O, et al. Combined electroacoustic stimulation in conventional candidates for cochlear implantation. Audiol Neurootol 2006; 11(Suppl 1):57–62.
51. Gifford RH, Dorman MF, McKarns SA, et al. Combined electric and contralateral acoustic hearing: word and sentence recognition with bimodal hearing. J Speech Lang Hear Res 2007;50:835–43.
52. Dorman MF, Gifford RH, Spahr AJ, et al. The benefits of combining acoustic and electric stimulation for the recognition of speech, voice and melodies. Audiol Neurootol 2008;13:105–12.
53. Turner CW, Reiss LA, Gantz BJ. Combined acoustic and electric hearing: preserving residual acoustic hearing. Hear Res 2008;242:164–71.
54. Gfeller KE, Olszewski C, Turner C, et al. Music perception with cochlear implants and residual hearing. Audiol Neurootol 2006;11(Suppl 1):12–5.
55. Pau HW, Just T, Bornitz M, et al. Noise exposure of the inner ear during drilling a cochleostomy for cochlear implantation. Laryngoscope 2007;117:535–40.
56. James C, Albegger K, Battmer R, et al. Preservation of residual hearing with cochlear implantation: how and why. Acta Otolaryngol 2005;125:481–91.

57. Dahm M, Xu J, Tykocinski M, et al. Post mortem study of the intracochlear position of the Nucleus Standard 33 electrode array. Proc 5th Eur Symp Paediatr Cochlear Implantat. Antwerp; Belgium, June 6, 2000.

58. Briggs RJ, Tykocinski M, Saunders E, et al. Surgical implications of perimodiolar cochlear implant electrode design: avoiding intracochlear damage and scala vestibuli insertion. Cochlear Implants Int 2001;2:135–49.

59. Briggs RJ, Tykocinski M, Xu J, et al. Comparison of round window and cochleostomy approaches with a prototype hearing preservation electrode. Audiol Neurootol 2006;11(Suppl 1):42–8.

60. Li PM, Wang H, Northrop C, et al. Anatomy of the round window and hook region of the cochlea with implications for cochlear implantation and other endocochlear surgical procedures. Otol Neurotol 2007;28:641–8.

61. Roland PS, Wright CG, Isaacson B. Cochlear implant electrode insertion: the round window revisited. Laryngoscope 2007;117:1397–402.

62. Skarzynski H, Lorens A, Piotrowska A, et al. Partial deafness cochlear implantation in children. Int J Pediatr Otorhinolaryngol 2007;71:1407–13.

63. Todt I, Basta D, Ernst A. Does the surgical approach in cochlear implantation influence the occurrence of postoperative vertigo? Otolaryngol Head Neck Surg 2008;138:8–12.

64. MED-EL surgical manual, version 1. Durham (NC): US MED-EL Corp; 1998:15.

65. Cohen LT, Xu J, Xu SA, et al. Improved and simplified methods for specifying positions of the electrode bands of a cochlear implant array. Am J Otol 1996;17:859–65.

66. Copeland BJ, Pillsbury HC, Buchman CA. Prospective evaluation of intraoperative cochlear implant radiographs. Otol Neurotol 2004;25:295–7.

67. Todd NW, Ball TI. Interobserver agreement of coiling of Med-El cochlear implant: plain x-ray studies. Otol Neurotol 2004;25:271–4.

68. Coelho DH, Waltzman SB, Roland JT Jr. Implanting common cavity malformations using intraoperative fluoroscopy. Otol Neurotol 2008;29:914–9.

69. Fishman AJ, Roland JT Jr, Alexiades G, et al. Fluoroscopically assisted cochlear implantation. Otol Neurotol 2003;24:882–6.

Bilateral Cochlear Implantation

George B. Wanna, MD[a],*, René H. Gifford, PhD[b],
Theodore R. McRackan, MD[a], Alejandro Rivas, MD[a],
David S. Haynes, MD[c]

KEYWORDS

- Cochlear implantation • Bilateral • Sensorineural hearing loss

UNILATERAL COCHLEAR IMPLANTATION

Unilateral cochlear implants (CIs) have provided significant benefit to adult and pediatric patients with severe-to-profound sensorineural hearing loss. When compared with children with hearing aids, CI recipients have shown significant language and literacy improvements and a much steeper trajectory of receptive and expressive language development.[1] Half or more of pediatric CI recipients obtain language scores within normal for age range.[2–6] Although both children and adults typically perform well with open-set word and sentence recognition in quiet listening situations, these results can decrease dramatically (20–80 percentage points) in the presence of even moderate levels of background noise.[7–13] Speech recognition in noise and other performance variables may improve with the addition of a second CI.

PERIPHERAL AND CENTRAL AUDITORY PROCESSING

Alteration in auditory processing pathways, measured by cortical and brainstem responses, is required for hearing and speech recognition improvement with bilateral CI. This alteration has been evaluated in multiple studies, and bilateral central auditory processing and development occur from birth to 3 years of age.[14–17]

Significant differences are recognized in cortical auditory evoked potentials in those implanted before and after 3 years of age.[18,19] Those children implanted early showed

[a] Department of Otolaryngology–Head and Neck Surgery, Division of Otology-Neurotology and Skull Base Surgery, Vanderbilt University Medical Center, 1215 21st Avenue South, 7209 Medical Center East, South Tower, Nashville, TN 37232, USA
[b] Department of Hearing and Speech Sciences, Vanderbilt Bill Wilkerson Center, Vanderbilt University, 1215 21st Avenue South, Room 8310, Medical Center East-South Tower, Nashville, TN 37232-8242, USA
[c] Otology Group of Vanderbilt, Department of Otolaryngology–Head and Neck Surgery, Vanderbilt Bill Wilkerson Center, Vanderbilt University, 1215 21st Avenue South, 7209 Medical Center East, South Tower, Nashville, TN 37232, USA
* Corresponding author.
E-mail address: george.wanna@vanderbilt.edu

Otolaryngol Clin N Am 45 (2012) 81–89
doi:10.1016/j.otc.2011.08.018
0030-6665/12/$ – see front matter © 2012 Elsevier Inc. All rights reserved.

oto.theclinics.com

normal wave morphology and P1 latency, whereas those implanted later showed atypical wave morphology and longer P1 latency compared with both normal hearing and children implanted at a younger age.[18,19] Also, 2 studies revealed that patients who were implanted sequentially (compared with simultaneously) had prolonged auditory brainstem responses and wave latencies in the second implanted ear.[17,20] Those implanted before 3 years of age showed normalized wave latencies over a shorter period.[17,20,21]

Appropriate alterations in auditory processing patterns are necessary for the bilateral CI recipients to have improved speech recognition and hearing outcomes. However, there are limits to auditory pathway plasticity because more significant changes are seen in those implanted before 3 years of age. What remains to be seen, however, is whether unilateral implantation before 3 years of age will suffice for auditory cortical maturation, given that electrical stimulation from the implanted ear transmits neural information to both the contralateral (primary) and ipsilateral (secondary) pathways. Galvin and colleagues[22] showed significant benefit from a second implant obtained with up to 16 years following the first implant for adolescents and/or young adults with congenital sensorineural hearing loss.

At the peripheral level to the auditory brainstem, pediatric recipients of simultaneous CI show a minimal interaural difference in latency between EABRs. Gordon and colleagues[20] studied 3 groups of bilateral pediatric CI recipients:

- The first group had a delay of more than 2 years between the first and second CIs
- The second group had a delay of less than 1 year between the first and second CIs
- The third group had no delay between implants.

This study concluded that the group with sequential implantation and long delay (more than 2 years) had a significantly longer latency in neural conduction between the 2 sides. The group with short delay also showed longer latency, but with trends decreasing in the first few months following the second implant. Finally, the group with simultaneous bilateral implants showed no clear difference between the 2 sides.

Another study by Sparreboom and colleagues[23] examined EABR in 30 prelingually deafened children at 6, 12, and 24 months following sequential bilateral implantation. The mean surgical interval time between CI1 and CI2 was 41 months (range 18–86 months). Their data showed no significant interaural differences in EABR wave III at any time points. Also, wave V latencies on the CI2 side were initially prolonged compared with the CI1 side; however, after 12 months, these interaural latency differences were no longer significant.

Based on their results, they suggested that age and time between CI2 and CI1 do not affect auditory brainstem development at the side of the second implant, and auditory brainstem maturation occurred despite the long delay of implantation to the other side.

BINAURAL SUMMATION

Binaural summation is defined as the sensation that a signal is perceptually louder when hearing with 2 ears compared with 1. Binaural summation yields a benefit of approximately 2 dB for listeners with normal hearing.[24] A recently published meta-analysis on bilateral CI including 349 patients with summation data revealed 21% improvement ($P<.0001$) in binaural summation in bilateral CI recipients,[7] affording an improvement of 14.6% to 27.4% in speech recognition in noise.

This study also suggests that a bilateral CI recipient would have a 14% improvement in speech recognition in noise compared with a unilateral CI recipient.[7] Several other studies on bilateral CI have shown significant binaural summation effects. Dorman and colleagues[25] pooled data from Litovsky and colleagues,[41] Buss and colleagues,[33] and Koch and colleagues[36] and showed that for 82 adult bilateral CI recipients, the mean binaural summation was significant 11 percentage points for monosyllabic word recognition.

BINAURAL SQUELCH

Binaural squelch refers to an effect in which an improvement in the signal-to-noise ratio results from a central comparison of time and intensity differences for signals and noise arriving at the 2 ears. Squelch has been shown to offer an improvement in the signal-to-noise ratio of 2 to 5 dB for individuals with normal hearing.[24] Data on binaural squelch in bilateral CI recipients are varied, with some recipients reporting improvements[26–28] whereas others reporting none.[29–32] Some studies have demonstrated the presence of binaural squelch with bilateral CIs after an extended period of implant experience including 1 year[33] and 4 years[34] of bilateral electrical stimulation. A meta-analysis of 251 bilateral CI recipients showed significantly greater suppression of noise 8.5% to 22.1% ($P<.0001$) compared with unilateral CI recipients. Comparing bilateral CI recipients with those implanted unilaterally and using a hearing aid on the contralateral ear (ie, bimodal hearing), no statistical significance was obtained.[7] These results suggest that the use of a contralateral hearing aid has similar effects regarding binaural squelch as a second CI; however clearly, further research is needed.

HEAD SHADOW EFFECT

The attenuation of a sound that occurs when it travels around the listener's head to the opposite ear is known as the head shadow effect. For normal-hearing listeners, head shadow ranges from 9 to 11 dB.[25,35] Having a present and *equal* head shadow across ears is one of the most robust and early benefits of bilateral CI.[33,36] Multiple studies have reported marked improvements in head shadow effects when comparing single versus bilaterally implanted patients.[26–28,32,37] This is primarily because unilateral CI recipients will have head shadow for just a single ear, provided that noise originates from side of the nonimplanted ear. There is also no statistical difference in head shadow effect in pediatric versus adult bilateral CI patients.[7,38]

SPATIAL RELEASE FROM MASKING

In contrast to the other binaural cues discussed, spatial release from masking describes the phenomenon of improved speech understanding—when listening with 2 ears—for conditions in which the target signal and background noise are spatially separated.[24] Spatial release from masking is thought to be a combination of head shadow and squelch and has been shown to yield a benefit of 3 to 4 dB for both adults and children with bilateral CIs.[38–41] Given that the evidence surrounding the presence of squelch for bilateral implant recipients is not unequivocal, it is thought that most spatial release from masking observed for individuals with bilateral implants comes from head shadow.

SOUND LOCALIZATION

The improved ability of bilateral CI recipients to localize sound in a quiet environment has been previously established.[42–47] There seems to be a necessary period of binaural hearing adaptation that occurs before recovery of spatial hearing. The first signs of spatial hearing recovery in bilateral CI recipients occur around 3 months after activation,[45] with 1 report of return of spatial hearing as early as 1 month.[47] It has been proposed by many authors that spatial hearing recovery is linked to the amount of auditory experience acquired by the recipient before the onset of deafness.[42,43,48]

More recent literature has investigated the increased localization ability in noisy environments. In a study by Mosnier and colleagues,[49] simultaneously implanted patients' ability to localize sound in a noisy environment was compared with 1 or both implants activated. A statistically significant increased ability in those patients was noted with both implants activated independent of the patient's speech performance.

SPEECH RECOGNITION IN NOISE

Another proposed advantage of bilateral CI over unilateral CI is improved speech recognition in a variety of different noisy environments. Although not all studies have shown this advantage,[50] the overwhelming majority have shown benefit hearing in noise with the addition of the second CI.[25,32,48,51–55] However, those with a prolonged period of deafness in the second ear are associated with poorer speech recognition in noise. Similarly, in 2 studies that reported no improvement in speech recognition in noise, the bilateral CI recipients had protracted periods between the time of the first and second implantations.[49,50] These data suggest that integration of the electrical signals across ears plays a significant role in improved hearing in noise.

Similar to spatial hearing improvement, there also seems to be a lag period for improved hearing in noise with bilateral CI, with performance improvements noted over time. In a recent study by Wolfe and colleagues,[56] there were statistically significant improvements in HINT scores in the bilateral CI condition compared with the unilateral CI condition at 3, 6, and 8 months. There were also statistically significant improvements in comparing individual HINT scores at 3 versus 8 months and 6 versus 8 months.[56]

QUALITY OF LIFE FOR BILATERAL VERSUS UNILATERAL COCHLEAR IMPLANTATION

There seems to be a significant improvement in patients' quality of life (QOL) for bilateral versus unilateral CIs. A recently published article by Bichey and Miyamoto[57] compared QOL measurements before the first CI, after the first CI, and again after the second CI. There were statistically significant improvements in QOL scores after the first CI and after the second CI. In fact, each individual's QOL score showed a statistically significant increase after both the first and second implants. As a group, however, the greatest average gain in QOL was after the first CI.

There are prior data showing no significant QOL difference between the unilateral and bilateral CI recipients.[45] However, the within-subject design of Bichey and Miyamoto controlled for many variables such that patients were able to personally experience both unilateral and bilateral implantations.

SIMULTANEOUS VERSUS SEQUENTIAL SURGERY FOR BILATERAL COCHLEAR IMPLANTATION

Once bilateral implant is decided, then the question will be whether to perform the surgery simultaneously (at the same operative setting) or sequentially (during a planned second surgery). CI teams who are proponents of the sequential bilateral implantation argue that bilateral simultaneous implantation can prolong the procedure or lead to hospital admission; can increase the risk of complications such as operative-site hematoma, deep venous thrombosis, and atelectasis/pneumonia; and has more potential of blood loss in small children. Furthermore, simultaneous bilateral implantation is argued to provide a poorer rate of reimbursement than sequentially staged operations.

Proponents of simultaneous implantation argue that sequential implantation requires a second procedure, with the associated additional anesthesia risks, recovery period, and time off from work or school. Sequential bilateral implantation is also argued to serve as a nonjudicious use of health care dollars if staged purely for reimbursement purposes.

In a study of 50 bilateral simultaneous CIs, Ramsden and colleagues[58] showed that the overall hospital stay is shorter with simultaneous implantation and that there is no extra complication or morbidity in experienced hands, there is a possibly better speech and language outcome, and maybe simultaneous implantation is the optimum rehabilitation of profoundly deaf children. Both sequential and bilateral CIs have merit and the decision should be made by the implant team based on the best interests of the patient.

It is fair to say from the literature that the optimal timing of the second implant has not yet been determined. Gordon and colleagues[20] showed that children recipient of simultaneous CI had a minimal interaural difference in EABR latency. However, Sparreboom and colleagues[23] suggested that auditory brainstem maturation will occur despite the long delay of implantation to the other side.

More research is required to evaluate the critical time before which the second CI should be implanted and what is the actual impact on overall performance by delaying the second implant via sequential implantation.

SURGICAL PROCEDURE FOR BILATERAL COCHLEAR IMPLANTATION

As with unilateral implantation, attention to detail is paramount to successful outcome. At the Vanderbilt University Medical Center, a surgical checklist is performed before surgery:

- All patients undergo a full candidacy evaluation before surgery and are reviewed by the CI team before scheduling surgery.
- Full medical and anesthesia evaluations are performed before surgery and re-confirmed as surgery approaches.
- All these evaluations are reviewed before surgery.
- Device type is confirmed with the patient, and the operating room confirms that the correct devices and backups are available the day before surgery (or earlier).
- Appropriate meningitis vaccinations are confirmed.
- Images (computed tomography [CT]/magnetic resonance imaging, or both) are obtained, reviewed, and confirmed. Outside films are scanned into our medical records system to ensure availability during surgery. At present, intraoperative CT scanning exists for the confirmation of difficult placement (malformations, osteogenesis), and this technology is invaluable in selected cases.

In addition to the above preoperative preparation, an additional time-out procedure is performed while the patient is in the room, confirming all patient information.

The surgical procedure for bilateral implantation has evolved over time at the Vanderbilt University Medical Center. The original study protocols specified for sterile prepping and draping the patient simultaneously, using 1 set of instruments, sterile drapes, and microscope drapes, which has now evolved into the senior author's current protocol:

- The patient is prepped and draped on 1 side, and surgery is performed unilaterally.

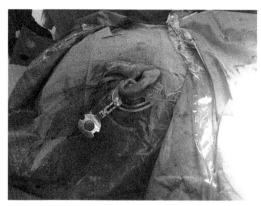

Fig. 1. Bilateral tool to aid in the symmetric placement of the contralateral CI.

- A dressing is applied, and the head is turned to the contralateral side and is prepped and draped in a similar fashion.
- The surgical team changes gloves and gowns, but the microscope drape and instrument from the previous side are used unless there is concern for contamination.
- All surgery is performed with intraoperative facial nerve monitoring.
- No monopolar cautery is used on the second side (bipolar cautery is used on the second side).
- The second side should be placed specifically to match the location of the first to give symmetric appearance of the telecoil. A specifically designed tool is used to aid in this symmetric placement (**Fig. 1**).
- All patients receive intravenous antibiotics and steroids, and the procedures are performed mostly treating the patients as outpatients.

SUMMARY

Bilateral CI is used increasingly to improve overall patient performance. Benefits of bilateral over unilateral implantation are argued on many levels including patient performance, resource use, cost benefit, and safety. Benefits achieved in special hearing, hearing in noise, sound localization, and head shadow effect seem to be consistent in children and adults. Several studies have advocated for bilateral CI to be considered the standard-of-care treatment option for adults and children with bilateral severe-to-profound sensorineural hearing loss.[59,60] More research into the effects of simultaneous versus sequential implantation and the potential for the negative impact on delayed second side implantation is needed.

REFERENCES

1. Hayes H, Geers AE, Treiman R, et al. Receptive vocabulary development in deaf children with cochlear implants: achievement in an intensive auditory-oral educational setting. Ear Hear 2009;30(1):128–35.
2. Moog JS, Geers AE. Epilogue: major findings, conclusions and implications for deaf education. Ear Hear 2003;24:121–5.
3. Geers AE, Nicholas JG, Sedley AL. Language skills of children with early cochlear implantation. Ear Hear 2003;24:46–58.

4. Moog JS, Geers AE. Early educational placement and later language outcomes for children with cochlear implants. Otol Neurotol 2010;31(8):1315–9.
5. Wie OB. Language development in children after receiving bilateral cochlear implants between 5 and 18 months. Int J Pediatr Otorhinolaryngol 2010;74(11):1258–66.
6. Niparko JK, Tobey EA, Thal DJ, et al, CDaCI Investigative Team. Spoken language development in children following cochlear implantation. JAMA 2010;303(15):1498–506.
7. Schafer EC, Amlani AM, Seibold A, et al. Meta-analytic comparison of binaural benefits between bilateral cochlear implants and bimodal stimulation. J Am Acad Audiol 2007;18:760–76.
8. Hamzavi J, Franz P, Baumgartner WD, et al. Hearing performance in noise of cochlear implant patients versus severely-profoundly hearing-impaired patients with hearing aids. Audiology 2001;40:26–31.
9. Fetterman BL, Domico EH. Speech recognition in background noise of cochlear implant patients. Otolaryngol Head Neck Surg 2002;126:257–63.
10. Garnham C, O'Driscoll M, Ramsden AR, et al. Speech understanding in noise with a Med-El COMBI 40+ cochlear implant using reduced channel sets. Ear Hear 2002;23:540–52.
11. Schafer EC, Thibodeau LM. Speech recognition performance of children using cochlear implants and FM systems. J Educ Audiol 2003;11:15–26.
12. Eisenberg LS, Kirk KI, Martinez AS, et al. Communication abilities of children with aided residual hearing. Arch Otolaryngol Head Neck Surg 2004;130:563–9.
13. Schafer EC, Thibodeau LM. Speech recognition abilities of adults using cochlear implants interfaced with FM systems. J Am Acad Audiol 2004;15:678–91.
14. Brown KD, Balkany TJ. Benefits of bilateral cochlear implantation: a review. Curr Opin Otolaryngol Head Neck Surg 2007;15:315–8.
15. Ching TY, van Wanrooy E, Dillon H. Binaural-bimodal fitting or bilateral implantation for managing severe to profound deafness: a review. Trends Amplif 2007;11:161–92.
16. Murphy J, O'Donoghue G. Bilateral cochlear implantation: an evidence-based medicine evaluation. Laryngoscope 2007;117:1412–8.
17. Gordon KA, Valero J, Papsin BC. Auditory brainstem activity in children with 9-30 months of bilateral cochlear implant use. Hear Res 2007;233:97–107.
18. Bauer PW, Sharma A, Martin K, et al. Central auditory development in children with bilateral cochlear implants. Arch Otolaryngol Head Neck Surg 2006;132:1133–6.
19. Sharma A, Dorman MF, Kral A. The influence of a sensitive period on central auditory development in children with unilateral and bilateral cochlear implants. Hear Res 2005;203:134–43.
20. Gordon KA, Valero J, Van Hoesel R, et al. Abnormal timing delays in auditory brainstem responses evoked by bilateral cochlear implant use in children. Otol Neurotol 2008;29:193–8.
21. Gordon KA, Valero J, Papsin BC. Binaural processing in children using bilateral cochlear implants. Neuroreport 2007;18:613–7.
22. Galvin KL, Hughes KC, Mok M. Can adolescents and young adults with prelingual hearing loss benefit from a second, sequential cochlear implant? Int J Audiol 2010;49(5):368–77.
23. Sparreboom M, Beynon AJ, Snik AF. Electrically evoked auditory brainstem responses in children with sequential bilateral cochlear implants. Otol Neurotol 2010;31:1055–61.
24. Bronkhorst AW, Plomp R. The effect of head-induced interaural time and level differences on speech intelligibility in noise. J Acoust Soc Am 1988;83(4):1508–16.

25. Dorman MF, Gifford RH. Combining acoustic and electric stimulation in the service of speech recognition. Int J Audiol 2010;49(12):912–9.
26. Müller J, Schön F, Helms J. Speech understanding in quiet and noise in bilateral users of the MED-ELCOMBI 40/40+ cochlear implant system. Ear Hear 2002;23:198–206.
27. Dunn CC, Tyler RS, Witt SA. Benefit of wearing a hearing aid on the unimplanted ear in adult users of a cochlear implant. J Speech Hear Res 2005;48:668–80.
28. Morera C, Manrique M, Ramos A, et al. Advantages of binaural hearing provided through bimodal stimulation via a cochlear implant and a conventional hearing aid: a six month comparative study. Acta Otolaryngol 2005;125:596–606.
29. Gantz BJ, Tyler RS, Rubinstein JT, et al. Binaural cochlear implants placed during the same operation. Otol Neurotol 2002;23:169–80.
30. Tyler RS, Gantz BJ, Rubinstein JT, et al. Three-month results with bilateral cochlear implants. Ear Hear 2002;23:80S–9S.
31. Ramsden R, Greenham P, O'Driscoll M, et al. Evaluation of bilaterally implanted adult subjects with the Nucleus 24 Cochlear Implant System. Otol Neurotol 2005;26:988–98.
32. Senn P, Kompis M, Vischer MW, et al. Minimum audible angle, just noticeable interaural differences and speech intelligibility with bilateral cochlear implants using clinical speech processors. Audiol Neurootol 2005;10:342–52.
33. Buss E, Pillsbury HC, Buchman CA, et al. Bilateral MED-EL cochlear implantation study: speech perception over the first year of use. Ear Hear 2008;29(1):20–32.
34. Eapen RJ, Buss E, Adunka MC, et al. Hearing-in-noise benefits after bilateral simultaneous cochlear implantation continue to improve 4 years after implantation. Otol Neurotol 2009;30(2):153–9.
35. Arsenault MD, Punch JL. Nonsense-syllable recognition in noise using monaural and binaural listening strategies. J Acoust Soc Am 1999;105(3):1821–30.
36. Koch DB, Soli SD, Downing M, et al. Simultaneous bilateral cochlear implantation: prospective study in adults. Coch Impl Int 2010;11(2):84–99.
37. Laszig R, Aschendorff A, Stecker M, et al. Benefits of bilateral electrical stimulation with the Nucleus Cochlear Implant in adults: 6-month postoperative results. Otol Neurotol 2004;25:958–68.
38. Van Deun L, van Wieringen A, Wouters J. Spatial speech perception benefits in young children with normal hearing and cochlear implants. Ear Hear 2010;31(5):702–13.
39. van Hoesel RJ, Tyler RS. Speech perception, localization, and lateralization with bilateral cochlear implants. J Acoust Soc Am 2003;113(3):1617–30.
40. Schleich P, Nopp P, D'Haese P. Head shadow, squelch, and summation effects in bilateral users of the MED-EL COMBI 40/40+ cochlear implant. Ear Hear 2004;25(3):197–204.
41. Litovsky R, Parkinson A, Arcaroli J, et al. Bilateral cochlear implants in adults and children. Arch Otolaryngol Head Neck Surg 2004;130:648–55.
42. Grantham W, Ashmead DH, Ricketts TA, et al. Horizontal-plane localization in noise and speech signals by postlingually deafened adults fitted with bilateral cochlear implants. Ear Hear 2007;28:524–41.
43. Grantham DW, Ashmead DH, Ricketts TA, et al. Interaural time and level difference thresholds for acoustically presented signals in post-lingually deafened adults fitted with bilateral cochlear implants using CIS+ processing. Ear Hear 2008;29(1):33–44.
44. Neuman AC, Haravon A, Sislian N, et al. Sound-direction identification with bilateral cochlear implants. Ear Hear 2007;28:73–82.

45. Nopp P, Schleich P, D'Haese P. Sound localization in bilateral users of MED-EL COMBI 40/40+ cochlear implants. Ear Hear 2004;25:205–14.
46. Schoen F, Mueller J, Helms J, et al. Sound localization and sensitivity to interaural cues in bilateral users of the Med-El Combi 40/40+ cochlear implant system. Otol Neurotol 2005;26:429–37.
47. Verschuur CA, Lutman ME, Ramsden R, et al. Auditory localization abilities in bilateral cochlear implant recipients. Otol Neurotol 2005;26:965–71.
48. Nava E, Bottari D, Portioli G, et al. Hearing again with two ears: recovery of spatial hearing after bilateral cochlear implantation. Neuropsychologia 2009;47:928–32.
49. Mosnier I, Sterkers O, Bebear JP, et al. Speech performance and sound localization in a complex noisy environment in bilaterally implanted adult patients. Aud Neuro 2009;14:106–14.
50. Schafer EC, Thibodeau LM. Speech recognition in noise in children with cochlear implants while listening in bilateral, bimodal, and FM-system arrangements. Am J Audiol 2006;15:114–26.
51. Galvin KL, Mok M, Dowell RC, et al. 12-month post-operative results for older children using sequential bilateral implants. Ear Hear 2007;28:S19–21.
52. Galvin KL, Mok M, Dowell RC. Perceptual benefit and functional outcomes for children using sequential bilateral cochlear implants. Ear Hear 2007;28:470–82.
53. Kuhn-Inacker H, Shehata-Dieler W, Muller J, et al. Bilateral cochlear implants: a way to optimize auditory perception abilities in deaf children? Int J Pediatr Oto 2004;68:1257–66.
54. Peters BR, Litovsky R, Lake J, et al. Sequential bilateral cochlear implantation in children. Intl Congress Series 2004;1273:462–5.
55. Steffens T, Lesinski-Schiedat A, Strutz J, et al. The benefits of sequential bilateral cochlear implantation for hearing-impaired children. Acta Oto-Laryngologica 2007;128:164–76.
56. Wolfe J, Baker S, Caraway T, et al. 1-Year postactivation results for sequentially implanted bilateral cochlear implant users. Otol Neurotol 2007;28:589–96.
57. Bichey BG, Miyamoto RT. Outcomes in bilateral cochlear implantation. Oto-HNS 2008;138:655–61.
58. Ramsden DJ, Papsin CB, Leung R, et al. Bilateral simultaneous cochlear implantation in children: our first 50 cases. Laryngoscope 2009;119:2444–8.
59. Balkany T, Hodges A, Telischi F, et al. William House Cochlear Implant Study Group: position statement on bilateral cochlear implantation. Otol Neurotol 2008;29(2):107–8.
60. Papsin BC, Gordon KA. Bilateral cochlear implants should be the standard for children with bilateral sensorineural deafness. Curr Opin Otolaryngol Head Neck Surg 2008;16(1):69–74.

Implanting Obstructed and Malformed Cochleae

Daniel H. Coelho, MD[a],*, J. Thomas Roland Jr, MD[b]

KEYWORDS

- Cochlear implant • Malformation • Dysplasia • Ossification
- Obstruction

Implantation of the ossified and dysplastic cochlea presents many unique challenges to both the surgeon and programming team. Altered embryology and physiology of these labyrinthine dysplasias may result in forms and functions unfamiliar to those casually involved with cochlear implants. However, with a thorough understanding of the specific issues attendant to this fascinating and varied patient population, the goal of successful implantation and performance can become a reality.

THE OSSIFIED COCHLEA
Introduction

In the earlier days of cochlear implantation, ossification was considered a contraindication to implantation. This belief was based on concerns that even if the anatomic obstructions that preclude electrode insertion were properly addressed, the damage caused to the spiral ganglion cells by ossification would be too great to result in any significant auditory precept.[1] However, subsequent refinements in the understanding of pathophysiology, early diagnosis, electrode design, processing strategies, and surgical techniques have allowed cochlear implantation to significantly benefit patients previously considered inoperable. In patients with partial ossification, performance may even equal those observed in patients with normal cochleae.[2–4]

Disclosures: J.T. Roland: Member of Surgical Advisory Board, Advanced Bionics; Member of Surgical Advisory Board, Cochlear Corporation; Member of Surgical Advisory Board, Med-el. D.H. Coelho: Member of Surgical Advisory Board, Med-el.
a Department of Otolaryngology–Head & Neck Surgery, Virginia Commonwealth University Cochlear Implant Center, Virginia Commonwealth University School of Medicine, PO Box 980146, Richmond, VA 23298-0146, USA
b Department of Otolaryngology, New York University Cochlear Implant Center, New York University School of Medicine, 660 First Avenue, 7th Floor, New York, NY 10016, USA
* Corresponding author.
E-mail address: dcoelho@mcvh-vcu.edu

Otolaryngol Clin N Am 45 (2012) 91–110
doi:10.1016/j.otc.2011.08.019
0030-6665/12/$ – see front matter © 2012 Elsevier Inc. All rights reserved.

Pathophysiology

Ossification of the labyrinth can occur following infection via 3 main pathways: meningogenic, tympanogenic, or hematogenic. Irrespective of the pathway, a sequence of inflammatory-mediator migration, fibroblast proliferation, and ossification can begin within days and may continue for decades. Ossification itself may directly destroy spiral ganglion cells, ultimately leading to poorer outcomes in cochlear implant recipients.[5] In these patients, auditory brainstem implants may be the only means to access auditory information.[6]

Infectious and inflammatory mediators enter the inner ear via the internal auditory canal or cochlear aqueduct (meningogenic) or by traversing the cochlear fenestra (tympanogenic). These two most common routes both result in ossification that progresses from the base to the apex, and in the scala tympani more commonly than the scala vestibuli. Therefore, the scala tympani of the basal cochlea is the most commonly affected area of labyrinthine ossification. This fact has important clinical implications, as the degree of cochlear ossification affects both surgical technique and hearing outcomes.

Although the incidence has decreased significantly over the last 30 years, bacterial meningitis remains one of the leading causes of hearing loss in children.[7] Severe to profound hearing loss occurs in 10% of children following bacterial meningitis.[8] Although *Streptococcus pneumoniae* is more likely to result in postmeningitis hearing loss, different bacteriology has not been shown to predict the severity of ossification.[9–11] Fibrosis can begin within days of infection, but can also slowly progress over years, often making diagnosis challenging.[12] Ossification following other less common causes of cochlear ossification have been reported, including otosclerosis, chronic otitis media, trauma (including iatrogenic), labyrinthine artery occlusion, ototoxic medications, leukemia, temporal bone tumors, viral infection, Wegener granulomatosis, and autoimmune and idiopathic processes.

Evaluation

A thorough history of all patients with severe to profound hearing loss, irrespective of age, is essential to elicit processes that may lead to labyrinthine ossification. A high-resolution computed tomography (HRCT) scan is necessary to assess the preoperative bony anatomy of the temporal bone (**Fig. 1**). However, its use alone may not provide sufficient detail regarding the degree of ossification, as a wide variance of sensitivities for identifying ossified cochlea has been reported.[13] Attenuation of intracochlear fluid signal seen on T2-weighted magnetic resonance imaging (MRI) has proved to be a more sensitive method of assessing blockage.[14,15] Similarly, contrast-enhanced T1-weighted images can detect early fibrosis and may aid the decision to implant earlier.[16] The routine of both HRCT and T2-weighted MRI is the authors' method of choice for all patients with suspicion of labyrinthine ossification. Despite advances in imaging, the true extent of ossification is determined intraoperatively.

Preoperative Planning

Given the potential for extremely early onset of intracochlear fibrosis, timing of implantation becomes a critical decision. Animal studies have shown that ossification of the basal cochlea can occur within 72 hours of meningitis.[17] Aschendorff and colleagues[18] verified intraoperative ossification of the scala tympani 4 weeks after meningitis. Such ossification may impede full electrode insertion, leaving precious little time in which to achieve ideal insertion and outcomes. Timely identification of postmeningitic bilateral deafness may be difficult. Patient age and/or general medical condition may delay

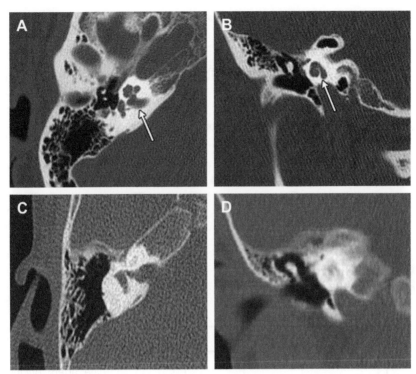

Fig. 1. (*A*) Noncontrast axial high-resolution computed tomography of normal right cochlea. The arrow is pointing to the internal auditory canal and cochlea to demonstrate similar fluid hypodensity. (*B*) Coronal view of normal cochlea. The arrow indicates the hypodense fluid-filled area of the pars ascendens at the end of the basal turn. (*C*) Axial view of severe cochlear ossification. (*D*) Coronal view of severe cochlear ossification.

recognition. Even if recognized, the concomitant morbidities of meningitis may leave the patient as a suboptimal candidate for general anesthesia. Furthermore, the patient must be completely free of the infectious agent that caused the meningitis in the first place. Once acute infectious and neurologic sequelae are stabilized, audiologic evaluation and (if necessary) immediate amplification should be implemented. As not all patients experience rapid onset of severe or profound hearing loss, serial audiometric evaluations are performed. If hearing deteriorates to severe to profound levels, the implant team should be ready to implant swiftly, as hearing loss is likely a reflection of progressive fibrosis and ossification. This implantation should be done even if the patient is younger than 12 months. All postmeningitis patients should ideally receive their pneumococcal vaccination before implantation.

Surgical Technique

Scala tympani insertion
The goal of all cochlear implantations, including for postmeningitic patients, is atraumatic full insertion of all electrodes into the scala tympani of the basal turn (**Fig. 2**). One hundred percent cochlear ossification leads to deafness, though not all deafness has 100% ossification. As a result, full insertion can often be achieved despite a history suggestive of labyrinthine fibrosis or ossification.

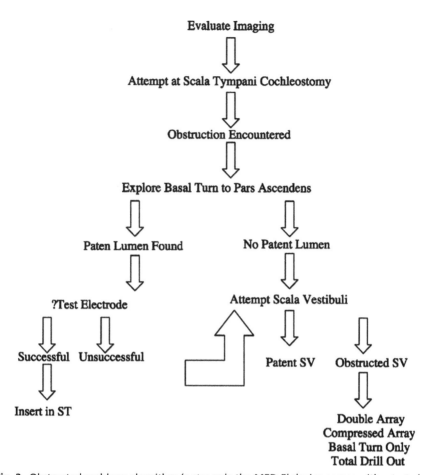

Fig. 2. Obstructed cochleae algorithm (note: only the MED-El device comes with a test electrode). (*From* Cosetti M, Roland JT Jr. Cochlear implant electrode insertion. Operat Tech Otolaryngol Head Neck Surg 2010;21(4):223–32; with permission.)

For those patients in whom full scala tympani insertion of a multichannel device is not possible, several options exist.

- If only limited basal cochlear ossification had occurred, drilling is continued along the basal turn until a lumen is visualized or encountered. The obstructing bone is often whiter and softer than the surrounding otic capsule, and serves as a guide to the axis of the cochlea.
- The basilar obstruction can also consist of uncalcified osteoid or fibrous tissue, which can be removed with picks, rasps, or drills to open into a lumen.
- If a patent lumen of the scala tympani is found before or at the ascending turn of the cochlea, a full insertion is performed.
- The judicious use of a test electrode or depth gauge can assist the surgeon with luminal patency determination, especially when the obstructive ossification or fibrosis extends beyond the lower basal turn into the pars ascendens.

Occasionally the lumen is extensively filled with hard bone, and no space can be visualized, necessitating a basal-turn drill-out procedure. Drilling with a 1-mm diamond burr is performed in the anteromedial direction for not more than 9.5 mm or until the internal carotid artery is visualized. This procedure allows for the placement of enough electrodes (7.5- to 10.5-mm drill-out) to obtain multichannel performance.[19]

As the number of electrodes implanted generally corresponds to performance, attention has been focused on design modifications of standard, long arrays.[20] At present, Cochlear Ltd (Sydney, Australia) offers the straight (ST) electrodes and Med-El (Innsbruck, Austria) offers the Medium and Compressed electrodes, in which the same number of electrodes are compressed into a shorter electrode array.

Scala vestibuli insertion

Early surgical techniques attempted to insert as much of a multichannel implant in the basal turn as possible, with the understanding that results might be limited.[21] Steenerson and colleagues[22] suggested attempted full insertion into the scala vestibuli as an alternative, though many of these patients had similar obstruction in that scala as well. This lumen is often patent in otosclerosis and postmeningitis cases, and full scala vestibuli insertion is desirable when the scala tympani is occluded.[23] Before the introduction of the double-array device, when the scala vestibuli was obstructed the surgeon settled for a partial insertion of whichever basal scala resulted in the most intracochlear electrodes. Subsequent, basal drill-out procedures of the neo-ossified cochlea (discussed later) allowed for further, though partial insertion.[24] Results were mixed. Cohen and Waltzman[19] found a wide range of performance in 8 patients, and Parisier and Chute[25] found only 2 of 5 partially implanted children with limited open-set speech understanding. More recently, Kirk and colleagues[26] found substantial improvements in speech with both closed-set and open-set speech perceptions, similar to the majority of matched full-insertion control subjects. Rotteveel and colleagues[27] reported no relation between speech perception and number of active electrodes (between 8 and 13) for a group of partially inserted implants.

Total cochlear drill-out

In cases of complete cochlear obliteration, total circum-modiolar drill-out has been described.[2,28] In this technique the tunnel of the basal turn is created, in similar fashion to that already described. A smaller drill bit is used to enter the anterior aspect of the pars ascendens; this requires unroofing the bone overlying the distal/anterior basal turn. The abnormal white, chalky bone is encountered and followed posteriorly to the anterior edge of the oval window. Further drilling can open a channel in the inferiorly bending second turn of the cochlear, but great care must be taken not to enter the modiolus or injure the horizontal/labyrinthine facial nerve. To achieve adequate visualization, a radical mastoidectomy (with or without obliteration) can be performed. Once the receiver-stimulator is securely situated, the electrode is passed through the cochleostomy, guided into the trough, and secured with bony spicules. The entire promontory is then packed with muscle or fascia. This procedure is technically demanding, and has been abandoned in many centers in favor of double-array electrode insertion, even in cases of second-turn obliteration. Despite the use of these techniques for some patients with subjective auditory precept, there are insufficient objective long-term patient data to support total drill-out as a superior method for implantation of the totally ossified cochlea.

Double/split-array implantation

To address the possible shortcomings of partial insertion, attention was given to the design of the electrode itself. The Nucleus Double Array (Cochlear Ltd, Sydney, Australia) cochlear implant was designed for the obliterated or surgically inaccessible cochlea, and was first implanted in 1995. The double array is based on the belief that there is a positive correlation between the number of activated intracochlear electrodes and speech recognition.[29] Similarly, two electrode arrays in different areas of the cochlea allow for a potentially greater number of spiral ganglion neurons stimulated. The number of activated intracochlear electrodes is higher than when only partial (basal) insertion is performed. Currently manufactured with the Nucleus 24 technology, the device has 11 active electrodes on each lead with two references electrodes—one on an additional electrode lead and one in the casing of the receiver/stimulator. The Med-El Corporation (Innsbruck, Austria) also markets a split-electrode array (C40 + GB), which has 5 and 7 pairs of electrode contacts, respectively (**Fig. 3**).

A basal array is placed in the inferior basal-turn tunnel as previously described. After the incus bar, the incus, and the stapes superstructure are removed, a second cochleostomy is placed in the second turn by drilling immediately adjacent to the anterior oval window ligament (**Fig. 4**). Care is taken to direct the 1-mm diamond burr parallel to the tensor tympani muscle below the cochleariform process to avoid damaging the facial nerve. The drilling is performed with irrigation to avoid heating. The more apical array can be placed in either a retrograde or an anterograde orientation, if a lumen is encountered, depending on the recommendations of the manufacturer (Cochlear Ltd prefers anterograde and Med-El prefers retrograde). In a totally obstructed second turn, retrograde drilling and insertion is preferred to avoid damage to the modiolus. Fluoroscopy can serve as a valuable adjunct in the insertion of electrode array(s) in ossified cochleae.[30]

For speech performance, Lenarz and colleagues[31] have demonstrated that both arrays of a double-array electrode lead to marked improvement compared with the basal array only, including pitch discrimination. The contribution of the apical electrodes seems to be limited when compared with the basal array, for several reasons:

1. The number of active electrodes in the basal turn is greater because the basal turn is larger in diameter than in the second turn, and insertion may be less traumatic
2. The density of neurons is lower at the apex than at the base
3. Apical neurons lie more centrally in the modiolus than those at the base
4. Many apical electrodes may need to be programmed off because of facial nerve stimulation or pain

Of note, the article by Lenarz and colleagues[31] also reported several patients with cerebrospinal fluid (CSF) leaks, likely caused by entering the modiolus, and thus affecting performance because of spiral ganglion cell damage. Although apical electrodes provide reduced pitch discrimination than basal electrodes, they do provide important information for speech recognition.[31] Roland and colleagues[32] found the double array allows for more usable electrodes than the partially inserted cochlear

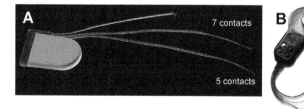

Fig. 3. (*A*) MED-El Split-electrode device. (*B*) Cochlear Corporation double-electrode device. (*From* Cosetti M, Roland JT Jr. Cochlear implant electrode insertion. Operat Tech Otolaryngol Head Neck Surg 2010;21(4):223–32; with permission.)

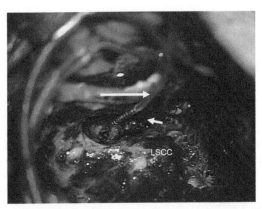

Fig. 4. Intraoperative view through facial recess of the left ear depicting double-array cochlear implant. The basal array (*long arrow*) is observed entering anteroinferior to the round window. The apical array (*short arrow*) is observed at the second-turn cochleostomy just anterior the oval window. Asterisk indicates the head of Malleus; LSCC, lateral semicircular canal. (*From* Roland JT Jr, Coelho DH, Pantelides H, et al. Otol Neurotol 2008;29(8):1068–75; with permission.)

implant, and compared with adults, children with ossified cochlea do well both in partial standard and double-array insertion.

Auditory brainstem implant

For patients with complete ossification, the decision may be made preoperatively to forgo cochlear implantation altogether in favor of auditory brainstem implant (ABI) insertion (**Fig. 5**). Originally used in patients with bilateral vestibular schwannomas (neurofibromatosis type II), the ABI has been described with varying degrees of success for nontumor patients.[6,33–35] Colletti and colleagues[6] published a 10-year experience of 31 ABI patients with "altered cochlear patency" (including both labyrinthine ossification and otosclerosis), demonstrating significant improvements in open-set speech recognition. The rationale for ABI lies in the belief that even after cochlear implantation the ossification process persists and ultimately affects the remaining spiral ganglion cells. This factor may explain the decrease in performance over time of some cochlear postmeningitic cochlear implant recipients, and the poorer

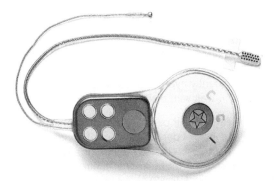

Fig. 5. Auditory brainstem implant. (Photo provided *courtesy of* Cochlear™ Americas, © 2009 Cochlear Americas.)

performance seen in adults implanted many years after the onset of meningitis-induced deafness.

DYSPLASTIC COCHLEAE
Introduction

As comfort and experience with implantation in patients with normal cochleovestibular anatomy has grown, currently more and more patients with abnormal anatomy are considered as candidates for this life-changing technology. Approximately 20% of all children with sensorineural hearing loss will have associated radiologic abnormalities of the temporal bone.[36] These abnormalities are associated with disparate clinical presentation including the severity and duration of hearing loss, and are associated with nonotologic abnormalities.[37] In general, the more dysplastic the deformity, the worse is the hearing expected.[38]

Nomenclature of cochleovestibular anomalies has historically confounded adequate classification. "Mondini dysplasia," for example, had been widely and incorrectly used for 200 years to describe any inner ear malformation. Mondini's original description detailed incomplete apical turn partitioning, enlarged vestibular aqueduct, and bulbous medial IAC. The authors caution against the use of the term "Mondini" deformity for any other inner ear anomaly.

In 1987, Jackler and colleagues[36] proposed a classification system, facilitated by advances in computed tomography (CT) resolution, and based on the theory that different deformities were the result of arrest of specific developmental stages in inner ear embryogenesis. Though a landmark scheme adopted widely by otologists, Jackler's classification does not completely address the possibility of multiple, isolated, independent arrests in development leading to unique phenotypes.[39] To address this, several investigators subsequently proposed new or modified classifications systems.

- Phelps[40] described a system based on the appearance of the basal turn of the cochlea, believed to correspond better with cochlear implant outcomes. Patients with abnormal cochleae, including abnormal basal turns, were grouped as "severe labyrinthine dysplasia," whereas those with normal basal turns were grouped as "Mondini dysplasia."
- Zheng and colleagues[41] further modified this classification depending on presence (type A) or absence (type B) of the bony modiolar base. This modification attempted to correlate increased risks of intraoperative complications as a result of altered intracochlear fluid pressure dynamics.
- In 2002, Sennaroglu and Saatci[42] revisited the concept of arrested development at different stages leading to specific dysplasias (**Fig. 6**). Unlike Jackler, these investigators considered cystic cochleovestibular anomaly as a severe form of incomplete partition that occurred before differentiation into cochlear and vestibular elements.
- In 2005, Papsin[39] eloquently hypothesized several distinct anomalous pathways of development that fit well with distinct clinical presentations observed.

The difficulty seen in creating a simple, linear, and widely accepted system of classification for cochlear dysplasias underlies the current notion that such malformations are the result of more than just arrested embryogenesis. For example, certain described genetic inactivations (single and/or multiple) result in clear genotype/phenotype relationships (eg, Hmx3, Pax2).[43] Despite significant advances, there is still much work to be done in the genetics of cochleovestibular development before complete understanding of dysmorphology can be achieved.

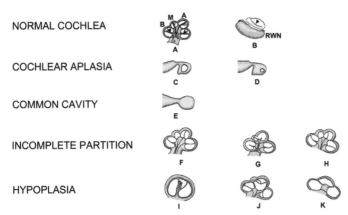

NORMAL COCHLEA

COCHLEAR APLASIA

COMMON CAVITY

INCOMPLETE PARTITION

HYPOPLASIA

Fig. 6. The normal cochlea and cochlear malformations. (*A*) Normal cochlea, midmodiolar section. Mo, modiolus; CA, cochlear aperture; B, basal turn; M, middle turn; A, apical turn; arrowheads, interscalar septa. (*B*) Normal cochlea, inferior section passing through the round window niche (RWN). Arrowhead, interscalar septum between middle and apical turns. (*C*) Cochlear aplasia with normal vestibule. (*D*) Cochlear aplasia with enlarged vestibule. (*E*) Common cavity. (*F*) Incomplete partition type I. (*G*) Incomplete partition type II. (*H*) Incomplete partition type III. (*I*) Cochlear hypoplasia, bud type (type I). (*J*) Cochlear hypoplasia, cystic cochlea type (type II). (*K*) Cochlear hypoplasia, with less than 2 turns (type III). (*Modified from* Sennaroglu L. Cochlear implantation in inner ear malformations—a review article. Cochlear Implants International 2009; doi: 10.1002/cii.416; with permission.)

Evaluation

Despite controversies in nomenclature, inner ear dysplasias are readily identifiable by thin-section HRCT. As mentioned, 20% of patients with sensorineural hearing loss have osseous abnormalities of the cochleovestibular complex.[36] However, not all patients have hearing loss severe enough to warrant cochlear implantation, and those with more severe dysplasia usually have worse hearing. Therefore, the percentage of patients who require cochlear implantation with osseous dysplasia is higher.[39] In general, the index of suspicion of inner ear malformations should be higher in patients whose hearing loss is part of a syndrome. T2-weighted MRI can be helpful evaluating cochlear patency, and can be particularly useful in determining the presence of septations within a cavity. MRI is especially important when no reliable auditory thresholds are obtainable with behavioral/play audiometry. In these patients, the presence or absence of a cochlear nerve can be ascertained by evaluating high-quality sagittal views of the IAC in the CISS (constructive interference into steady state) or FIESTA (fast imaging with steady-state acquisition) sequences.

Surgical Technique

Patients with cochlear abnormalities were initially precluded from implantation over concerns of electrode placement, array stability, and perceived risks to surrounding structures (including facial nerve, modiolus, and carotid artery). Advances in radiologic accuracy as well as surgical technique prompted implant centers to offer implantation to those with cochlear dysplasia. Coupled with reports of beneficial outcomes of speech perception, this further bolstered support.[38,44–48]

The type of cochlear malformation dictates the surgical approach. Nearly all cochlear dysplasias can be implanted, with the exception of complete inner ear aplasia (Michel deformity—see previous section on ABI). For the vast majority of implantable inner ear malformations, a standard transmastoid facial-posterior tympanostomy (facial recess) approach to the middle ear can be applied. The main exception to this is the common cavity malformation, which is best approached through a transmastoid labyrinthotomy.

Posterior tympanotomy

Cochlear implantation via the posterior tympanotomy can be accomplished in the vast majority of dysplastic cochleae. It is a standard approach with which otologists and those experienced in routine cochlear implantation are quite comfortable.

- The mastoidectomy is performed using conventional burrs.
- The superior and posterior cortical bony margins are not saucerized, allowing for later stable coiling of the electrode within the mastoid cavity.
- The short process of the incus is identified, and serves as a valuable landmark for the development of the posterior tympanotomy.
- The posterior bony external auditory canal is thinned.
- Confirmation of normal facial nerve anatomy by preoperative imagine is critical. If normal, the facial nerve is identified at the second genu and followed inferiorly while taking care to preserve a thin layer of bone over the nerve.
- The chorda tympani is identified anterior to the facial nerve superiorly, but joins it laterally and inferiorly in the mastoid at the annular edge, thus creating a triangle of dissection that can be followed medially until the middle ear space is encountered. Often this is facilitated by an air cell tract between the mastoid and middle ear that runs through the posterior tympanotomy.
- The space is widened, taking care not to injure the facial nerve, chorda tympani, incus, ear canal, or fibrous annulus of the tympanic membrane. Smaller burrs will be necessary to accomplish this, as the recess itself rarely exceeds 2 or 3 mm.
- With the facial recess opened, one can easily visualize many structures of the middle ear, including the round window niche. The round window niche usually lies just inferior to the stapedius tendon and oval window, though the location may vary in dysplastic cochleae.
- The round window niche is removed, revealing the round window membrane.
- Gentle palpation of the ossicles may elicit a round window reflex, which can be helpful in confirming location.
- The cochleostomy is made just anteroinferior to the round window annulus. Size is determined by the type of electrode array inserted.
- The cochleostomy is then packed with fascia to make a tight seal.
- Intraoperative monitoring (impedances, telemetry) is performed.
- The incisions are closed, keeping the electrode lead array in the confines of the mastoid cavity.
- Conventional radiographs or fluoroscopy confirm electrode position after closure, making sure the array has not migrated.
- This image then serves as a record of the position of final placement.

Transmastoid labyrinthotomy

The posterior tympanostomy is not necessary for all inner ear malformations. For the common cavity malformation, the inner ear can be accessed directly on opening of the mastoid antrum, usually obviating the need a facial recess approach and/or extended incudal fossa approach and their attendant risk of complications.

Although the transmastoid approach to the common cavity is fairly straightforward, it is the actual implantation of common cavity malformations that presents unique challenges to the surgeon. The cavity lacks a central modiolus, hence the usual goal of perimodiolar electrode positioning does not apply. Histologic studies show that many rudimentary forms of normal cochlear structures are present in a common cavity malformation.[49] An equivalent to the organ of Corti is observed, as is a vascular equivalent to the stria vascularis. Most importantly for cochlear implantation consideration, the auditory neural tissue present lies peripherally, in the walls of the common cavity. Clusters of cell bodies (spiral ganglion cell equivalents) are present in the wall, as are many of the support cell structures. Reviews of histologic studies of malformed cochleae show that their spiral ganglion cell numbers are significantly lower than those in a normal ear.[49] This finding has not, however, been shown to correlate with a reduced performance using a cochlear implant. It has been suggested that a minimal number of spiral ganglion cells is needed for effective electrical stimulation of the auditory nerve.[50] Beyond this, the presence of additional spiral ganglion cell populations may not be essential for obtaining good outcomes from a cochlear implant, perhaps because the operating system of the implant is relatively simpler than the intricate functioning of the normal inner ear and its full complement of spiral ganglion cells. It is not only the number but the location of the neural elements that must be considered in common cavity cases.

Approach to the common cavity is determined based on preoperative images, and mostly can be approached directly via the mastoid antrum (**Fig. 7**). Using continuous facial nerve monitoring, the surgery commences.

- Well and tie-down holes are drilled, followed by the trough and mastoidectomy.
- Subperiosteal pockets are made for the receiver-stimulator package and ball electrode.
- Mastoid bone around the cavity is removed with the drill for adequate exposure of the posterior surface of the cavity in the antrum.
- Drilling the cochleostomy commences (approximately 1.0–1.5 mm in diameter), attempting to keep the endosteum intact.
- By using intraoperative imaging (plain film, fluoroscopy, CT) to better demonstrate common cavity architecture, a site directly opposite the IAC is avoided.

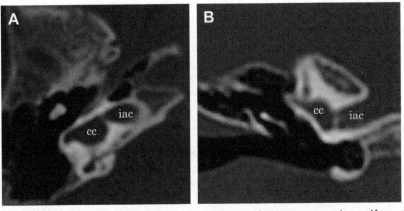

Fig. 7. Axial (*A*) and coronal (*B*) images of a patient with a common cavity malformation who was implanted under fluoroscopic guidance. Note the common cavity (cc) and internal auditory canal (iac). (*From* Fishman AJ, Roland JT Jr, Alexiades G, et al. Fluoroscopically assisted cochlear implantation. Otol Neurotol 2003;24(6):882–6; with permission.)

- The authors prefer to make the cochleostomy laterally, at the inferior portion of the cavity because it bulges into the mastoid, although others have described opening through the site of the remnant of the ampullated portion of the lateral semicircular canal.[45,51–54]
  - Both techniques allow for introduction of the electrode array and insertion of the full complement electrodes, although in the authors' experience the ampullated end of the lateral canal is usually poorly formed and not easily identified.
  - Other surgeons advocate a canal wall–down mastoidectomy to better visualize and approach the middle and inner ear structures.[45]
- These procedures are completed by obliterating the external meatus in one case and reconstructing and reinforcing the canal wall with temporal bone and temporalis muscle in the other.[47,54]
  - It is thought that these steps may also help in preventing a subsequent prolonged CSF leak.
  - To stabilize the electrode within the cavity and avoid intrameatal placement, Beltrame and colleagues[55] developed a "double posterior labyrinthotomy" technique in which a customized implant array is fed through one labyrinthotomy and manipulated/secured through a second. Manolidis and colleagues[56] described the addition of a third labyrinthotomy that is used to endoscopically confirm placement of the electrode array. However, with fewer than 2% of all cochlear implant recipients having common cavities, insufficient data exist to support the impact of these techniques.[57]
- The receiver/stimulator is placed in the well and tied down.
- The ground electrode (if separate) is placed under the temporalis muscle.
- After copious irrigation, the cochlear endosteum is opened.
- At the authors' institution, fluoroscopic guidance is used to insert the electrode along the lateral wall, preventing kinking and bending, so that intrameatal (IAC) placement is avoided.
- Intraoperative use of CT has also been described.[58]
- The electrode array can be manipulated with gentle rotation if insertion is impeded by a septation.
- The insertional stop point is reached when the outer wall of the cavity is covered by electrodes. Further insertion will initiate kinking or bending or fold over in the cavity, resulting in shorting of electrodes. This distortion is unnecessary and might be detrimental to performance and number of usable electrodes.
- The authors currently implant a straight array with concentric banded electrodes so that outer wall contact can be achieved. Newer perimodiolar electrode arrays would not appose the neuroepithelium and might affect performance.
- After the electrode is securely in place, the remainder of the procedure is exactly as is performed during traditional posterior tympanostomy cochlear implantation.

Special Surgical Considerations

CSF leaks

For many inner ear malformations, the bony cochlear lamina cribrosa is either missing or replaced by a fibrous band, thus increasing markedly the risk of CSF leak. Defects of the modiolus (as seen in incomplete partition) and the lamina cribrosa at the fundus of the IAC are responsible for the mixing of perilymph and CSF. True leaks almost certainly contain CSF in addition to perilymph, as the inner ear only contains a few milliliters of perilymph.[59] Leakage of perilymph/CSF is commonly seen following cochleostomy; however, degree of dysplasia does not necessarily correlate with risk of leakage. Likewise, when it does occur the rate of leakage, pressure of the fluid, and time until cessation is highly variable. As a result, the reported incidence of CSF leak may be overestimated. Nonetheless, published rates vary widely.[39,44,47–49,52,59–62] Of all the inner ear dysplasias, perilymph/CSF leakage is seen most frequently in patients with common cavity deformities.[39]

Rates of CSF leak can be decreased first by recognizing the risk from preoperative imaging, which will help prepare the surgeon for a suspected CSF leak at the time of cochleostomy. Wider cochleostomies allows for more packing material (the authors prefer fascia or periosteum) to be inserted between the electrode and the bony edge. Trendelenburg or head-down positioning coupled with Valsalva maneuvers can be useful in confirming the cessation of leakage. Rarely, continuous CSF diversion by lumbar drain becomes necessary. The decision to place a lumbar drain should not be taken lightly, as it is associated with its own risks and complications as well as significant inconvenience to patients and family.

All cochlear implant recipients with inner ear malformation are at increased risk for developing meningitis postoperatively, particularly those associated with CSF leakage (adjusted odds ratio of 9.3).[63] The importance of preoperative pneumococcal vaccination cannot be overemphasized, and must not be overlooked.

IAC implantation

In addition to CSF leakage, absence of the cochlear lamina cribrosa predisposes to inadvertent implantation of the IAC (**Fig. 8**). If unrecognized, this can lead to continued CSF leakage, vertigo, facial nerve stimulation, and suboptimal hearing outcomes. Several techniques have been described to avoid this complication. Tucci and colleagues[47] and, later, Sennaroglu and colleagues[60] both recommend insertion only of active electrodes (and few, if any, stiffening rings) to avoid IAC implantation. Short or compressed electrode arrays can limit, but not necessarily eliminate, risk of entry into the IAC. Coelho and colleagues[64] and Fishman and colleagues[65] both described the use of intraoperative fluoroscopy to confirm optimal electrode placement and to avoid insertion into the IAC. The use of intraoperative fluoroscopy eliminated this complication.[64]

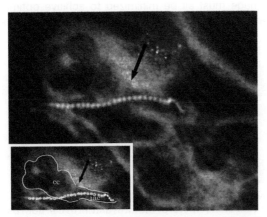

Fig. 8. Transorbital plain radiograph, intraoperative view. Note that the array has passed into the internal auditory canal (iac). The arrow denotes the junction between the common cavity and the iac as seen in this orientation. Inset outlines the lumen of the common cavity (cc) and the iac. (*From* Fishman AJ, Roland JT Jr, Alexiades G, et al. Fluoroscopically assisted cochlear implantation. Otol Neurotol 2003;24(6):882–6; with permission.)

Facial nerve

Increased surgical difficulty can be expected for a variety of reasons. In approximately 15% of patients with cochleovestibular anomalies, the facial nerve courses aberrantly.[39,44] Typically the aberrant nerve in these patients runs anteriorly, from the first genu down across the promontory toward the round window. In some cases the nerve is split, with one branch in the normal position. Occasionally the nerve obscures the proposed cochleostomy site, and the cochleostomy must be placed more anteriorly, resulting in less cochlea available for implantation.

In situations where the facial nerve is more anterior or in abnormal locations, the authors recommend drilling along the tegmen mastoidae until the antrum is encountered and the incus is seen. The incus is then removed and the facial nerve can be easily located in its horizontal segment. The facial recess is then opened from a superior to inferior direction, all the while following the course of the facial nerve. Adequate visualization of the middle ear structures can be obtained, and a proper cochleostomy position determined and executed, avoiding facial nerve injury (**Fig. 9**). This technique is always used in patients with CHARGE syndrome and BOR syndrome as well as other situations where mastoid, labyrinthine, and facial nerve anatomy present challenges to the normal posterior tympanotomy technique.

Electrode choice

The ideal electrode in both normal and malformed cochlea is one that lies in closest proximity to the neuroepithelium. In malformed cochleae, these critical neuronal sensory cells do not necessarily lie in the normal perimodiolar location close to the scala tympani. Moreover, the cochlear neuronal count can in some cases be a fraction of the normal count of 20,000 and still provide meaningful auditory input.[5] The ideal electrode in such a cochlea would therefore be one that remains close to the outer walls of the common cavity chamber, and has a circumferential direction of stimulation so that the electrical fields are distributed toward the cell bodies. In addition, these delicate neural elements might be traumatized by electrode insertion, so great care must be taken to avoid trauma during the insertion procedure.

The increased risk of complications, including extracochlear placement, intrameatal array insertion, electrode kinking or bending, or insertional trauma resulting in cochlear neuroepithelial damage must all be minimized to achieve optimal placement and performance. Intrameatal arrays have been successfully removed and replaced within

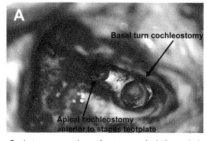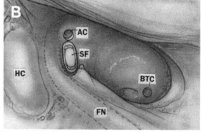

Fig. 9. Intraoperative photograph (*A*) and drawing (*B*) of a transmastoid view through the facial recess of a right ear after removal of the incus and incus bar. Both basal and apical cochleostomies are seen before insertion of a dual-electrode array. AC, apical cochleostomy; BTC, basal-turn cochleostomy; FN, facial nerve in descending (mastoid) portion; HC, horizontal (lateral) semicircular canal; SF, stapes footplate. (*From* Cosetti M, Roland JT Jr. Cochlear implant electrode insertion. Operat Tech Otolaryngol Head Neck Surg 2010;21(4):223–32; with permission.)

the primitive cochleae successfully by the authors on several occasions without complications using fluoroscopic guidance. The most common anomaly for which intrameatal electrode placement has occurred is the X-linked deafness cochlear anomaly where the normal modiolus architecture is absent.

Device programming

Clear communication between surgeon and implant audiologist is critical. Knowing electrode choice and implanted location are essential to successful programming and usage. The absence of normal tonotopic cochlear architecture can result in unpredictable frequency representation along the electrode (analogous to the ossified cochlear, for which the surgeon must know if the apical array is inserted in an anterograde or retrograde fashion). Just as with surgical considerations, there are several programming challenges that present as a result of the abnormal cochlear anatomy and, in particular, the location of neural elements. Successful usage of an implant is related to establishment of a usable program or "MAP." In patients with malformed cochlea, threshold and comfort levels fluctuate more; therefore, frequent adjustment in programming of these implants is necessary.[44,47,66] Likewise, wider stimulation pulse-width modes may be needed and hence more power consumed.[67] Stimulation of the facial nerve by the cochlear implant electrodes is common, and deactivation of the electrodes in question may be necessary to remove this problem. Though necessary, the deactivation can result in further degradation of the signal available to the neural elements. As a result, MAPping children with anomalous cochleovestibular systems is more difficult and takes longer to achieve. However, within the published literature there is a consensus that the speech perception results in malformed cochleae obtained over time can be in the same range as results observed in implant recipients with normally formed cochleae.[44,47,49,51,52,54,60,66,67] To more thoroughly compare recipients with malformed cavities with recipients with normal cochleae, a retrospective matched-pairs analysis of 17 patients with malformed cochleae (including 4 common cavities) and 17 controls was performed by Eisenman and colleagues.[67] The investigators showed that although eventual outcomes for 24 months after implantation were similar between the groups, the malformation cases took longer to reach this end point. For more on device programming issues in children with anomalous cochleovestibular anatomy, the reader is referred to an excellent discussion by Papsin.[39]

Performance

Ever since first being reported in 1983, patients with inner ear malformations have derived significant benefit from cochlear implantation.[46,47,61,62,68–72] However, there is a wide range in performance that does not always correlate directly with degree of dysplasia.[39,57,73] The relatively small number of patients implanted at any one given center coupled with rapid evolution in both implant design and processing strategies make reliable and reproducible outcome measurements a challenge. Furthermore, children with inner ear malformations may have very disparate patterns of hearing loss before implantation, ranging from congenital profound hearing loss to adults with excellent speech and postlingual progressive hearing loss. The vast majority of literature on this subject includes case reports and series, many reporting surgical outcomes only without specific mention of audiologic performance. Reports that do include outcomes frequently exclude patients too young for behavioral testing or those with developmental delays. With these caveats mentioned, the following paragraphs discuss speech performance in this small but diverse patient population.

Numerous published reports and series have included speech perception patients with incomplete partition (IP) of the cochlea.[38,44,47,59,71,72,74] The first known report, by

Miyamoto and colleagues,[46] describes a single patient whose electrical threshold measurements were similar to those seen in implanted patients without cochlear malformations, thus paving the way for future implantation in candidates with IP. In the largest study to date of IP, Papsin showed significant improvements in both closed-set (TAC, WIPI) and open-set (GASP-Word, PBK-Word, PBK-Phoneme) speech perception in 42 patients.[39] These patients performed better than patients with other malformations, and even better than patients with normal cochleae, though Weber and colleagues[75] report 8 implanted children of whom 6 had speech recognition. Of the 2 patients who did not, one had a device rejection and the other was autistic. Many other patients are included within larger series of inner ear malformations. Review of these studies shows that most patients have speech reception, with the majority obtaining closed-set reception and nearly half with open-set reception.[38,47,62] Buchman and colleagues[57] and Lee and colleagues[68] report results of implantation in patients with enlarged vestibular aqueduct with and without other temporal bone abnormalities. In these studies patients without associated abnormalities scored better postoperative pure-tone averages than those with abnormalities.

Children with hypoplastic cochleae (HC) or common cavities (CC) generally have worse performance than patients with IP.[39,76] This fact also holds true when older children and those with oral language preimplantation were included.[39] The anatomic and physiologic basis for this is apparent: fewer active electrodes implanted, narrower dynamic ranges, impaired neural synchrony, and lack of tonotopic organization and access all result in poorer speech perception outcomes. However, the vast majority of implanted patients with HC have some degree of speech reception, some with closed-set speech perception a and few with open-set speech perception.[38,39,47,62] The same holds true for CC malformations.[38,39,45,47,51–53,60,62,64,72,75] Other than age of implantation, no specific factors have been found to determine which patients with severely malformed cochlea will do well and which will do poorly.[76] For this predictive difficulty, careful preoperative counseling with patients and families is critical. Despite poorer performance in the population, implantation is still justified, as speech perception is still better than that in worse performing patients with normal cochlea.[39]

As the evidence mounts to clearly support bilateral implantation for candidates with normal cochlea, so too does it for patients with malformed cochleae. In fact, binaural implantation may serve an even more important role in patients with malformations, and the first side may not be performing optimally. Chadha and colleagues[77] report 10 children (aged 9–33 months) implanted bilaterally (5 IP, 3 HC, 2 CC) with a mean follow-up of 12 months. All 10 had speech reception, 8 of 8 tested had closed-set speech perception (>75% on WIPI, TAC, ESP tests), and 5 of 7 tested had open-set speech perception (>75% on PBK, GASP tests). The investigators also looked at balance function, as bilateral implantation may further degrade a congenital vestibular hypofunction.[78] Despite abnormal tests, in this study no patients had clinically significant long-term imbalance problems (though only 6 of 10 patients were tested). This finding supports previous reports that unilateral and bilateral implantation in normal cochlea does not clinically affect balance.[79,80]

To confirm and further explore the specific differences in performance requires larger multicenter studies. The impact of type and severity of malformation on outcome also warrants further investigation. To this end, initial counseling for a candidate with any cochlear malformation should always include mention of the potential challenges that may occur in maximizing the outcomes achieved with the device, and that outcomes may or may not be what one would expect in patients with normal cochleae.

SUMMARY

Implantation of obstructed and malformed cochleae presents a challenging yet rewarding endeavor for the implant team. Remarkable developments in diagnosis, surgical technique, electrode design, processing strategies, and programming have all contributed to the ability to successfully implant patient populations previously excluded from this life-changing intervention.

REFERENCES

1. Nadol JB Jr, Young YS, Glynn RJ. Survival of spiral ganglion cells in profound sensorineural hearing loss: implications for cochlear implantation. Ann Otol Rhinol Laryngol 1989;98(6):411–6.
2. Balkany T, Gantz B, Nadol JB Jr. Multichannel cochlear implants in partially ossified cochleas. Ann Otol Rhinol Laryngol Suppl 1988;135:3–7.
3. Gantz BJ, McCabe BF, Tyler RS. Use of multichannel cochlear implants in obstructed and obliterated cochleas. Otolaryngol Head Neck Surg 1988;98(1): 72–81.
4. Hodges AV, Balkany TJ, Gomez-Marin O, et al. Speech recognition after implantation of the ossified cochlea. Am J Otol 1999;20(4):453–6.
5. Otte J, Schunknecht HF, Kerr AG. Ganglion cell populations in normal and pathological human cochleae. Implications for cochlear implantation. Laryngoscope 1978;88(8 Pt 1):1231–46.
6. Colletti V, Shannon R, Carner M, et al. Outcomes in nontumor adults fitted with the auditory brainstem implant: 10 years' experience. Otol Neurotol 2009;30(5): 614–8.
7. Schuchat A, Robinson K, Wenger JD, et al. Bacterial meningitis in the United States in 1995. Active Surveillance Team. N Engl J Med 1997;337(14):970–6.
8. Shelton MM, Marks WA. Bacterial meningitis: an update. Neurol Clin 1990;8(3): 605–17.
9. Axon PR, Temple RH, Saeed SR, et al. Cochlear ossification after meningitis. Am J Otol 1998;19(6):724–9.
10. Dodge PR, Davis H, Feigin RD, et al. Prospective evaluation of hearing impairment as a sequela of acute bacterial meningitis. N Engl J Med 1984;311(14): 869–74.
11. Ozdamar O, Kraus N. Auditory brainstem response in infants recovering from bacterial meningitis. Neurologic assessment 1. Arch Neurol 1983;40(8):499–502.
12. Richardson MP, Reid A, Tarlow MJ, et al. Hearing loss during bacterial meningitis. Arch Dis Child 1997;76(2):134–8.
13. Gleeson TG, Lacy PD, Bresnihan M, et al. High resolution computed tomography and magnetic resonance imaging in the pre-operative assessment of cochlear implant patients. J Laryngol Otol 2003;117(9):692–5.
14. Laszig R, Terwey B, Battmer RD, et al. Magnetic resonance imaging (MRI) and high resolution computer tomography (HRCT) in cochlear implant candidates. Scand Audiol Suppl 1988;30:197–200.
15. Silberman B, Garabedian EN, Denoyelle F, et al. Role of modern imaging technology in the implementation of pediatric cochlear implants. Ann Otol Rhinol Laryngol 1995;104(1):42–6.
16. Isaacson B, Booth T, Kutz JW Jr, et al. Labyrinthitis ossificans: how accurate is MRI in predicting cochlear obstruction? Otolaryngol Head Neck Surg 2009; 140(5):692–6.

17. Tinling SP, Colton J, Brodie HA. Location and timing of initial osteoid deposition in postmeningitic labyrinthitis ossificans determined by multiple fluorescent labels. Laryngoscope 2004;114(4):675–80.
18. Aschendorff A, Klenzner T, Laszig R. Deafness after bacterial meningitis: an emergency for early imaging and cochlear implant surgery. Otolaryngol Head Neck Surg 2005;133(6):995–6.
19. Cohen NL, Waltzman SB. Partial insertion of the nucleus multichannel cochlear implant: technique and results. Am J Otol 1993;14(4):357–61.
20. Fishman KE, Shannon RV, Slattery WH. Speech recognition as a function of the number of electrodes used in the SPEAK cochlear implant speech processor. J Speech Lang Hear Res 1997;40(5):1201–15.
21. Miyamoto RT, Osberger MJ, Robbins AM, et al. Comparison of speech perception abilities in deaf children with hearing aids or cochlear implants. Otolaryngol Head Neck Surg 1991;104(1):42–6.
22. Steenerson RL, Gary LB, Wynens MS. Scala vestibuli cochlear implantation for labyrinthine ossification. Am J Otol 1990;11(5):360–3.
23. Lin K, Marrinan MS, Waltzman SB, et al. Multichannel cochlear implantation in the scala vestibuli. Otol Neurotol 2006;27(5):634–8.
24. Balkany T, Gantz BJ, Steenerson RL, et al. Systematic approach to electrode insertion in the ossified cochlea. Otolaryngol Head Neck Surg 1996;114(1):4–11.
25. Parisier SC, Chute PM. Multichannel implants in postmeningitic ossified cochleas. Adv Otorhinolaryngol 1993;48:49–58.
26. Kirk KI, Sehgal M, Miyamoto RT. Speech perception performance of nucleus multichannel cochlear implant users with partial electrode insertions. Ear Hear 1997;18(6):456–71.
27. Rotteveel LJ, Snik AF, Vermeulen AM, et al. Three-year follow-up of children with postmeningitic deafness and partial cochlear implant insertion. Clin Otolaryngol 2005;30(3):242–8.
28. Balkany T, Bird PA, Hodges AV, et al. Surgical technique for implantation of the totally ossified cochlea. Laryngoscope 1998;108(7):988–92.
29. Hartrampf R, Dahm MC, Battmer RD, et al. Insertion depth of the Nucleus electrode array and relative performance. Ann Otol Rhinol Laryngol Suppl 1995; 166:277–80.
30. Roland JT Jr, Fishman AJ, Alexiades G, et al. Electrode to modiolus proximity: a fluoroscopic and histologic analysis. Am J Otol 2000;21(2):218–25.
31. Lenarz T, Buchner A, Tasche C, et al. The results in patients implanted with the nucleus double array cochlear implant: pitch discrimination and auditory performance. Ear Hear 2002;23(Suppl 1):90S–101S.
32. Roland JT Jr, Coelho DH, Pantelides H, et al. Partial and double-array implantation of the ossified cochlea. Otol Neurotol 2008;29(8):1068–75.
33. Colletti V, Carner M, Miorelli V, et al. Auditory brainstem implant in posttraumatic cochlear nerve avulsion. Audiol Neurootol 2004;9(4):247–55.
34. Grayeli AB, Kalamarides M, Bouccara D, et al. Auditory brainstem implant in neurofibromatosis type 2 and non-neurofibromatosis type 2 patients. Otol Neurotol 2008;29(8):1140–6.
35. Sanna M, Khrais T, Guida M, et al. Auditory brainstem implant in a child with severely ossified cochlea. Laryngoscope 2006;116(9):1700–3.
36. Jackler RK, Luxford WM, House WF. Congenital malformations of the inner ear: a classification based on embryogenesis. Laryngoscope 1987;97(3 Pt 2 Suppl 40):2–14.
37. Park AH, Kou B, Hotaling A, et al. Clinical course of pediatric congenital inner ear malformations 380. Laryngoscope 2000;110(10 Pt 1):1715–9.

38. Jackler RK, Luxford WM, House WF. Sound detection with the cochlear implant in five ears of four children with congenital malformations of the cochlea. Laryngoscope 1987;97(3 Pt 2 Suppl 40):15–7.

39. Papsin BC. Cochlear implantation in children with anomalous cochleovestibular anatomy. Laryngoscope 2005;115(1 Pt 2 Suppl 106):1–26.

40. Phelps PD. The basal turn of the cochlea. Br J Radiol 1992;65(773):370–4.

41. Zheng Y, Schachern PA, Cureoglu S, et al. The shortened cochlea: its classification and histopathologic features. Int J Pediatr Otorhinolaryngol 2002;63(1):29–39.

42. Sennaroglu L, Saatci I. A new classification for cochleovestibular malformations. Laryngoscope 2002;112(12):2230–41.

43. Represa J, Frenz DA, Van De Water TR. Genetic patterning of embryonic inner ear development. Acta Otolaryngol 2000;120(1):5–10.

44. Hoffman RA, Downey LL, Waltzman SB, et al. Cochlear implantation in children with cochlear malformations. Am J Otol 1997;18(2):184–7.

45. McElveen JT Jr, Carrasco VN, Miyamoto RT, et al. Cochlear implantation in common cavity malformations using a transmastoid labyrinthotomy approach. Laryngoscope 1997;107(8):1032–6.

46. Miyamoto RT, Robbins AJ, Myres WA, et al. Cochlear implantation in the Mondini inner ear malformation. Am J Otol 1986;7(4):258–61.

47. Tucci DL, Telian SA, Zimmerman-Phillips S, et al. Cochlear implantation in patients with cochlear malformations. Arch Otolaryngol Head Neck Surg 1995;121(8):833–8.

48. Weber BP, Dillo W, Dietrich B, et al. Pediatric cochlear implantation in cochlear malformations. Am J Otol 1998;19(6):747–53.

49. Graham JM, Phelps PD, Michaels L. Congenital malformations of the ear and cochlear implantation in children: review and temporal bone report of common cavity. J Laryngol Otol Suppl 2000;25:1–14.

50. Schmidt JM. Cochlear neuronal populations in developmental defects of the inner ear. Implications for cochlear implantation. Acta Otolaryngol 1985;99(1–2):14–20.

51. Ito J, Sakota T, Kato H, et al. Surgical considerations regarding cochlear implantation in the congenitally malformed cochlea. Otolaryngol Head Neck Surg 1999;121(4):495–8.

52. Luntz M, Balkany T, Hodges AV, et al. Cochlear implants in children with congenital inner ear malformations. Arch Otolaryngol Head Neck Surg 1997;123(9):974–7.

53. Molter DW, Pate BR Jr, McElveen JT Jr. Cochlear implantation in the congenitally malformed ear. Otolaryngol Head Neck Surg 1993;108(2):174–7.

54. Shintani T, Himi T, Homma T, et al. Cochlear implant in children with common cavity deformity. Adv Otorhinolaryngol 2000;57:90–2.

55. Beltrame MA, Bonfioli F, Frau GN. Cochlear implant in inner ear malformation: double posterior labyrinthotomy approach to common cavity. Adv Otorhinolaryngol 2000;57:113–9.

56. Manolidis S, Tonini R, Spitzer J. Endoscopically guided placement of prefabricated cochlear implant electrodes in a common cavity malformation. Int J Pediatr Otorhinolaryngol 2006;70(4):591–6.

57. Buchman CA, Copeland BJ, Yu KK, et al. Cochlear implantation in children with congenital inner ear malformations. Laryngoscope 2004;114(2):309–16.

58. Bloom JD, Rizzi MD, Germiller JA. Real-time intraoperative computed tomography to assist cochlear implant placement in the malformed inner ear. Otol Neurotol 2009;30(1):23–6.

59. Janssens S, Govaerts PJ, Casselman J, et al. The LAURA multichannel cochlear implant in a true Mondini dysplasia. Eur Arch Otorhinolaryngol 1996;253(4–5): 301–4.
60. Sennaroglu L, Sarac S, Ergin T. Surgical results of cochlear implantation in malformed cochlea. Otol Neurotol 2006;27(5):615–23.
61. Silverstein H, Smouha E, Morgan N. Multichannel cochlear implantation in a patient with bilateral Mondini deformities. Am J Otol 1988;9(6):451–5.
62. Slattery WH III, Luxford WM. Cochlear implantation in the congenital malformed cochlea. Laryngoscope 1995;105(11):1184–7.
63. Reefhuis J, Honein MA, Whitney CG, et al. Risk of bacterial meningitis in children with cochlear implants 1. N Engl J Med 2003;349(5):435–45.
64. Coelho DH, Waltzman SB, Roland JT Jr. Implanting common cavity malformations using intraoperative fluoroscopy. Otol Neurotol 2008;29(7):914–9.
65. Fishman AJ, Roland JT Jr, Alexiades G, et al. Fluoroscopically assisted cochlear implantation. Otol Neurotol 2003;24(6):882–6.
66. Firszt JB, Reeder RM, Novak MA. Multichannel cochlear implantation with inner ear malformation: case report of performance and management. J Am Acad Audiol 1995;6(3):235–42.
67. Eisenman DJ, Ashbaugh C, Zwolan TA, et al. Implantation of the malformed cochlea. Otol Neurotol 2001;22(6):834–41.
68. Lee KH, Lee J, Isaacson B, et al. Cochlear implantation in children with enlarged vestibular aqueduct. Laryngoscope 2010;120(8):1675–81.
69. Luxford WM, House WF. Cochlear implants in children: medical and surgical considerations. Ear Hear 1985;6(Suppl 3):20S–3S.
70. Mangabeira-Albernaz PL. The Mondini dysplasia—from early diagnosis to cochlear implant. Acta Otolaryngol 1983;95(5–6):627–31.
71. Turrini M, Orzan E, Gabana M, et al. Cochlear implantation in a bilateral Mondini dysplasia. Scand Audiol Suppl 1997;46:78–81.
72. Woolley AL, Jenison V, Stroer BS, et al. Cochlear implantation in children with inner ear malformations. Ann Otol Rhinol Laryngol 1998;107(6):492–500.
73. Dettman S, Sadeghi-Barzalighi A, Ambett R, et al. Cochlear implants in forty-eight children with cochlear and/or vestibular abnormality. Audiol Neurootol 2010; 16(4):222–32.
74. van Wermeskerken GK, Dunnebier EA, van Olphen AF, et al. Audiological performance after cochlear implantation: a 2-year follow-up in children with inner ear malformations. Acta Otolaryngol 2007;127(3):252–7.
75. Weber BP, Lenarz T, Dillo W, et al. Malformations in cochlear implant patients. Am J Otol 1997;18(Suppl 6):S64–5.
76. Kim LS, Jeong SW, Huh MJ, et al. Cochlear implantation in children with inner ear malformations. Ann Otol Rhinol Laryngol 2006;115(3):205–14.
77. Chadha NK, James AL, Gordon KA, et al. Bilateral cochlear implantation in children with anomalous cochleovestibular anatomy 5. Arch Otolaryngol Head Neck Surg 2009;135(9):903–9.
78. Licameli G, Zhou G, Kenna MA. Disturbance of vestibular function attributable to cochlear implantation in children. Laryngoscope 2009;119(4):740–5.
79. Brey RH, Facer GW, Trine MB, et al. Vestibular effects associated with implantation of a multiple channel cochlear prosthesis. Am J Otol 1995;16(4):424–30.
80. Das S, Buchman CA. Bilateral cochlear implantation: current concepts. Curr Opin Otolaryngol Head Neck Surg 2005;13(5):290–3.

Cochlear Implant Programming

William H. Shapiro, AuD[a],*, Tamala S. Bradham, PhD[b]

KEYWORDS

- Cochlear implant • Device programming
- Intraoperative monitoring • Programming parameters

Cochlear implants have become a viable treatment for individuals who present with severe to profound hearing loss. This technology allows them to access sound in their environment and communicate more effectively with their peers. Despite the substantial benefit this treatment can provide recipients, cochlear implantation is an underutilized service. One of the Public Health Application and Outreach goals from Healthy People 2020, Objective ENT-VSL-3, is to increase the number of people who are deaf or very hard of hearing who use cochlear implants.[1] The NIDCD's Healthy Hearing Progress Report noted that in 2004 only 2 of every 1000 adults who are deaf or very hard of hearing received a cochlear implant.[2] For children, Bradham and Jones[3] reported that only 55% of children between the ages of 1 and 6 years who were appropriate for cochlear implantation were recipients of this technology.

To address this national health care issue, there has been significant emphasis on educating practitioners on candidacy criteria for cochlear implants, advancing cochlear implant device designs, surgical techniques, and programming of the device. Children who meet the Food and Drug Administration (FDA) guidelines and receive an implant early enough often develop age-appropriate language skills.[4,5] Adults who are postlingually deafened and meet the FDA guidelines often receive open-set speech recognition.[6] These successes are greatly dependent on a variety of issues, including the quality of the programming of the cochlear implant system.

The ultimate goal of device programming is to adjust a device so that it can effectively convert acoustic input into a usable electric signal for each electrode stimulated. Although this conversion varies across devices, the more accurate the process, the greater the potential for open-set speech perception.[7] This review focuses on general (traditional) device programming, programming techniques specific to children, objective programming techniques, a brief overview of the programming parameters of the currently commercially available multichannel systems in the United States—Harmony

[a] Department of Otolaryngology, NYU Langone Medical Center, 550 First Avenue, New York, NY 10016, USA
[b] Department of Hearing and Speech Sciences, Vanderbilt Bill Wilkerson Center, Medical Center East, South Tower, Room 6209, 1215 21st Avenue South, Nashville, TN 37232-8718, USA
* Corresponding author.
E-mail address: William.Shapiro@nyumc.org

Otolaryngol Clin N Am 45 (2012) 111–127
doi:10.1016/j.otc.2011.08.020
0030-6665/12/$ – see front matter © 2012 Elsevier Inc. All rights reserved.

device (Advanced Bionics Corporation, Valencia, CA), Med-El combi 40+ (Innsbruck, Austria), and the Nucleus Freedom and N5 device (Cochlear Corporation, Sydney Australia)—as well as managing patient programming complaints, device failures, and what the authors believe the future may hold for new programming techniques.

GENERAL DEVICE PROGRAMMING

Programming a cochlear implant is a process that can be divided into 4 time periods: preprogramming, the operating room (OR), initial stimulation, and follow-up. In order for a patient to achieve maximum benefit from the cochlear implant experience, all 4 phases need to be maximized.

Preprogramming

The goal of preprogramming is to prepare the patient for the initial stimulation. This preparatory phase is spent training auditory concepts in young children or adults who are prelingually or perilingually impaired and therefore have limited exposure to auditory stimuli. The goal is twofold:

1. Establish a clear and rapid response to auditory stimulation
2. Familiarize the patient with the task/procedure.

The responsibility for training these tasks typically lies with the speech pathologist working with the patient, the audiologist evaluating the patient, and occasionally the parent of the child. It is critical, at this juncture, that the type of amplification in use be appropriate; this can range from a powerful in the ear hearing aid to a postauricular aid to an FM system. The larger, more mature cochlear implant centers have instituted hearing aid loaner programs to defray the cost of purchasing expensive temporary amplification between identification and surgery, and to ensure that patients are using the most appropriate amplification during the evaluation period. Cross-modality training, using vibrotactile stimulation, has been used with some success in patients with total loss of hearing, limited exposure to auditory stimuli, and multiply handicapping conditions, for example, visual impairment. Over the last decade, as centers have gained experience with cochlear implants, the duration of preprogramming has decreased, which most likely is a result of improved hearing aid technology and facility with the overall evaluation process, especially in the pediatric population.

Intraoperative Monitoring

Over the last several years intraoperative monitoring has gained wider acceptance and, therefore, use among cochlear implant centers. Although intraoperative monitoring requires an inordinate amount of personnel time, is often not reimbursed by insurance companies, and out-of-the-box device failures are rare, it can provide the implant team with valuable information. Monitoring can confirm electrical output and patient stimulation, provide objective data that can be used as a starting point for behavioral testing (psychophysics), especially in the difficult to test, and can be a powerful counseling tool in assuaging the concerns of family members at the conclusion of the surgical procedure. The battery of tests typically performed by the audiologist in the OR include, but are not limited to, impedance telemetry, which confirms the integrity of the electrodes; and electrical stapedial reflex thresholds (ESRT) and measurement of the electrical compound action potential (ECAP), which confirm stimulation of the auditory nerve. There has been a significant amount of research on the relationship between these electrophysiological indices and psychophysical measures obtained during device programming.[8–16] Over the last 10 years, implant centers have begun to use the Internet to allow audiologists to monitor devices from remote locations. In a study by Shapiro and colleagues,[17] 8 patients were evaluated; 4 were monitored in situ and 4 from a remote location (cochlear implant center) in an effort to determine the feasibility and efficacy of remote monitoring compared with in situ monitoring. The results showed the average audiologist's time for remote testing was 9 minutes compared with 93 minutes required for performing in situ testing. In an example, based on 170 surgeries performed by New York University in 2006, the potential for 6.35 weeks of gained productivity for the audiology staff was demonstrated. This result represents a significant reduction in time required for testing and, consequently, cost. The only additional equipment needed was an Internet connection, additional commercially available software applications, and a telephone.

Finally, a plain film is obtained in the OR to assess electrode placement and to serve as a baseline in the event of device issues at a later date. If, during intraoperative monitoring, the device does not stimulate and/or impedance measures cannot be obtained, the backup device may be used to ensure proper functioning at initial stimulation.

Initial Stimulation

The initial stimulation typically begins 10 days to 4 weeks postoperatively and lasts for approximately 2 hours per day for 2 consecutive days. This timeframe should be reduced for both a device failure, as the need to get the patient back "on the air" is crucial, and bilateral simultaneous implantation, as the patient is typically without access to their auditory environment after surgery. If intraoperative monitoring was performed, either in situ or remotely, these data should have already been loaded on the programming computer before the initial stimulation. The audiologist uses the time period between surgery and initial stimulation to set up a programming plan. The objective data obtained, along with the results of the plain film and discussions with the surgeon, are crucial to an uneventful initial stimulation; that is, stimulating an electrode that is extracochlear, which may result in a nonauditory side effect, can be counterproductive. Many centers will use the data obtained in the OR to program a device (objective programming), and this has had a positive direct impact in streamlining the programming process.

Physical environment for stimulation
Maintaining a comfortable physical environment in which device programming is performed can be crucial to the overall success of the initial stimulation, especially for children.[18] In children a team approach, similar to traditional pediatric testing, is the preferred approach. This method will involve a primary audiologist and an audiologist, speech pathologist, or possibly a parent working with the child using either visual reinforcement auditory (VRA) or conditioned play audiometry (CPA) techniques to elicit behavioral responses to the electrical stimulation during programming. Often programming sessions may be videotaped to document a patient's progress and to provide information about a child's mode of response. These initial sessions are dedicated to both providing the patient with a comfortable and usable program and counseling the patient or parent about care, maintenance, and initial troubleshooting of the device. With the use of intraoperative device monitoring and streamlined programming techniques, the time required during the initial stimulation has been significantly reduced.

Psychophysical measures

Regardless of the device, traditionally two basic psychophysical measures need to be obtained on each intracochlear electrode: electrical thresholds (T level), defined as the softest level at which a patient is stimulated 100% of the time, and most comfortable loudness levels (C/M levels), defined as the loudest sound a patient can listen to comfortably for a sustained period of time. To confirm that recipients consistently hear at T levels, they may be asked to count the number of sounds they hear, referred to as "counted T level." The methods used and the degree of difficulty in obtaining these measures will vary considerably depending on several factors (eg, patient's chronologic age, mental status, length of deafness, other handicapping conditions, and so forth). The techniques used are similar to those used by pediatric audiologists. Using a wide range of techniques, both behaviorally and objectively, is especially important with expanded patient criteria.

Fundamental parameters

Before obtaining psychophysical measures, certain parameters typically need to be chosen (device-specific parameters are discussed later in this article). Fundamental among these parameters is the speech-processing (encoding) strategy. Encoding strategies can be defined as the method by which a given implant translates the incoming acoustic signal into patterns of electrical pulses, which then stimulate the existing nerve fibers. These strategies provide the listener with cues regarding spectral or envelope information, that is, spectral peak (SPEAK), temporal information (continuous interleaved sampling [CIS]/high resolution [high RES120]), temporal fine structure, or a combination of both, advanced combination encoder (ACE). Advances in speech-coding strategies have contributed to improved patient performance over the years. The typical device offers the audiologist more than one strategy, and there is no consensus on the most effective approach.

Historically, stimulation mode has been a parameter that requires prior choice. Stimulation mode refers to the electrical current flow, that is, the location of the indifferent (reference) electrode relative to the active electrode (stimulating) electrode. Monopolar stimulation refers to a remote ground (outside of the cochlea), whereas bipolar stimulation refers to both the active and ground electrode within the cochlea. The Nucleus device can be programmed in both monopolar and bipolar stimulation mode, and the Advanced Bionics and Med-El device can be programmed in a monopolar mode only. The wider the stimulation mode, the lower the threshold values, due to the greater physical separation of active and ground electrodes. Typically monopolar stimulation is the preferred mode, as this mode may extend battery life, allowing for a more consistent threshold and threshold value for adjacent electrodes due to a wider current spread. Therefore this mode will lend itself to interpolation of T and C/M levels in populations in whom obtaining psychophysical measure on every electrode implanted is not feasible. Research has suggested that individuals in a monopolar mode can pitch rank and perceive a monotonic decrease in pitch as the stimulating electrode is moved from the base to the apex of the cochlea.[19] After establishing T and C/M levels, clinicians may choose to balance loudness of the electrodes at 100% and possibly 50% of the dynamic range. Experience and research suggest that achieving an equal loudness contour across the electrode array can maximize speech perception. While not difficult for postlingually deafened adults, loudness balancing can be a problematic task for the early implanted, long-term deafened, multiply handicapped, and so forth. Nevertheless, high levels of speech perception have been obtained on early implanted patients, negating the need for loudness balancing.

Program creation

After all psychophysical tasks have been completed, a program can be created and the device can then be activated for live speech. Initial reactions to speech stimuli vary widely, ranging from no reaction to an adverse reaction. Of course, this will be dependent on the patient's previous exposure to auditory stimuli. There are several device-specific parameters that can be manipulated depending on initial reaction, discussed later.

Speech testing

Finally, informal speech testing, for example, Ling sounds, should be performed to ensure that the patient has access to various frequencies in the speech domain. In addition, Holden and colleagues[20] suggested the use of warbled tone stimuli in the soundfield following a programming session. These investigators postulated that soundfield thresholds needed to be at 30 dB or less for a patient to have adequate access to the critical elements of the speech signal.

Bilaterally implanted patients

As more patients receive bilateral cochlear implants, a protocol for device programming of these patients needs to be implemented. Bilaterally implanted individuals require additional programming time and therefore the need for streamlined fitting procedures is critical. As the majority of device-fitting strategies use a monopolar stimulation mode, which typically has consistent thresholds and C/M levels across the array, measuring select electrodes across the array (interpolation) can be performed without sacrifice of performance. It is not uncommon for cochlear implant centers to only program one cochlear implant at the initial activation and then introduce the second device on the next day for patients who have been simultaneously implanted. Individuals implanted sequentially require a different approach to programming. Before surgery for the second side, the patient's first device should be programmed to ensure optimal functioning, which will allow the clinician to focus programming efforts on the new side for the first 3 months (the initial phases of programming). At the 3-month interval the patient will then be scheduled as bilateral, affording the clinician more time at subsequent visits. It is likely that the second (new) side, depending on time between surgeries, will not, at least initially, function as the dominant side and it is therefore important to use a conservative approach to loudness levels on the second side. This approach will serve to reduce initial "dyssynchronization" between the ears. Finally, patients functioning in a bimodal mode (hearing aid + cochlear implant) will require similar caution during programming as well.

Counseling

Other than programming, a large part of the initial stimulation phases consists of counseling, that is, daily care, maintenance, and troubleshooting. Providing patients and parents with "front-end" counseling and a basic understanding of these concepts will reduce the time professionals need to spend on nonreimbursable activities over the long term, and streamline the process. As devices have become more sophisticated so have the patients' instructions for use. The manufacturers have responded by including instructional CDs, online instruction manuals, and telephone support. This information has been helpful to clinics in reducing the in-clinic workload, and further streamlining the fitting process.

OBJECTIVE PROGRAMMING TECHNIQUES
Evoked Stapedial Reflex Threshold

One objective measure for programming cochlear implants is setting the upper stimulation levels (C/M levels) based on the ESRT. An acoustic immittance probe is placed in the external ear canal in the contralateral ear of the ear being programmed. With a continuous 226-Hz probe tone in the contralateral ear, the programming stimulus is presented to the cochlear implant ear in an ascending manner until there is a decrease in admittance. The decrease in admittance is observed in the ear contralateral to the cochlear implant because the stapedial reflex is a bilateral response. Typically the audiologist will measure ESRT on as many channels as possible and then interpolate the remaining channels. Then during live speech they will gradually increase the stimulation levels globally. It is important to not set the global levels at or higher than the measured ESRT levels. The ESRT is a fairly reliable predictor of upper stimulation levels.[21–23]

Electrically Evoked Compound Action Potential

Not all patients can tolerate, or have absent, ESRT. The ECAP uses a lower stimulation rate than the stimuli used for programming, and thus may be more tolerated during the first 2 days of programming. The ECAP measurement system is referred to by many different names based on the manufacturer: auditory response telemetry (Med-El), neural response imaging (Advanced Bionics), and neural response telemetry (Cochlear Corporation). The ECAP is used to estimate both thresholds (T levels) and upper stimulation levels (C/M levels), and usually falls within the patient's electrical dynamic range. Using the cochlear implant system and the specialized manufacturer software, obtaining the ECAP for each electrode can be easily accomplished. Obtaining an ECAP response provides the audiologist with a confirmation of an audible stimulation level for a particular channel/electrode and provides a baseline objective measurement for comparison later on if there are reported problems. Due to the variability in responses, researchers suggest combining the ECAP with behavioral programming levels for 1 (ie, middle of the array) to 3 (ie, apical, middle, and basal ends of the array) channels/electrodes.[24] By measuring at least one T and C/M level, the audiologist can interpolate the remaining T and C/M levels with the ECAP responses obtained.

DEVICE-SPECIFIC PROGRAMMING PARAMETERS
Advanced Bionics

Advanced Bionics (AB) has two programming platforms for their cochlear implant systems. The SCLIN software platform is used with previous C1 internal devices (C1.0 and C1.2) and sound processors (Platinum Sound Processor body worn or Platinum BTE ear level). The newer CII and HiRes 90 K internal devices are programmed on the SoundWave 2.0 platform. While the Platinum Sound Processors are compatible with the new internal devices, the ear level sound processor is different. The ear level sound processor available for the internal implants is the Harmony.

The HiRes 90 K implant is a hermetically sealed titanium case with a telemetry coil attached and encased in silastic. A removable magnet is housed in a silastic sleeve in the center of the coil of the HiRes 90 K implant. The overall dimensions are approximately 28 mm wide by 56 mm long.[25] The HiFocus and the Helix electrode arrays have 16 platinum-iridium intracochlear electrodes with two extracochlear reference electrodes. Because each electrode has its own capacitor, there are 16 independent channels that could be potentially programmed.

The Harmony sound processor has several battery-pack options to reduce the weight at the ear and for overall comfort. These devices also have an optional battery pack for bilateral cochlear implant users. The sound processors can hold up to 3 programs and offer several coding strategies: ClearVoice, HiRes-Sequential, HiRes-Paired, HiRes-Sequential Fidelity 120, HiRes-Paired Fidelity 120 (default), MPS, and CIS. With Fidelity 120, audiologists can program up to 120 independent channels of stimulation for more specific frequency and pitch information. There are two telephone options, one a built-in telecoil and the other a T-mic. Users have found that the T-mic also improves speech understanding in noise in the T-mic-only mode versus the T-mic plus microphone.[26]

Using the SoundWave 2.0 software and the clinician's programming interface (CPI), the audiologist may begin programming the Harmony sound processor.

- Across the ribbon bar at the top, the software alerts the audiologist of the status of the CPI, the sound processor, and the internal device.
- If all the icons are green, the audiologist can begin to program.
- If any of the lights are red, the audiologist will need to troubleshoot the system before programming.
- When all the icons are green and the patient file is open, the software will automatically measure the impedance at each of the 16 intracochlear electrodes relative to the reference electrode. Values between 1 and 30 kiloohms are within normal limits.
- If the electrode impedance is out of range (ie, open circuit), then the electrode(s) should be disabled.
- In some cases, there may be a short in an electrode. If there is a short in 2 consecutive electrodes, the recipient may have a preference for those electrodes to remain on in their programs. If the shorted electrodes are not consecutive, it is recommended that the electrode(s) be disabled.
- Conditioning is another feature available with AB. Conditioning removes any buildup of substances present on the electrode contact and is usually completed at the initial stimulation.
- When programming the AB system, setting the "M-Level" is the most important measurement obtained. Because the M-Levels and volume control are tied together, the volume control first should be set to 0% unless disabled. The M-Levels are obtained using speech-burst stimulation instead of biphasic pulses. Making 4 primary measurements, the M-Levels are set for electrodes 1 to 4, 5 to 8, 9 to 12, and 13 to 16.
- To fine-tune the measurements, the audiologist may adjust the electrodes globally to live speech and environmental sounds. M-Levels are set to the patient's most comfortable listening level.
- The T-Levels, or thresholds, are not usually measured. Typically the audiologist will set the levels to 10% of the M-Levels. If the cochlear implant user complains of constant, low-level noise then the audiologist may want to measure the T-Levels or set them to zero charge units.
- For children, the audiologist may elect to measure T-Levels to ensure audibility. Because children usually provide minimal response levels, the audiologist should globally reduce the T-Levels by 6 to 8 charge units.[27]

Some other programming considerations for AB include Fidelity 120, input dynamic range (IDR), and clipping. The HiRes coding strategy now comes with the option of adding Fidelity 120. During clinical trials with Fidelity 120, most users reported better sound quality for speech and music than with conventional HiRes sound processing.[28]

The IDR is the recipient's electrical dynamic range that is mapped from the acoustic input. The default IDR is 60 dB, which is appropriate for most users. Decreasing the IDR may make soft sounds inaudible but the cochlear implant recipient may report better listening comfort, especially in noise. For improved quality with music, AB recommends allocating one program setting with a higher IDR, using a coding strategy with Fidelity 120, and disabling the automatic gain control (AGC). Clipping channels ensures that stimulation will never exceed the set M-Level for that electrode. Clipping is used primarily when facial nerve stimulation is observed. Clipping the electrode should eliminate any undesired response (**Table 1**).

Cochlear Corporation

The Nucleus system employs Custom Sound software to program the speech processor so that the cochlear implant delivers sound that is audible and comfortable to the recipient. This software supports the newest system, the Nucleus 5, as well as all legacy implant models (Nucleus 22 series, CI24R [CA], CI24R [CS], CI24 [ST], CI24 M, Freedom [CA], and the ABI24 M) and speech processors (ESPrit 22, ESPrit, ESPrit3 G, Spectra, Sprint, Freedom, CP810).

The CI512 implant, Cochlear Corporation's newest model, comprises 22 half-banded platinum electrodes molded in a perimodiolar shape and two extracochlear electrodes, one titanium plate at the implant receiver and a separate "ball" electrode inserted under the temporalis fascia to support different stimulation modes. The implant coil supports fully integrated electrophysiology telemetry modes neural response telemetry (NRT), AutoNRT, ESRT, ABR, CEP, and intraoperative NRT, which as previously mentioned allows for objective data collection. The Nucleus 5 sound processor (CP810) uses SmartSound 2 technology, which offers customized settings for 4 different listening environments. It is designed to function with either disposable or rechargeable batteries. It features a telecoil circuit as well as an AutoPhone option to allow for automatic telephone detection through the auto telecoil. The microphone technology has been upgraded from previous Nucleus devices to use a Dual Omni-Microphone that incorporates 2 calibrated, phased matched omnidirectional microphones for improved listening in noise. The Nucleus 5 remote assistant (CR110) uses bidirectional telemetry, which allows for communication with the sound processor as well as providing diagnostic and troubleshooting assistance. This option is especially important for young recipients who cannot provide feedback.

Custom sound programming software allows for 3 different streamlined programming methods (1 behavioral and 2 objective) to reduce programming time without compromising outcomes.[29] The behavioral streamlined programming approach involves measuring the threshold levels across 5 equidistant electrodes along the electrode array. As previously alluded to, this technique is valid because the default stimulation mode is monopolar, which allows for consistent T levels across the electrode array. The clinician can then go to the "go live" button and speak to the patient while globally increasing the C levels to a comfortably loud level. The NRT/objective Offset method offsets the T level profile from the objective measurement profile, and enables a single offset channel to be measured using psychophysics. Comfort levels are then measured using live voice. The NRT/objective preset method offsets the T-level and C-level profiles from the objective measurement profile. The clinician can then create additional maps with C levels set progressively higher, with the loudest MAP with C levels set to T-NRT. This method will result in the most conservative loudness level and is especially recommended in situations where reliable psychophysics is not possible. The behavioral approach can be used for adults and adolescents, and one of the objective methods may be used for young children and patients who may have difficulty responding to sound. One of these methods should be used at the initial stimulation to achieve a quick, comfortable, accurate, and wearable program.

Clinician-controlled primary parameters include:

- Stimulation mode
- Stimulation rate
- Speech-coding strategy (SPEAK, ACE, CIS).

Additional adjustable parameters are number of maxima, which are the frequency ranges in the audio signal that contain the greatest amounts of energy and therefore determine which electrode is stimulated; and frequency allocation table (FAT), the frequency bandwidth that is assigned to each active electrode. The FAT depends on the speech-processing strategy and the number of channels in the MAP, channel gain, the amount of gain applied to each channel before output stimulation levels are sent to the implant. IDR defined as the entire operating range of the speech processor including the AGC compression range. This range is adjustable. The Q value controls the steepness of the amplitude growth function and determines the percentage of a recipient's electrical output dynamic range that is allocated to the top 10 dB of the speech processor input dynamic range. As the clinician reduces the Q value, the amplitude growth function at the lower end of the speech processor's input range becomes steeper. Reducing the Q value can make soft sounds seem louder, increasing background noise. Increasing the Q value reduces the background noise but may result in decreased hearing at soft input levels. All of these parameters can be manipulated, with caution, to achieve a desired performance outcome.

The Nucleus 5 system uses 4 distinct input processing algorithms, ADRO (Adaptive Dynamic Range Optimization), a digital preprocessing signal algorithm designed to improve audibility of low-level sounds while reducing gain of higher-level sounds to keep the signal below C level. Research suggests that ADRO improves performance in quiet with no decrement in performance in noise.[30,31] Whisper is a fast-acting compression circuit that makes soft sounds easier to hear.[32] Beam is an adaptive beam-forming algorithm that uses spatial input processing and noise canceling to adjust microphone directionality.[33] Zoom uses a fixed directional pattern algorithm to allow for maximal attenuation of diffuse noise. Autosensitivity automatically adjusts microphone sensitivity based on the noise floor of the surrounding environment. These input-processing algorithms can be used separately or in combination to form 4 "smart sound listening environments," referred to as everyday, noise, focus, and music.

Basic patient controlled parameters include both volume and sensitivity functions, Unfortunately, these two controls are often either underutilized or misunderstood by many recipients. Microphone sensitivity determines the minimum input signal level required for stimulation. Raising the sensitivity means less acoustic energy is required for stimulation; conversely, on lowering the sensitivity setting more acoustic is required for stimulation, that is, recipients should lower, not raise the sensitivity in noisy situations. The volume simply controls the maximum amount of stimulation and is probably a control that is less useful. In addition, the Nucleus 5 system allows recipients to control accessory and telecoil mixing ratios with the use of a remote control (**Table 1**).

MED-EI

MED-EI Corporation has two Windows-based programming platforms for their cochlear implant systems. The CI.STUDIO+ platform is used with all MED-EI internal devices and TEMPO+ ear level or earlier sound processors. The new generation SONATATI[100], as well as PULSARCI[100] and COMBI 40+ internal devices, and OPUS 1 and OPUS 2 ear level sound processors use the MAESTRO System Software platform. The MAESTRO System Software is "backward compatible," in that it can be used to program OPUS ear level sound processors for previous generation MED-EI internal devices.

The SONATATI[100] has 12 channels, with 24 electrode contacts, and is made of titanium and silastic. It is available with a standard, compressed, or medium-length array. The PULSARCI[100] ceramic internal device is also available with those electrode configurations, as well as a split array for patients who have significantly ossified cochlea.

Two of the primary differences between the OPUS 1 and OPUS 2 include the housing design and controls. Like the TEMPO+, the OPUS 1 control switches are on the sound processor. The OPUS 2 has a new design with FineTuner Remote Control to adjust processor settings. Both processors have a variety of battery packs, making it ergonomically appropriate for young children or adults who are very athletic. The sound processors can hold multiple programs and offer two coding strategies called high-definition continuous interleaved sampling (HDCIS) and fine structure processing (FSP).

Before programming the MED-EI system, the audiologist measures electrode impedances. The voltages of 12 intracochlear electrode pairs, relative to the reference electrode, are measured independently. The results will indicate "OK"—electrode suitable for stimulation, "HI"—electrode voltage exceeds acceptable limits and cannot be programmed, "SC-x"—when there is a short circuit, "HSC-x" or "HSC?"—a short circuit with several HI electrodes.

When programming the MED-EI system the most comfortable level (MCL) is the most important measure for each channel. MCL in the MED-EI system is defined as the highest level of stimulation that is perceived to be loud but not uncomfortable. For children who are unable to provide traditional behavioral responses, MED-EI recommends the ESRT as an alternative for setting MCL levels. MCLs may also be measured behaviorally using traditional psychophysical approaches already described.

Once MCLs are set appropriately, the THRs (also known as electrical thresholds) may be programmed, if needed, or estimated quickly in several ways. Often, this is set at a percentage of the MCL, or at a minimum value, verses a measured THR. If the THR is measured, it should be set 1 or 2 steps below the measured response so that stimulation at THR is inaudible. If THR is at a level that is audible then the recipient may hear a buzzing sound, so it is important to set each THR slightly below audibility.

The Balance function stimulates pairs or groups of channels, and the Sweep function stimulates each channel sequentially. Balancing and Sweeping can both be used to verify appropriate MCL and THR levels. For children and adults, the audiologist should watch for any negative reactions during these tests. For adults, one can also have them report if the channels all sound equally loud across the electrode array. During live speech, the audiologist will typically start at a reduced electrical dynamic range. The goal is to confirm that the recipient is comfortable at 100% of the dynamic range for the program.

Some other programming considerations for MED-EI include the settings Frequency Bands, Maplaw, and Automatic Sound Management (ASM). Due to the length of the electrode array, the frequency range can be as low as 70 Hz up to as high as 8500 Hz. The Maplaw feature allows the audiologist to control how acoustical information is placed in the electrical dynamic range. Steeper Maplaw functions boost soft and medium sounds up a bit higher in the patient's dynamic range. ASM controls the compression ratio and the microphone sensitivity. These features automatically adjust the program to maximize audibility, without discomfort, based on the listening environment.

Both soundfield and speech perception measures are ways to verify the audibility of a cochlear implant system and to ensure an optimized program in the MED-El system. With common testing procedures, appropriate soundfield thresholds for MED-El recipients should show a flat configuration in the range of 25 to 35 dB HL. In general, narrow band noise stimuli provide better results than warbled tones in the sound field. Working to achieve thresholds softer than this range by adjusting the program or sensitivity settings may create a more desirable audiogram, but may not result in optimal speech perception in day-to-day life. Better examples for verifying audibility and map optimization include speech perception testing in quiet and noise, or, for a small child, a Ling sound detection audiogram (**Table 1**).

MANAGING PROGRAMMING CONCERNS

To diagnose any possible problems with the program, the audiologist must be aware of the typical progress an individual can achieve with a cochlear implant. In addition, the patient and/or the patient's family should be counseled on appropriate expectations. The preoperative counseling is essential to help guide the patient and his or her family as to realistic expectations and therefore overall performance over time with a cochlear implant. It is critical for the adult, who cannot hear during this counseling, to have access to written materials or captioned videos. Aural (re)habilitation therapy can be very helpful to the adult adjusting to their cochlear implant system. For children, aural (re)habilitation by a qualified speech-language pathologist and/or teacher of the deaf is necessary to learn how to make the sounds meaningful. Another simple, but very effective tool, is having the patient complete a guided journal (ie, Cochlear Implant Journal by Wagner and colleagues).[34] This personal journal will remind them of where they were and how far they have come. Also, videotaping patients preoperatively and having them give themselves a message about what they are expecting and then showing it to them on their 1-year anniversary can also be an effective counseling tool.

Most complaints about the sound quality (ie, echo, tinny sound, muffled, humming sound, and so forth) can easily be managed by manipulating the T and/or C/M levels, or the audiologist can refer to the manufacturer's support service system for assistance. When a patient plateaus, it may be time to make some aggressive changes to the programming parameters such as the speech-coding strategy, repetition rate, IDR, and so forth. Also, having the patient obtain a second opinion on the programming from another audiologist at the implant center can be helpful in this situation.

MANAGING DEVICE FAILURE

Although the reliability of data for the cochlear implant is very high, there are occasions when the internal device fails. Device failures can be divided into two categories: hard failures and soft failures. Before suspecting a device failure, the audiologist should check and replace the external hardware and reprogramming should be attempted. Hard failures are easily identifiable because the entire internal cochlear implant ceases to function. To confirm a hard failure, a device integrity test is typically performed, by either the audiologist or the manufacturer's representative. An integrity test measures

Table 1
Device specific information

	Advanced Bionics	Cochlear Corporation	Med-El Corporation
Product Name	Clarion	Nucleus	MED-EI
Implant	90 k with HiFocus Array	Nucleus 5 Contour Advance (CI512) Nucleus Freedom Straight Nucleus 24 Double Array	SONATA Standard PULSAR Standard PULSAR Split PULSAR Medium PULSAR Compressed
Casing	Titanium and silicone	Titanium and silicone	Titanium and silicone (PULSAR-ceramic)
Channels/Electrodes	Up to 31 channels with 16 electrodes	Up to 22 channels with 24 electrodes	Up to 12 channels with 24 electrodes
Stimulus rate	Up to 83,000 pps	Up to 32,000 pps	Up to 50,704 pps
Features	Neural response imaging (NRI) MRI compatible 1.5 T with removable magnet Fine structure coding	Neural response telemetry (NRT) MRI compatible 1.5 T with removable magnet Thinnest implant	Auditory nerve response telemetry (ART) Deep insertion with atraumatic electrode PULSAR: MRI compatible 2 T Fine structure coding
Behind-The-Ear (BTE)	Harmony	Nucleus 5	OPUS I or Opus II (with FineTuner)
Battery	1 rechargeable battery	2–675 power zinc air or Rechargeable	3–675 power zinc air or rechargeable
Battery life	16 h with extended size, 6 h with regular size	Between 24 (rechargeable) and 48 h (disposable) (varies with strategy)	2–3 days (rechargeable) to 3–5 days (disposable)
Colors	Beige, brown, silver, black with multiple colored cover	Black, Brown, Beige, Charcoal, White (colored covers available)	Black, gray, brown, beige, red, blue

Programs	2	4	4
Strategies	HiRes-S, HiRes-P, Fidelity 120, MPS, CIS	ACE, ACE (RE), SPEAK, CIS, CIS (RE)	FSP, HDCIS, CIS+
Features	ALD capabilities	ALD capabilities	ALD capabilities
	Optional battery packs	Water resistant	Lightest processor
	Volume control	Bodyworn option	Remote
	Indicator light on processor	Remote with troubleshooting features	Optional battery packs including baby worn option
	T-microphone	Indicator light on processor	Indicator light on processor
		Auto Telecoil, Situation settings, Blue tooth compatible	
Body Style			
Name	Platinum body processor	Freedom Bodyworn	Opus II: available with different battery packs
Battery	1 rechargeable battery	1 or 2 AA batteries	
Battery life	8 h	14 h	
Colors	Silver with color headpieces	Gray	
Programs	3	4	
Strategies	HiRes-S or HiRes-P	SPEAK, CIS, ACE	
Features	ALD capabilities	ALD capabilities	
	Large tactile buttons	ADRO	
	Aluminum casing	Autosensitivity button	
	Microphone listening capabilities	Lock button	

the voltages generated at the electrode array. A plain film may also be obtained to compare it with the one taken intraoperatively.

Soft failures are more elusive to diagnose. While the cochlear implant internal device may continue to provide sound, the patient may be hearing intermittency of sounds, extraneous sounds (ie, popping, crackling, static, clicking, and so forth), have poorer speech recognition abilities than expected, or a decline in speech recognition over a period of time. Integrity tests may not diagnose a soft failure, and the cochlear implant team may need to decide on whether to explant the device based on the absence of electrophysiologic data to support a device failure. For patients unable to provide feedback, such as young children, behavioral changes may be observed such as pulling the device off (after successfully wearing it for a period of time with no complaints), aggressive behavior, unexplained crying when wearing the cochlear implant system, and/or refusal to put the device on. Reimplantation should occur as quickly as possible following device failure so that performance is not compromised.[35]

FOLLOW-UP PROGRAMMING

Regardless of age, accurate psychophysical measures appear to be the main contributing factor to maintaining consistent patient performance. Research has shown that electrical thresholds can fluctuate during the first year following initial stimulation, underscoring the need for comprehensive follow-up.[36] The first-year schedule for children after initial stimulation includes stimulation at:

- 7 to 10 days
- 4 to 5 weeks
- 3 months
- 4 to 5 months, if needed
- 6 months
- Twice between 6 months and 12 months, if needed
- At 12 months post initial stimulation.

Subsequent visits usually occur at 3-month intervals. Of course additional programming sessions should occur if a child demonstrates a change in auditory responsiveness or a decrement in speech production. These changes may include changes in auditory discrimination, increased requests for repetition, addition and/or omission of syllables, prolongation of vowels, and a change in voice quality. As the programming audiologist does not spend as much time with the child as do his or her other caretakers, reliance on the parents, therapists, and teachers for feedback is a critical component in the programming process. The programming timetable for postlingually deafened adults is not as rigorous as for children, as adults typically are more accurate responders at initial stimulation.

FUTURE OF COCHLEAR IMPLANT PROGRAMMING

Until recently there has been a common lethargy among cochlear implant audiologists to consider changes in device programming and a willingness to accept the status quo. Manufacturers, researchers, and cochlear implant clinics are, however, beginning to realize that there are too many external pressures that require a "rethink" of the present technique of cochlear implant programming. Reimbursement for device programming is poor, and in order for clinics to be financially viable they need to reduce the overall time spent with a patient during a programming session, without compromising patient performance and satisfaction. This goal needs to be accomplished by all concerned parties. Manufacturers will need to continue to streamline the programming process by offering innovative software that allows devices to be programmed quicker and more efficiently. This aspect is particularly vital for two reasons: the increased numbers of both simultaneously and sequentially bilateral implantations, and the fact that recent data suggest that this technology is severely underpenetrated because only 2% to 3% of individuals who could benefit from this technology use it. If the industry is successful in capturing more of the market that will put further strain the delivery system. Clinics may need to hire individuals to serve in a "supporting role" to the primary audiologist, for example i-techs. These individuals can perform nonreimbursable activities, that is, counseling, troubleshooting, setup, and so forth, and free up the audiologist for direct programming time. Remote device programming (tele-medicine) has begun to make some inroads in certain areas where direct access to a programming audiologist is not feasible and may serve, in some way, to streamline the process. The absolute goal for device programming is to provide the patient with a comfortable, wearable program, obtained via a variety of techniques, which ensures maximum performance. Although consistent programming is integral to patient success, it is by no means the sole determinant of patient performance. Age of implantation, family support, duration of deafness, communicative approach, cognitive ability, and duration of device usage are among the other variables to affect performance.

REFERENCES

1. Healthy People 2020: hearing and other sensory or communication disorders. Washington, DC: United States Department of Health and Human Services; 2011.
2. Healthy People 2010 hearing health progress review. National Institute for Health, Washington, DC: National Institute on Deafness and Other Communication Disorders; 2010.
3. Bradham T, Jones J. Cochlear implant candidacy in the United States: prevalence in children 12 months to 6 years of age. Int J Pediatr Otorhinolaryngol 2008;72(7):1023–8.
4. Geers AE, Nicholas JG, Moog J. Estimating the influence of cochlear implantation on language development in children. Audiol Med 2007;5(4):262–73.
5. Nicholas JG, Geers AE. Will they catch up? The role of age at implantation in cochlear implantation in spoken language development of children with severe to profound hearing loss. J Speech Lang Hear Res 2007;50(4):1048–62.
6. Gifford RH, Shallop JK, Peterson AM. Speech recognition materials and ceiling effects: considerations for cochlear implant programs. Audiol Neurootol 2008; 13(3):193–205.
7. Shapiro WH. Device programming. In: Waltzman SB, Roland JT, editors. Cochlear implants. New York: Thieme Medical Publishers, Inc; 2005. p. 133–45.
8. Brown CJ, Abbas PJ. Electrically evoked whole nerve action potentials: data from human cochlear implant. J Acoust Soc Am 1990;88:1385–91.
9. Brown CJ, Abbas PJ, Fryauf-Bertschy H, et al. Intraoperative and postoperative electrically evoked auditory brainstem responses in Nucleus cochlear implant users: implications for the fitting process. Ear Hear 1994;15:168–76.
10. Brown CJ, Abbas PJ. Electrically evoked whole-nerve action potentials in Ineraid Cochlear implant users: responses to the different stimulating electrode configurations and comparison to psychophysical responses. J Speech Hear Res 1996; 39:453–67.

11. Brown CJ, Hong SH, Hughes M, et al. Comparisons between electrically evoked whole nerve action potential (EAP) thresholds and the behavioral levels used to program the speech processor of the Nucleus C124M cochlear implant. Presented at the 7th Symposium on Cochlear Implants in Children. Iowa City (IA); 1997.

12. Brown CJ, Hughes M, Luk B, et al. The relationship between EAP and EABR thresholds and levels used to program the Nucleus 24 speech processor: data from adults. Ear Hear 2000;21:151–63.

13. Buckler L, Overstreet E. Relationship between electrical stapedial reflex thresholds and HiRes program settings: potential tool for pediatric cochlear-implant fitting. Valencia (CA): Advanced Bionics; 2003.

14. Gordon K, Gilden J, Ebinger K, et al. NRT in 12 to 24 month old children. Ann Otol Rhinol Laryngol Suppl 2002;189:42–8.

15. Gordon K, Papsin BC, Harrison RV. Toward a battery of behavioral and objective measures to achieve optimal cochlear implant stimulation levels in children. Ear Hear 2004;25(5):447–63.

16. Gordon K, Papsin BC, Harrison RV. Programming cochlear implant stimulation levels in infants and children with a combination of objective measures. Int J Audiol 2004;43(Suppl 1):28–32.

17. Shapiro WH, Huang T, Shaw T, et al. Remote intraoperative monitoring during cochlear implant surgery is feasible and efficient. Otol Neurotol 2008;29(4): 495–8.

18. Shapiro WH, Waltzman SB. Cochlear implant programming for children: the basics. In: Estabrooks W, editor. Cochlear implants for kids, vol. 4. Washington, DC: A.G. Bell; 1998. p. 58–68.

19. Technical report: cochlear implants. Rockville (MD): American Speech-Language Hearing Association; 2004. ASHA Supplement 24.

20. Holden LK, Skinner MW, Fourakis MS, et al. Effect of increased IIDR in the Nucleus Freedom Cochlear Implant System. J Am Acad Audiol 2007;18:778–91.

21. Brickly G, Boyd P, Wyllie F, et al. Investigation into electrically evoked stapedius reflex measures and subjective loudness percepts in the MED EL COMBI 40+ cochlear implant. Cochlear Implants Int 2005;6(1):31–42.

22. Jerger J, Oliver TA, Chmiel RA. Prediction of dynamic range from stapedious reflex in cochlear implant patients. Ear Hear 1988;9(1):4–8.

23. Lorens A, Walkowiak A, Piotrowska A, et al. ESRT and MCL correlations in experienced pediatric cochlear implant users. Cochlear Implants Int 2004;5(1):28–37.

24. Franck K. A model of a Nucleus 24 cochlear implant fitting protocol based on the electrically evoked whole nerve potential. Ear Hear 2002;23(1):67S–71S.

25. HiRes 90K surgeon's manual for HiFocus Helix and HiFocus 1j Electrode. Sylmar (CA): Advanced Bionics Corporation; 2004. USA.

26. Gifford RH, Revit U. Speech perception for adult cochlear implant recipients in a realistic background noise: effectiveness of preprocessing strategies and external options for improving speech recognition in noise. J Am Acad Audiol 2010;2(17):441–51.

27. Wolfe J, Schafer EC. Programming cochlear implants. San Diego (CA): Plural Publishing; 2010. p. 69.

28. HiRes with Fidelity 120 clinical results. Sylmar (CA): Advanced Bionics Corporation; 2009.

29. Plant K, Whitford L, Psarros C. Strategy comparison for Nucleus 24 recipients with a limited number of available electrodes. Cochlear White Paper, N94317F Iss1. Centennial (CO): Cochlear Americas; 2000.

30. Dawson PW, Decker JA, Psarros CE. Optimizing dynamic range in children using the Nucleus cochlear implant. Ear Hear 2004;25(3):230–41.
31. James CJ, Blamey PJ, Martin L, et al. Adaptive dynamic range optimization for cochlear implants: a preliminary study. Ear Hear 2002;23(Suppl 1):49S–58S.
32. McDermott HJ, Henshall KR, McKay CM. Benefits of syllabic input compression for users of cochlear implants. J Am Acad Audiol 2002;13(1):14–24.
33. Van den Berghe J, Wouters J. An adaptive noise canceller for hearing aids using two nearby microphones. J Acoust Soc Am 1998;103:3621–6.
34. Wagner DS, Abrahamson JE, Casterton SF. Better communication and cochlear implants: a personal journal in learning to hear again with a cochlear implant. Austin (TX): Hear Again; 1998.
35. Waltzman S, Roland JT, Waltzman M, et al. Cochlear reimplantation in children: soft signs, symptoms and results. Cochlear Implants Int 2004;5(4):138–45.
36. Shapiro WH, Waltzman SB. Changes in electrical thresholds over time in young children implanted with the Nucleus cochlear implant prosthesis. Otol Rhinol Laryngol 1995;104(Suppl 166):177–8.

Current Research on Music Perception in Cochlear Implant Users

Charles J. Limb, MD[a],*, Jay T. Rubinstein, MD, PhD[b]

KEYWORDS

• Melody • Rhythm • Pitch • Timbre

Cochlear implantation has undergone tremendous evolution over the past 5 years, with advances in processing strategies, electrode design, and a greater push toward bilateral implantation. Despite these many advances, however, music perception in cochlear implant (CI) users remains essentially limited, with severe deficits observed in pitch and timbre perception. Although rare individual examples can be found who demonstrate high-level music performance through a cochlear implant, even users with excellent speech understanding typically display major limitations in their ability to perceive (much less perform) music. Recent research has led to a more rigorous development of psychophysical test methods and parameters to assess music perception in implant users. These methods have enabled the analysis of perceptual difficulties experienced by implant users for increasingly complex (and realistic) musical stimuli. Furthermore, neuroimaging experiments have helped characterize the central neural correlates in implant-mediated music perception in comparison with individuals with normal hearing (NH). This article reviews some of the notable recent advances in music perception for CI users.

OVERVIEW OF RECENT STUDIES
Exposure to Music

A growing body of literature over the past decade has contributed to a thorough characterization of the limitations of music perception demonstrated by CI users. Many of the early studies described significant impairment in melody perception for CI users, whereas rhythmic stimuli seemed to remain relatively intact. Recent studies have both confirmed and extended these initial findings.[1,2] Migirov and colleagues[3] used

[a] Department of Otolaryngology–Head and Neck Surgery, Peabody Conservatory of Music, Johns Hopkins University School of Medicine, 601 North Caroline Street, Baltimore, MD 21287, USA
[b] Department of Otolaryngology–Head and Neck Surgery, Virginia Merrill Bloedel Hearing Research Center, University of Washington Medical Center, Box 357923, Seattle, WA 98195, USA
* Corresponding author.
E-mail address: climb@jhmi.edu

Otolaryngol Clin N Am 45 (2012) 129–140
doi:10.1016/j.otc.2011.08.021
0030-6665/12/$ – see front matter © 2012 Elsevier Inc. All rights reserved.

a simple questionnaire method to assess listening habits in postlingually deafened CI users, demonstrating that about 50% of the subjects tested described lesser enjoyment of music following implantation. Much of this difficulty is attributable to implant user difficulty following melodic contours, an ability that deteriorates significantly in the presence of competing instrumentation.[4,5] Unfortunately, these abilities do not seem to improve over time as a result of regular auditory exposure, as demonstrated in a longitudinal study of music perception and appraisal.[6] Instead, a growing number of studies have shown the importance of musical training for the improvement of pitch perception. These studies have included prelingually deaf children with CI's[7] who lack a great deal of prior music experience and, rather than finding music disconcerting, tend to find it enjoyable and interesting while also showing improvements over time.[8] During pitch tasks, it seems increasingly clear that musical experience leads to better performance in implant users in comparison with individuals without musical experience, with near equivalent performance on some tasks (eg, melodic contour identification) in comparison with NH listeners.[4] These trends are supported by results showing that NH listeners can display improved music performance during perception of implant simulations.[9]

Auditory Training Programs for Music Perception

The implications of improved performance as a result of musical experience point obviously to the need for further development of auditory training programs directed toward music perception. Looi and She[10,11] used a questionnaire approach to 100 CI users that focused on obtaining information germane to the development of a training program specifically oriented toward music. Thus far, music plays a minor role (if any) during routine postimplant rehabilitation, which is typically focused toward speech perception. Music is regarded in this sense as a lower-priority objective. However, it should be emphasized that music remains an acoustically richer and, therefore, more challenging stimulus than speech, and consequently, improved performance on music tasks (through music rehabilitation) is likely to have a broad beneficial impact on implant-mediated listening well beyond musical stimuli per se. In conjunction with the need to develop rehabilitation strategies and programs, individual filter strategies aimed at improving pitch mapping,[12] technological advances in sound processing strategies,[13] and bilateral CI[6,14] all show great promise regarding improving music perception in implant users.

METHODS OF ASSESSMENT: THE DEVELOPMENT OF MUSIC PERCEPTION TESTS FOR CI LISTENERS

Many recent studies have focused on the fact that few standardized measures of music performance exist for CI users. It seems ironic that although studies of the mechanisms of temporal and place pitch perception with electrical stimulation of the cochlea represent some of the earliest experiments performed on implant recipients,[15–18] subsequent interest in music perception with these devices would take more than a decade to develop[19–21] and would not truly flourish until the following decade. The reason for this is, of course, that once pitch perception with CI was documented, speech perception became the next target of both clinicians and scientists in the field. Interest in music perception only had the opportunity to arise once it became clear that speech perception was not only possible but was an expected clinical outcome in most implant recipients. From the beginning of interest in music perception with implants, testing could be divided into the more psychophysical approach whereby performance was rigorously tested on a variety of materials and questionnaire-based assessments of music appreciation. This review focuses on the former, although it is clear that enjoyment and appreciation of music as measured by a questionnaire may have little relationship to the accuracy of musical perception as measured by a perceptual test battery. This consideration may lead some to appropriately question the relevance of perceptual testing; however, it is difficult for these authors to imagine that restoration of normal musical perceptual ability in CI users would not ultimately lead to normal appreciation. In addition, perceptual testing correlates highly with speech perception in quiet and noise as well as a variety of clinically important psychophysical tasks.[22-26] Maximizing hearing benefit from CI requires perceptual testing to measure the effects, or lack thereof, of a given intervention, whether it be training or technology.

Perceptual Results

Early perceptual results (see McDermott[1] for review) made it clear that CI users performed comparably with NH listeners on rhythmic tasks; extremely poorly, indeed near chance, on melody tasks when deprived of lyrics or rhythmic cues; and poorly, although typically better than chance, on timbre tasks as assessed by musical instrument identification. These results have been confirmed in a later series.[27] It was also clear that musical training has the potential to improve music perception, although the potential limits of training benefits were unknown and remain so today.[4,5,9] Lastly, addition of low-frequency acoustic information seems to be substantially beneficial for melody perception either through hybrid or electroacoustic hearing in the ipsilateral ear or bimodal hearing via the contralateral, unimplanted ear.

Basic Metrics

Music is a complex language involving a rich and diverse interplay of pitch, timbral, rhythmic, harmonic, lyrical, and interval-based perceptual features. As the limitations of CI in representing some of these features have become clear, appropriate methods for the development of music perception test materials can be better defined. These definitions do involve certain testing trade-offs, but determination of basic performance metrics for CI users is critical to the future development of speech processing strategies as well as to understand. As in speech testing, open-set song identification would seem the most clinically pertinent test; however, because songs potentially include lyrics, speech perception ability will artifactually enhance performance and potentially allow patients with no melody perception but excellent speech discrimination to score at 100% on such a task. Because rhythmic perception is normal or near normal in most implant users, rhythmic cues can have a similar effect and, thus, need to be removed if the goal of testing is to measure melody discrimination.[28] Such isochronous melody perception is extremely challenging for most implant users and, therefore, a closed-set test is necessary to minimize floor effects. Such tests have been developed and used by a wide variety of investigators and typically consist of nursery rhymes and other simple and highly familiar melodies. Across-language versions of such tests have also been described.[29]

Isochronous Melody Perception

Although isochronous melody perception is a central component of many musical test batteries, it has significant limitations. Because many CI users are able to discriminate pitch direction for 1-semitone stimuli,[27] isochronous melody testing is necessary to avoid the ceiling effects of pitch testing alone; however, as mentioned, the test is too difficult for many CI users, is closed-set, and depends on familiarity with the melody corpus. Recently proposed alternatives that potentially avoid some of these issues include a Melodic Contour Identification test[30] and a Modified Melodies test.[31] These tests attempt to assess the interval perception that underlies the discrimination of melodies. Failure to accurately assess intervals likely explains why melody perception with implants is so poor despite many users being readily able to discriminate 1-semitone pitch changes; however, it can be difficult to directly assess interval perception when one is not working with a musically trained patient. Use of melodies and melodic contours as test materials also successfully sidesteps potential uncertainties and complexities in the definition of pitch as obtained with a CI by intrinsically defining it as the capacity to represent melodic sequences.[32] Elimination of floor effects through the use of the Melodic Contour Identification test has permitted measuring the effects of competing instruments on melody perception, a test arguably similar in concept to a speech perception test in noise.[4,5]

Music Timbre Perception

Musical timbre perception is another critical piece of any music perception test battery. It is typically based on closed-set identification of commonly recognized musical instruments.[10,28,33,34] The development of such materials is complicated by the difficulty in controlling for loudness and other cues introduced by whatever musical sources make up the test corpus. Some of these problems could potentially be solved through recent efforts to vary timbre electronically[35] but that remains to be proven. Complex interplay between timbre and melody perception have been identified[36] and provides a sense for just how intricate the assessment of polyphonic music perception with CI could become. This point argues for the continued use of the simplest validated test materials available when testing in a clinical environment,[27] assuming the materials adequately encompass the breadth of clinical performance. Although a wide variety of other music test materials have been developed,[37,38] few have the combined attributes of being simple and fast and having undergone the validation studies needed for robust clinical trials.

TOWARD A MORE SPECIFIC CHARACTERIZATION OF MUSICAL DEFICITS

In addition to the large number of studies confirming deficits in melody and timbre perception and the preservation of rhythm perception in CI users, 2 studies were recently performed specifically to address the perception of polyphony[39] and rhythmic clocking[40] in CI users. These studies were motivated by the need to study pitch perception beyond melody recognition in a way that was musically relevant and not previously examined and also to study rhythm perception using an ostensibly more difficult task to avoid ceiling effects observed in most studies of rhythm.

CI Users Demonstrate Perceptual Fusion of Polyphonic Pitch

Most studies of pitch perception in CI users have focused on pitch discrimination (in which subjects are asked to detect whether 2 sounds differ in pitch) and pitch ranking (in which subjects are asked to identify which of 2 presented pitches is higher). Relatively little research, however, has been done on the perception of polyphony (or harmony) in CI patients. In a recent study,[39] the investigators sought to evaluate the ability of postlingually deafened adult CI users to perceive the number of pitches in acoustically presented polyphonic stimuli. Subjects listened to stimuli consisting of 1, 2, or 3 simultaneous tones with different fundamental frequencies within a single octave. Both pure tones and piano tones were used for stimuli. The investigators hypothesized that CI users would show decreased ability to differentiate between single versus multiple tones in comparison with NH controls. It was further hypothesized that the ability of CI users to detect polyphony would increase as a function of interval distance between pitches.

Pitch Study Methods

Twelve CI users and 12 NH controls participated in the study. Each CI user had at least 1 year of experience using their implant system and none of the subjects had musical training beyond an amateur level. All stimuli consisted of pitches from within a central octave ranging in f_0 from 261 Hz (C4) to 523 Hz (C5). Single-pitch stimuli consisted of either pure tones or piano tones from C4 to B4 (12 unique pitches, 24 total stimuli). Two-pitch stimuli consisted of either pure tone or piano tone representations of all 12 possible intervals within the range of C4 to C5 (1–12 semitones interval distance, 24 total stimuli). Three-pitch stimuli consisted of either pure tone or piano tone representations of 6 unique symmetric chords (equal interval spacing between lower/ middle and middle/higher pitches) within the range of C4 to C5.

Stimuli were randomly presented in a soundproof booth through a calibrated loudspeaker. Stimuli were presented in a 3-alternative, single-interval, forced-choice procedure in which the subjects were instructed to choose whether the given stimuli consisted of 1, 2, or 3 pitches. Subjects were familiarized with the stimuli and the procedure before formal testing. No feedback was given regarding the correctness of responses. The number of correct responses for each subject was averaged across the separate tone and pitch-number conditions to obtain an overall mean score.

Pitch Study Results

The CI group scored significantly lower than the NH group for all conditions. The overall mean scores for each subject group were 43.1 ± 12.3% for CI users and 66.9 ± 9.4% for NH subjects ($P<.001$, unpaired t-test). The CI group scored close to chance levels when identifying 2- and 3-pitch stimuli. In comparison, the NH group was much more successful at distinguishing single from multiple pitches but had greater difficulties at distinguishing between 2- and 3-pitch stimuli. Although NH subjects often identified 3-pitch stimuli as having 2 pitches, CI subjects often identified both 3-pitch and 2-pitch stimuli as a single pitch. For 3-pitch conditions, there was no apparent relationship between interval spacing and the ability to detect polyphony in CI users. For 2-pitch conditions, increased interval spacing did not lead to better performance for detection of polyphony. In fact, an inverse relationship was suggested for identification of the 1-semitone interval spacing in 2-pitch conditions (minor second interval) for which CI users were nearly as accurate as NH subjects.

The results from this study show that CI users obtain significantly lower average scores than NH subjects when asked to distinguish between single and multiple acoustically presented tones. Although a listener's ability to identify the number of components in a polyphonic stimulus does not necessarily correspond to one's ability to perceive differences between polyphonic stimuli, perceptual fusion of polyphonic pitch likely impairs CI users in accurately perceiving many features of music that are polyphonic in nature, such as harmony, consonance, dissonance, and tonality. No statistically significant difference was found between average scores for pure tones and piano tones across both subject groups. This finding indicates that the presence of additional pitch information in complex tones may not aid either subject group in the resolution of polyphonic pitch. Because most music is polyphonic in nature rather than monophonic, these findings underscore the need for further research and development of processing strategies directed toward the perception of polyphony.

Rhythmic Clocking Ability Remains Intact in CI Users

Although many studies suggest that CI-mediated rhythmic perception is normal,[22,41–43] it must be emphasized that these studies have used simple tasks, such as rhythmic pattern identification, that may not have been sensitive enough to reveal limitations in rhythmic perception for CI users. In a recent study,[40] the investigators sought to design a task of rhythm perception for CI users that exceeded the temporal processing requirements for simple pattern recognition or tempo differentiation by focusing on the concept of internal rhythmic clocking. Rhythmic clocking deals with the capacity of a regular interval stimulus to induce a temporal clock in a listener.[44] Also known as beat perception or synchronization, rhythmic clocking refers to the extrapolative expectancy that is established with as few as 3 isochronous beats when internal rhythmicity is intact.[45] Rhythmic clocking is an integral concept in both music and spoken language.[22,46]

Rhythm Study Methods

In this study, the investigators devised a test of rhythmic clocking in which subjects were presented with 4 percussive beats, the first 3 of which were perfectly regular in temporal interval spacing. The fourth beat was presented either isochronously or anisochronously, slightly before or after the anticipated downbeat. Subjects were asked to identify whether the fourth beat occurred early, late, or in perfect timing with respect to the expected rhythmic clock produced by the first 3 isochronous beats. A subject group of highly trained conservatory musicians (MUS) was also included in the study because it was hypothesized that individuals with significant musical training would perform superiorly in rhythmic clocking tasks in comparison.

Twelve NH individuals, 12 cochlear implant users, and 7 highly trained musicians with NH participated in the study. No CI subjects had significant musical experience before or after implantation. Each category of auditory stimuli consisted of 4 percussive beats, presented as either snare drum hits or white noise bursts. The first 3 beats were perfectly isochronous, followed by a fourth beat that was either slightly early, isochronous, or slightly late. The 4 beats were presented at tempos of 60 (slow), 120 (medium), and 180 (fast) beats per minute. For the fourth beat, deviations were introduced before (early) or after (late) the isochronous position; $3°$ of deviation were tested (1/16, 1/8, or 3/16 fractions of a beat). Each subject was presented with a set of 84 stimuli in a soundproof booth through a single calibrated loudspeaker. Stimuli were presented in a single-interval, 3-alternative, forced-choice procedure in which the subjects were required to indicate whether the fourth beat in the given stimulus was early, isochronous, or late.

Rhythm Study Results

The results of the rhythmic clocking tasks show that CI users performed comparably with NH participants across all tempos, sound sources, and degrees of deviation (overall mean scores for correct identification of the final beat: CI users [56.4 $\pm$ 13.93%] and NH subjects [51.5% $\pm$ 13.82%]; $P = .143$, unpaired t-test). However, the musician group scored significantly higher than either group, with a mean score of 70.9% $\pm$ 5.95% ($P<.0001$ for both MUS vs CI and MUS vs NH). An ANOVA of the subject group and tempo as factors showed statistically significant differences among the NH, CI, and MUS groups at all tempos (tempo 60 beats per minute [bpm], $F_{(2,28)} = 4.55$, $P = .019$; tempo 120 bpm, $F_{(2,28)} = 3.71$, $P = .037$; tempo 180 bpm, $F_{(2,28)} = 4.60$, $P = .019$). Although faster tempos were harder for all groups, performance differences between the groups were also preserved at these faster tempos. Surprisingly, no significant differences between NH and CI subjects were noted when early and late stimuli were separated according to degree of deviation, suggesting that CI subjects performed as well as NH subjects for even the most difficult stimuli. MUS significantly outperformed NH subjects in the $\pm 1/8$ and $\pm 3/16$ final beat deviations, suggesting that musical experience and training may be related to improved performance.

It is important to note that the task used here differed significantly from the identification of beat patterns, a task that can be performed successfully even with impaired rhythmic clocking because minor temporal irregularities on the scale of milliseconds do not distort basic rhythmic patterns and rhythmic patterns are robust to temporal degradation. Because of the small degree of temporal deviation used in these stimuli and responses were based on only 3 preceding isochronous beats, it was thought that this test would be sensitive enough to identify any true performance differences for the CI and NH groups. Interestingly, the authors found that CI subjects performed as well as NH controls during this task, with no difference in performance along any parameter. These results lend strong support to the growing body of literature that suggests that rhythm perception is largely intact in CI users. It should be emphasized here that although the present study used a more difficult rhythmic task than other studies (NH subjects averaged only 51.49% correct), it is still possible that an even more complex task, such as polyrhythm detection, could indeed reveal subtle differences in rhythmic performance for CI users and NH groups.

NEURAL MECHANISMS OF MUSIC PERCEPTION IN CI USERS

The study of the cortical mechanisms that underlie music perception in CI users remains an unexplored area of research. A recent study by Sandemann and colleagues[47] used a paradigm based on the measurement of cortical responses (by electroencephalography) to mismatch negativity as an objective measure of the ability of CI users to perceive differences between stimuli. In this study, the investigators concluded that there is objective evidence (in brain patterns for mismatch negativity analysis) that CI users do indeed demonstrate impairments in music perception. This study adds important information to the scant electrophysiologic literature on music perception in CI users[48] and may encourage the development of an important new tool for the analysis of complex stimuli perception in implant users.

In 2010, Limb and colleagues[49] described the first neuroimaging results of CI users in response to musical stimuli.[49] Previous to this study, several positron emission tomography (PET) neuroimaging studies have examined cortical activity during language-based tasks in implant users. These studies have examined basal metabolism in auditory cortices of deaf individuals using ^{18}F-fluoro-2-deoxy-D-glucose,[49–51] and have also used $H_2{}^{15}O$ as a tracer of cerebral blood flow.[52–58] Nonimplanted deaf individuals display decreased levels of metabolic activity in auditory cortices in comparison to NH individuals.[50,51,59] Studies of experienced cochlear implant users suggest that the degree of activation of auditory cortex corresponds to the degree of success in speech perception.[54,55,59,60] In the study by Limb and colleagues,[49] the investigators used $H_2{}^{15}O$ PET scanning to examine cortical activity in postlingually deafened CI subjects and NH control subjects during the perception of melodic, rhythmic, and language stimuli. It was hypothesized that implant users would demonstrate activations of auditory cortex that exceed those of NH control subjects for all categories of stimuli.

Neuroimaging Study Methods

Ten NH controls and 10 postlingually deafened CI users with more than 1 year of implant experience participated in the study. None of the subjects had greater than amateur level musical experience before implantation. Three categories of auditory stimuli were presented to each subject (melody, rhythm, and language). In the melody condition, 18 songs were taken from a source list of popular melodies (eg, "Row, Row, Row Your Boat," "Twinkle, Twinkle Little Star," "Star-Spangled Banner," "Mary Had a Little Lamb") found to be easily recognized by the general American population.[61,62] A high-quality sampled piano was used to present all melodies, which were prerecorded isochronously (quarter notes only) to eliminate rhythmic cues. After listening to each melody, subjects were asked to identify the song title from a list of 3 choices. In the rhythm condition, 5 rhythmic patterns were presented at a fixed tempo (120 bpm) using a high-quality snare drum sample, each derived as a permutation of a basic 4 beats per bar pattern. The percussive snare sound had a temporal envelope that matched that of the piano quarter notes used in the melody condition. After the stimulus presentation, subjects were asked to reproduce the core rhythmic pattern using a Musical Instrument Digital Interface (M-Audio Ozone, Irwindale, CA, USA) keyboard. In the language condition, a series of Central Institute of the Deaf sentences were presented to each subject. Following the stimulus presentation, subjects were given a closed-set list of 3 sentences from which they were asked to select 1 sentence that they heard in the presented series.

During the stimulus presentation, PET scan images were acquired using 10 mCi of $H_2^{15}O$ as an intravenous tracer. A thermoplastic mask was used to immobilize the head in the scanner. The subjects closed their eyes during the rest intervals and during the auditory stimuli presentation. Following image acquisition and data processing, contrast analyses were performed between subject groups and between conditions. Local maxima of activation clusters were identified using the Montreal Neurological Institute stereotactic brain coordinate system.

Neuroimaging Study Results

In both groups, the subjects scored highest on rhythm tasks (100% in both groups), second highest on language tasks (controls 98.0 ± 6.3%; CI 82.0 ± 31.9%) and poorest on melody (controls 88.0 ± 21.5%; CI 46.0 ± 28.4%). Implant subjects scored significantly poorer on melody than on the other two conditions, just more than chance. In this study, the investigators never observed greater activity in auditory cortex in control subjects than in implant users, regardless of the nature of the stimulus. Instead, implant users demonstrated greater auditory cortical activity than control subjects for all conditions. This observation may reflect either successful recruitment or more intense activation of neuronal substrates to assist in processing sensory information received through an implant, and such recruitment may be a prerequisite for high-level CI use. These data support the hypothesis that activity in the temporal cortices is greater in CI subjects in comparison with NH subjects regardless of the stimulus category (language, melody, or rhythm here). Overall, implant subjects demonstrated the greatest difference in activity in comparison with control subjects during language perception. This finding is particularly relevant because CI are essentially designed for speech processing rather than music processing. This finding may represent the underlying neural mechanism of the typically excellent speech performance observed in many postlingually deafened CI users. Interestingly, the authors observed left-hemispheric lateralization in CI users when comparing cortical responses for language with responses for melody or rhythm, which likely reflects the idea that cortical responses to language rely on a left-lateralized network of auditory cortex that is specialized for language even in the CI user population.

FUTURE DIRECTIONS

The progressive improvement in technology and new research efforts directed toward improving music perception should translate into clinical benefits for CI users. As a result of the improvements in psychophysical assessment methods, the authors anticipate broader acceptance of standard tests of music perception for CI users and a more detailed understanding of the limitations faced by CI users. In turn, this trend should lead to greater emphasis on the development of music rehabilitation programs for inclusion as a basic component of postimplantation auditory rehabilitation. Further research on neural mechanisms of music perception will allow objective identification of differences in music perception in implant-mediated versus normal hearing. A series of studies have shown the importance of low-frequency hearing for music perception,[63–65] an area known to be poor in CI users that may receive further attention in the future. In addition, CI users have demonstrated limitations in auditory stream segregation,[66] a feature that is critically important for music perception[67] and also dependent on musical timbre. Further research toward characterization of stream segregation, improvement of musical timbre, and effects of bilateral implantation are, therefore, critically important. In the aggregate, it is hoped that these kinds of data will contribute toward a basic improvement not only in the perception of discrete musical elements but in overall musical sound quality, which remains the ultimate goal for patients with CI.

REFERENCES

1. McDermott HJ. Music perception with cochlear implants: a review. Trends Amplif 2004;8(2):49–82.
2. Gfeller K, Woodworth G, Robin DA, et al. Perception of rhythmic and sequential pitch patterns by normally hearing adults and adult cochlear implant users. Ear Hear 1997;18(3):252–60.
3. Migirov L, Kronenberg J, Henkin Y. Self-reported listening habits and enjoyment of music among adult cochlear implant recipients. Ann Otol Rhinol Laryngol 2009;118(5):350–5.
4. Galvin JJ 3rd, Fu QJ, Oba SI. Effect of a competing instrument on melodic contour identification by cochlear implant users. J Acoust Soc Am 2009;125(3): EL98–103.
5. Galvin JJ 3rd, Fu QJ, Shannon RV. Melodic contour identification and music perception by cochlear implant users. Ann N Y Acad Sci 2009;1169:518–33.
6. Gfeller K, Jiang D, Oleson JJ, et al. Temporal stability of music perception and appraisal scores of adult cochlear implant recipients. J Am Acad Audiol 2010; 21(1):28–34.
7. Chen JK, Chuang AY, McMahon C, et al. Music training improves pitch perception in prelingually deafened children with cochlear implants. Pediatrics 2010; 125(4):e793–800.
8. Trehub SE, Vongpaisal T, Nakata T. Music in the lives of deaf children with cochlear implants. Ann N Y Acad Sci 2009;1169:534–42.
9. Driscoll VD, Oleson J, Jiang D, et al. Effects of training on recognition of musical instruments presented through cochlear implant simulations. J Am Acad Audiol 2009;20(1):71–82.

10. Looi V, She J. Music perception of cochlear implant users: a questionnaire, and its implications for a music training program. Int J Audiol 2010;49(2): 116–28.

11. Looi V, McDermott H, McKay C, et al. Music perception of cochlear implant users compared with that of hearing aid users. Ear Hear 2008;29(3):421–34.

12. Kasturi K, Loizou PC. Effect of filter spacing on melody recognition: acoustic and electric hearing. J Acoust Soc Am 2007;122(2):EL29–34.

13. Chang YT, Yang HM, Lin YH, et al. Tone discrimination and speech perception benefit in Mandarin-speaking children fit with HiRes fidelity 120 sound processing. Otol Neurotol 2009;30(6):750–7.

14. Veekmans K, Ressel L, Mueller J, et al. Comparison of music perception in bilateral and unilateral cochlear implant users and normal-hearing subjects. Audiol Neurootol 2009;14(5):315–26.

15. Eddington DK, Dobelle WH, Brackmann DE, et al. Place and periodicity pitch by stimulation of multiple scala tympani electrodes in deaf volunteers. Trans Am Soc Artif Intern Organs 1978;24:1–5.

16. Fujiki N, Naito Y, Hirano S, et al. Influence of speech-coding strategy on cortical activity in cochlear implant users: a positron emission tomographic study. Acta Otolaryngol 1998;118(6):797–802.

17. Simmons FB. Electrical stimulation of the auditory nerve in man. Arch Otolaryngol 1966;84(1):2–54.

18. Singh S, Kong Y, Zeng FG. Cochlear implant melody recognition as a function of melody frequency range, harmonicity, and number of electrodes. Ear Hear 2009; 30(20):160–8.

19. Gfeller K, Lansing CR. Melodic, rhythmic, and timbral perception of adult cochlear implant users. J Speech Hear Res 1991;34(4):916–20.

20. McDermott HJ, McKay CM. Musical pitch perception with electrical stimulation of the cochlea. J Acoust Soc Am 1997;101(3):1622–31.

21. Pijl S, Schwarz DW. Melody recognition and musical interval perception by deaf subjects stimulated with electrical pulse trains through single cochlear implant electrodes. J Acoust Soc Am 1995;98(2 Pt 1):886–95.

22. Gfeller K, Turner C, Oleson J, et al. Accuracy of cochlear implant recipients on pitch perception, melody recognition, and speech reception in noise. Ear Hear 2007;28(3):412–23.

23. Won JH, Drennan WR, Kang RS, et al. Psychoacoustic abilities associated with music perception in cochlear implant users. Ear Hear 2010;31(6):796–805.

24. Won JH, Drennan WR, Rubinstein JT. Spectral-ripple resolution correlates with speech reception in noise in cochlear implant users. J Assoc Res Otolaryngol 2007;8(3):384–92.

25. Drennan WR, Longnion JK, Ruffin C, et al. Discrimination of Schroeder-phase harmonic complexes by normal-hearing and cochlear-implant listeners. J Assoc Res Otolaryngol 2008;9(1):138–49.

26. Drennan WR, Rubinstein JT. Music perception in cochlear implant users and its relationship with psychophysical capabilities. J Rehabil Res Dev 2008;45(5): 779–89.

27. Kang R, Nimmons GL, Drennan W, et al. Development and validation of the University of Washington Clinical Assessment of Music Perception test. Ear Hear 2009;30(4):411–8.

28. Nimmons GL, Kang RS, Drennan WR, et al. Clinical assessment of music perception in cochlear implant listeners. Otol Neurotol 2008;29(2):149–55.

29. Jung KH, Cho YS, Cho JK, et al. Clinical assessment of music perception in Korean cochlear implant listeners. Acta Otolaryngol 2010;130(6): 716–23.

30. Galvin JJ 3rd, Fu QJ, Nogaki G. Melodic contour identification by cochlear implant listeners. Ear Hear 2007;28(3):302–19.

31. Swanson B, Dawson P, McDermott H. Investigating cochlear implant place-pitch perception with the Modified Melodies test. Cochlear Implants Int 2009;10(Suppl 1): 100–4.

32. Burns EM, Viemeister NF. Played-again SAM: further observations on the pitch of amplitude-modulated noise. J Acoust Soc Am 1981;70:1655–60.

33. Gfeller K, Knutson JF, Woodworth G, et al. Timbral recognition and appraisal by adult cochlear implant users and normal-hearing adults. J Am Acad Audiol 1998; 9(1):1–19.

34. Leal MC, Shin YJ, Laborde ML, et al. Music perception in adult cochlear implant recipients. Acta Otolaryngol 2003;123(7):826–35.

35. Rahne T, Böhme L, Götze G. Timbre discrimination in cochlear implant users and normal hearing subjects using cross-faded synthetic tones. J Neurosci Methods 2011;199(2):290–5.

36. Galvin JJ 3rd, Fu QJ, Oba S. Effect of instrument timbre on melodic contour identification by cochlear implant users. J Acoust Soc Am 2008;124(4): EL189–95.

37. Brockmeier SJ, Peterreins M, Lorens A, et al. Music perception in electric acoustic stimulation users as assessed by the Mu.S.I.C. test. Adv Otorhinolaryngol 2010;67:70–80.

38. Spitzer JB, Mancuso D, Chengt MY. Development of a clinical test of musical perception: appreciation of music in cochlear implantees (AMICI). J Am Acad Audiol 2008;19(1):56–81.

39. Donnelly PJ, Guo BZ, Limb CJ. Perceptual fusion of polyphonic pitch in cochlear implant users. J Acoust Soc Am 2009;126(5):EL128–33.

40. Kim I, Yang E, Donnelly PJ, et al. Preservation of rhythmic clocking in cochlear implant users: a study of isochronous versus anisochronous beat detection. Trends Amplif 2010;14(3):164–9.

41. Cooper WB, Tobey E, Loizou PC. Music perception by cochlear implant and normal hearing listeners as measured by the Montreal battery for Evaluation of Amusia. Ear Hear 2008;29(4):618–26.

42. Gfeller K, Christ A, Knutson JF, et al. Musical backgrounds, listening habits, and aesthetic enjoyment of adult cochlear implant recipients. J Am Acad Audiol 2000; 11(7):390–406.

43. Kong YY, Cruz R, Jones JA, et al. Music perception with temporal cues in acoustic and electric hearing. Ear Hear 2004;25(2):173–85.

44. Szelag E, Kolodziejczyk I, Kanabus M, et al. Deficits of non-verbal auditory perception in postlingually deaf humans using cochlear implants. Neurosci Lett 2004;355(1–2):49–52.

45. Patel AD, Iversen JR, Chen Y, et al. The influence of metricality and modality on synchronization with a beat. Exp Brain Res 2005;163(2):226–38.

46. Patel AD. Rhythm in language and music: parallels and differences. Ann N Y Acad Sci 2003;999:140–3.

47. Sandemann P, Kegel A, Eichele T, et al. Neurophysiological evidence of impaired musical sound perception in cochlear implant users. Clin Neurophysiol 2010; 121(12):2070–82.

48. Koelsch S, Wittfoth M, Wolf A, et al. Music perception in cochlear implant users: an event-related potential study. Clin Neurophysiol 2004;115(4):966–72.
49. Limb CJ, Molloy AT, Jiradejvong P, et al. Auditory cortical activity during cochlear implant-mediated perception of spoken language, melody and rhythm. J Assoc Res Otolaryngol 2010;11(1):133–43.
50. Ito J, Sakakibara J, Iwasaki Y, et al. Positron emission tomography of auditory sensation in deaf patients and patients with cochlear implants. Ann Otol Rhinol Laryngol 1993;102(10):797–801.
51. Lee HJ, Giraud AL, Kang E, et al. Cortical activity at rest predicts cochlear implantation outcome. Cereb Cortex 2007;17(4):909–17.
52. Giraud AL, Truy E. The contribution of visual areas to speech comprehension: a PET study in cochlear implant patients and normal-hearing subjects. Neuropsychologia 2002;40(9):1562–9.
53. Giraud AL, Truy E, Frackowiak R. Imaging plasticity in cochlear implant patients. Audiol Neurootol 2001;6(6):381–93.
54. Giraud AL, Price CJ, Graham JM, et al. Cross-modal plasticity underpins language recovery after cochlear implantation. Neuron 2001;30(3):657–63.
55. Miyamoto RT, Wong D. Positron emission tomography in cochlear implant and auditory brainstem implant recipients. J Commun Disord 2001;34(6):473–8.
56. Wong D, Miyamoto RT, Pisoni DB, et al. PET imaging of cochlear-implant and normal-hearing subjects listening to speech and nonspeech. Hear Res 1999;132(1–2):34–42.
57. Wong D, Pisoni DB, Learn J, et al. PET imaging of differential cortical activation by monaural speech and nonspeech stimuli. Hear Res 2002;166(1–2):9–23.
58. Fujiki N, Naito Y, Hirano S, et al. Influence of speech-coding strategy on cortical activity in cochlear implant users: a positron emission tomographic study. Acta Otolaryngol 1998;118(6):797–802.
59. Green KM, Julyan PJ, Hasings DL, et al. Auditory cortical activation and speech perception in cochlear implant users: effects of implant experience and duration of deafness. Hear Res 2005;205(1–2):184–92.
60. Nishimura H, Doi K, Iwaki T, et al. Neural plasticity detected in short- and long-term cochlear implant users using PET. Neuroreport 2000;11(4):811–5.
61. Drayna D, Manichaikul A, de Lange M, et al. Genetic correlates of musical pitch recognition in humans. Science 2001;291(5510):1969–72.
62. Drennan WR, Won JH, Dasika VK, et al. Effects of temporal fine structure on the lateralization of speech and on speech understanding in noise. J Assoc Res Otolaryngol 2007;8(3):373–83.
63. Gifford RH, Dorman MF, Brown CA. Psychophysical properties of low-frequency hearing: implications for perceiving speech and music via electric and acoustic stimulation. Adv Otorhinolaryngol 2010;67:51–60.
64. Sucher CM, McDermott HJ. Bimodal stimulation: benefits for music perception and sound quality. Cochlear Implants Int 2009;10(Suppl 1):96–9.
65. Singh S, Kong YY, Zeng FG. Cochlear implant melody recognition as a function of melody frequency range, harmonicity, and number of electrodes. Ear Hear 2009;30(2):160–8.
66. Cooper HR, Roberts B. Auditory stream segregation in cochlear implant listeners: measures based on temporal discrimination and interleaved melody recognition. J Acoust Soc Am 2009;126(4):1975–87.
67. Oxenham AJ. Pitch perception and auditory stream segregation: implications for hearing loss and cochlear implants. Trends Amplif 2008;12(4):316–31.

Rehabilitation and Educational Considerations for Children with Cochlear Implants

Uma G. Soman, MED, LSLS Cert AVEd[a], Dana Kan, MA, NBCT[a],
Anne Marie Tharpe, PhD[a,b],*

KEYWORDS

- Rehabilitation • Education • Cochlear implants
- Pediatric deafness

Cochlear implants improve numerous outcomes for children with hearing loss. They make spoken language a viable communication option for those with severe-to-profound losses,[1] improve speech perception[2,3] and speech production skills,[4] and contribute to improved reading outcomes for school-aged students.[5] Moreover, the use of cochlear implants increases the likelihood that children with hearing loss can be included in general education settings.[6] These findings are encouraging; however, the device is rarely the sole contributor to these positive outcomes. Systematic rehabilitation and educational programming are necessary for cochlear implant recipients to reach their full potential.[7]

This article focuses on rehabilitation and educational considerations for children with cochlear implants. Although distinctly different, the goals of rehabilitation and education overlap considerably in good practice. The term rehabilitation is typically used to refer to an individualized model of therapy, such as one-on-one training

The authors have nothing to disclose.

[a] Department of Hearing and Speech Sciences, Vanderbilt University School of Medicine, 1215 21st Avenue South, Room 8310, Nashville, TN 37232-8242, USA

[b] Vanderbilt Bill Wilkerson Center, Nashville, TN, USA

* Corresponding author. Department of Hearing and Speech Sciences, Vanderbilt University School of Medicine, 1215 21st Avenue South, 6308 Medical Center East, Nashville, TN 37232-8718.

E-mail address: anne.m.tharpe@vanderbilt.edu

Otolaryngol Clin N Am 45 (2012) 141–153

doi:10.1016/j.otc.2011.08.022

0030-6665/12/$ – see front matter © 2012 Elsevier Inc. All rights reserved.

oto.theclinics.com

with a speech-language pathologist or auditory-verbal therapist[1]; education typically refers to learning facilitated by a teacher in a school-based environment. Children with cochlear implants benefit from the intentional collaboration of these 2 practices. For example, teachers should integrate speech and language goals into academic lessons and speech-language pathologists should integrate academic content into speech and language activities. This article uses the terms interchangeably as a reminder of their ideal interconnectedness.

OVERVIEW OF DEAF EDUCATION

The roots of deaf education date back to the early sixteenth century in Western Europe. However, it was not until the nineteenth century that deaf education came to the United States. Thomas Hopkins Gallaudet, a graduate of Yale University and an ordained minister, helped establish the first permanent school for the deaf in 1817. Now called The American School for the Deaf, the institute's first teacher was a deaf man Gallaudet met while studying manual education methods in France. This teacher, Laurent Clerc, is credited with the development of American Sign Language (ASL) and was responsible for training many of the first teachers of the deaf. Fifty years later, oral education was introduced. These programs were designed for children who were adventitiously, and postlingually, deafened. Shortly after World War II, transistors were invented, which greatly reduced the size of hearing aids. This miniaturization of hearing aids permitted more practical use of the devices, especially in children. As amplification devices became more sophisticated, oral communication expanded to children who were congenitally deaf. Educational recommendations were subsequently based on degree of hearing loss. Children with adequate residual hearing were considered candidates for the oral approach; manual education programs were recommended for children with limited residual hearing. However, approval of the use of cochlear implants in children in the 1990s expanded the option of oral communication to those with profound hearing loss. Today, children with diverse types and degrees of hearing loss are served by a wide variety of educational approaches.

Historically, the educational program chosen for children with hearing loss has been linked with their communication modality. Although the dichotomy of spoken (oral) versus signed (manual) language is predominant, there are a variety of communication modalities that span across a continuum:

1. ASL. ASL is often referred to as the language of the Deaf community (ie, people who affiliate themselves with deaf culture). It is a rich and vibrant language, complete with unique syntactical and morphologic elements that are distinct from English. Deaf children of deaf parents, who receive exposure to ASL from infancy, develop linguistic competence comparable with hearing children of hearing parents, albeit not in English.[8] ASL is used in residential and day schools for the deaf, as well as in classrooms located in both public and private institutions.
2. Total communication (TC). TC refers to a diverse group of communication options that combines manual signs with spoken language. Sign systems, such as Signing

---

[1] An auditory-verbal therapist is a speech-language pathologist, audiologist, or teacher of the deaf who specializes in teaching children with hearing loss to develop spoken language through the development of audition. The auditory-verbal therapist also guides and coaches the family. The Alexander Graham Bell Academy for Listening and Spoken Language oversees the certification of auditory-verbal therapists.

Exact English (SEE) and pidgin signs, are typically used because of their compatibility with English word structure. This approach also includes the bilingual-bicultural method, which treats English instruction as a second language for students whose first language is ASL.
3. Auditory/oral. Oral communication options rely on amplification and use of residual hearing to develop audition and spoken language. This modality is used in both public and private schools, including special schools designed for children with hearing loss. Cued speech, a visual system used to improve speech reading, is also in this category.

Although these 3 categories simplify the variety of communication types and educational programming options available to children with hearing loss, they provide a framework for the common approaches that have resulted from the selection of communication modality. These categories are not mutually exclusive; children with hearing loss might participate in any or all of these programs at various times throughout their education.

Approximately 90% of children with hearing loss are born to parents who have normal hearing,[9] so the number of parents choosing oral methods for their children's education is increasing.[10] From the 1999 to 2000 until the 2007 to 2008 school years, students relying exclusively on spoken language as their primary method of instruction increased from 44% to 52%.[11,12] Moreover, 87% of children with hearing loss are using some degree of spoken language in educational settings.[12]

Cochlear implants have allowed the education of students with hearing loss to follow the national trend toward educating students with disabilities alongside their typically developing peers. Instead of attending residential schools, children with hearing loss are increasingly being educated in their neighborhood schools.[13] During the 2007 to 2008 school year, approximately 60% of students with hearing loss were included in general education classrooms. Regardless of communication modality, early identification and intervention for hearing loss facilitates the development of language skills that lead to increased participation in general education classrooms.

Educational Legislation

The education of students with hearing loss is governed by federal legislation. In 1975, Public Law 94-142, the Education of All Handicapped Children Act, radically changed the concept of special education. The primary provisions mandated that students with disabilities receive a free, appropriate, public education; be educated in the least restrictive environment; and receive an Individualized Education Program (IEP). In 1990, this law was amended by the Individuals with Disabilities Education Act (IDEA), which was divided into 4 parts[14]:

A. General provisions
B. Special education services for children and youth
C. Early intervention services for infants and toddlers
D. National activities for improving the education of students with disabilities.

Parts B and C relate directly to educating students with hearing loss.

Part C of IDEA covers infants and toddlers from birth until age 3 years. The provisions are designed to improve long-term outcomes for children with disabilities through early intervention. The focus of early intervention is to empower families to meet their children's developmental needs. Several professionals are involved in this process, including audiologists who assess the child's hearing, otologists who assess the cause of the hearing loss, and early interventionists who provide family-centered therapy. Similar to an IEP, an Individualized Family Service Plan (IFSP) is a legal document developed to guide the rehabilitation process for children and their families. The provisions in part C, along with the rest of IDEA, enable the development of effective educational plans for children with cochlear implants.

Part B of IDEA addresses school-aged children and youth (aged 3–21 years) and provides specific guidelines for educational services. Before the mandate of free, appropriate, public education, children with hearing loss, as well as those with other 1 exceptionalities, were systematically denied access to individualized rehabilitation. The law does not guarantee services to every child with a disability, or to every child with a hearing loss. Students must show a need, resulting from the disability, for specialized educational programming. Although disagreements exist about what constitutes appropriate services, students with hearing loss often have delayed language skills that negatively affect their educational performance, thus qualifying them for services under IDEA.

When a child qualifies for services, the educational team develops an IEP based on the student's current functioning level. The team is typically composed of a special educator, a general educator, a local education agency representative, and the parents/guardians of the child. Other members might include school administrators, related service providers (eg, speech-language pathologists, audiologists, occupational therapists, psychologists), and the students themselves. The IEP team makes numerous educational decisions, including which services are needed, how often and in which settings the services will be provided, and how progress on selected goals will be evaluated. The IEP is updated at least annually and serves as a unique blueprint for each child's specific educational needs.

An important task for the IEP team is to determine the least restrictive environment in which rehabilitation should occur. A continuum of possible placements is shown in **Fig. 1**. The specific needs of each individual student also need to be considered. These needs include academic supports (eg, teacher of the deaf, interpreters, hearing technology) as well as opportunities for socialization. The child's environment should be continuously evaluated to reflect the child's development and to achieve the family's desired outcome.

FACTORS INFLUENCING REHABILITATION AND EDUCATION

Several studies have documented the variability of outcomes for children with cochlear implants.[15–17] A cochlear implant, even when provided at a young age, does not guarantee the acquisition of age-appropriate listening and spoken language skills, general educational placement, or successful academic and social outcomes. Some factors that influence outcomes are age of implantation,[18] participation in early intervention,[19] and presence of additional disabilities.[20] Evidence of the impact of underlying neurocognitive processes is also emerging.[21]

A rehabilitation plan developed through collaboration among professionals is necessary to meet the child's needs and facilitate desired outcomes. Each of the professionals involved (the otologist, the audiologist, the speech-language pathologist, and the teacher of the deaf) makes a distinct and essential contribution to the rehabilitation process. For example, the teacher of the deaf might report a child's difficulty with auditory discrimination in noise. The audiologist can then create a separate speech-in-noise program in the implant for use in adverse listening conditions. Purposeful collaboration at different stages of rehabilitation, including candidacy decisions and periodic evaluation of performance (**Table 1**), identifies changing needs expediently, allows for ongoing adaptation of the rehabilitation plan, and helps maintain realistic expectations for families.

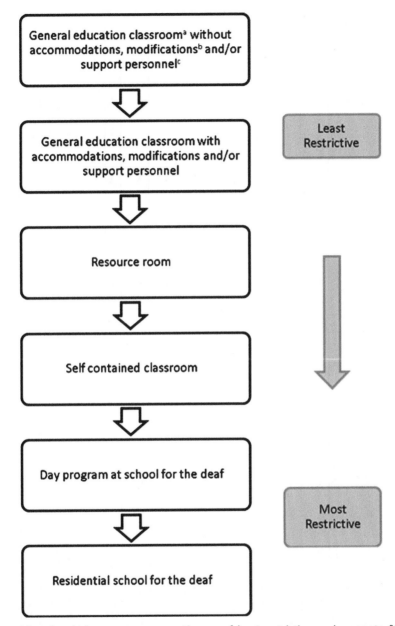

Fig. 1. Educational placements on a continuum of least restrictive environments. [a]Often referred to as mainstreaming. [b]Modifications refer to changes (eg, modified test of listening comprehension); accommodations refer to supports (eg, assistive listening devices, pre-teaching of vocabulary). [c]Often referred to as inclusion.

Table 1
A collaborative model for rehabilitation of cochlear implant recipients

Steps in the Rehabilitation Process	Parent	Otologist	Audiologist	Speech-Language Pathologist	Teacher of the Deaf	General Education Teacher
1. Determine candidacy for cochlear implantation	✓	✓	✓	✓	✓	✓
2. Assess physiologic structures/function for implant compatibility	—	✓	✓	—	—	—
3. Implant the device and monitor the internal device function in the operating room	—	✓	✓	—	—	—
4. Program the implant for maximum auditory access	—	—	✓	—	—	—
5. Assist with maintenance and troubleshooting of cochlear implant	✓	✓	✓	✓	✓	✓
6. Develop age-appropriate speech, language, and auditory skills	✓	—	✓	✓	✓	✓
7. Develop age-appropriate academic and social skills	✓	—	—	✓	✓	✓
8. Evaluate and monitor progress	✓	✓	✓	✓	✓	✓
9. Develop goals and objectives for Individualized Education Plan/IFSP	✓	—	✓	✓	✓	✓
10. Facilitate opportunities for meaningful interaction with normal-hearing peers	✓	—	—	✓	✓	✓
11. Educate parents and other professionals about cochlear implants	✓	✓	✓	✓	✓	✓

The rehabilitation plan should take into account the various mitigating factors related to:

1. The child receiving the implant
2. The family of the recipient
3. The rehabilitation supports

Reed and colleagues[22] identified the unique contributions of each of these factors to the academic success of children with hearing loss. Each is described later in relation to the rehabilitation of children with cochlear implants.

Child Receiving the Implant

Rehabilitation teams consider the individual characteristics of the child, especially the present level of performance on academic, speech-language, and auditory tasks, and the presence of additional disabilities. Input from all professionals regarding the child's abilities before implantation is necessary to develop a plan that builds on the child's current level of skills. For example, the rehabilitation plan for a 3-year-old with profound hearing loss who has limited auditory and language skills should be distinctly different than that for a 6-year-old who has a progressive hearing loss and age-appropriate language skills.

The presence of an additional disability adds a new dimension to the rehabilitation plan. The unique impact of the additional disability on overall development will likely require the team to develop a plan and establish benchmarks for measuring progress that are different from the ones used for children with hearing loss only.

Family Involvement and Expectations

Discussion regarding the parents' desired outcomes after implantation is essential for setting realistic expectations, planning rehabilitation, and recommending educational options. For example, the rehabilitation plan for a 12-month-old whose parents want him to develop listening and spoken language and go to a mainstream school along-side his hearing peers is vastly different than that for a 12-month-old whose parents want her to learn spoken English and ASL and be part of the deaf community.

Parental involvement and expectations are positively correlated with academic achievement. That is, children of parents who have high expectations, maintain consistent communication with the school, help with homework, and enroll their children in extracurricular activities have better academic outcomes.[22,23] Educating parents to be active participants in the rehabilitation process is critical to their children's successful use of cochlear implants. Typically, parents of children with cochlear implants are responsible for:

- Maintaining and troubleshooting the equipment
- Providing transportation to 1 or more therapies
- Providing academic support beyond the level typical of hearing children
- Facilitating opportunities for social skill development
- Advocating for education and rehabilitation services
- Educating school personnel about cochlear implants and the impact of hearing loss on development

Parents need to understand the importance of their continued involvement in the rehabilitation process and receive support from the rehabilitation team to follow through with the recommendations. The following questions should be addressed by the rehabilitation team before cochlear implantation and throughout the rehabilitation process:

- What is the family's desired outcome for the child?
- What are the recommendations for rehabilitation and education?
- What types of support are available through the implant center, local early intervention system, and school system?
- What resources (physical, social, financial) does the family have to follow these recommendations?
- What is the role of the family in the rehabilitation process?

As noted previously, there is wide variation in outcomes for children who receive cochlear implants. It is rare, but not impossible, for some children to receive minimal or no benefit from the implant and the rehabilitation process. However, 87% of parents report wanting their children to use spoken language to communicate after receiving an implant.[24] Although all the factors influencing outcome variability are not yet fully understood, professionals have a responsibility to provide parents with appropriate and adequate information about all potential outcomes.

Rehabilitation Supports

Achievement of desired outcomes requires a rehabilitation plan that meets the needs of the child and facilitates development of auditory, language (spoken and/or signed), and academic skills. At a minimum, supports in the following areas should be considered as necessary supplements to educational intervention:

Audiological management

Access to an implant center is essential to ensure the maintenance of the cochlear implant. Being far away from an implant center is stressful for parents and can have a negative impact on the language and academic outcomes of children.[25] Experience suggests that children who have difficulty accessing the services of an implant center might experience longer periods of time between mapping sessions, spend more days waiting for equipment to be replaced or serviced, and lose valuable listening time as a result of damaged or malfunctioning equipment. Although all families cannot be expected to move their homes to be close to implant centers, it is becoming increasingly common for cochlear implant programming and troubleshooting to be available via telehealth options. Implant manufacturers and cochlear implant teams should be able to advise families of such options.

Speech and language therapy

When the desired outcome of cochlear implantation is to develop listening and spoken language skills, intensive speech and language therapy is necessary. Although services differ based on each child's current level of performance, it is recommended that children receive auditory-based therapy after implantation to maximize benefit from the cochlear implant. The speech-language pathologist focuses on developing listening skills to facilitate language acquisition. The teacher of the deaf complements the speech-language pathologists by focusing on language through academic development. However, few speech-language pathologists are currently trained to work with children with hearing loss who are developing listening and spoken language.[26] Thus, the rehabilitation team should collaborate with the speech-language pathologist and provide information and resources.

Academic services

Teachers of the deaf are trained to develop language skills (spoken or signed) to support academic instruction and social development. Some teachers of the deaf work at one specific school; others are itinerant teachers who serve numerous students at multiple locations. Because the inclusion of children with hearing loss in general education classrooms is increasing, teachers of the deaf are often responsible for collaborating with general education teachers. A factor that contributes to academic success is the willingness of general education teachers to support the child with hearing loss, but maintain appropriate academic expectations.[22] That is, a general education teacher should provide the tools for learning (eg, study guides, modified tests) but expect children to participate to the best of their abilities.

COMMON SCENARIOS AND REHABILITATION PLANS

The following scenarios illustrate case examples commonly experienced by implant teams. They show the variability in the rehabilitative process and conclude with possible recommendations. For each of these examples, it is assumed that the child is receiving audiological and otologic management, and that teachers and professionals are included in rehabilitation planning.

Case Example 1: Isabella

Case history

Isabella is a 14-month-old girl who failed her newborn hearing screening. She was diagnosed with a congenital severe-to-profound bilateral sensory hearing loss by 3 months of age and received hearing aids by 4 months. Isabella's family was referred to the local early intervention agency by her pediatrician and was found eligible for speech and language services provided through part C funding. The parents chose spoken language as the primary mode of communication for Isabella and started working with an early interventionist. Isabella met the candidacy requirements for a cochlear implant and is scheduled for surgery next month. Speech and language evaluations indicate that Isabella functions like a 6- month-old to 9-month-old in the areas of speech, receptive language, and expressive language, and a 9-month-old to 12-month-old in the areas of play skills and social-emotional development. Her parents have indicated that Isabella will attend a full-time community childcare program after the cochlear implant surgery.

Rehabilitation recommendations

- Early intervention services
  - Work with an early interventionist or speech-language pathologist who is trained to develop listening and spoken language with infants and young children who have a hearing loss.
  - Review the current IFSP and include objectives that facilitate development of age-appropriate auditory, language, speech, and cognitive skills.
  - Consider a community childcare program that follows a developmental curriculum and has peers who can serve as language models.
- School-based rehabilitation
  - Request a developmental evaluation through the early intervention agency when Isabella is 30 months old.
  - Arrange an IEP meeting with the local school system to assess eligibility for special education services. If Isabella shows any delays and qualifies for services, consider the following recommendations:
    - Receive services from a teacher of the deaf and speech-language pathologist to develop age-appropriate listening, language, and academic skills.

- Evaluate acoustics of the classroom environment and make modifications to maximize auditory access.
- Assess the need for assistive listening devices (eg, frequency modulated systems and soundfield systems).

The rehabilitation team should review these recommendations at least annually. Updates should be made based on Isabella's progress and the family's current desired outcomes.

Case Example 2: Marcus

Case history

Marcus is a 6-year-old boy who passed the newborn hearing screening and was not diagnosed until age 2 years with a severe-to-profound bilateral sensory hearing loss. He received hearing aids within 1 month following the diagnosis and qualified for early intervention services through part C funding. Marcus received early intervention from a teacher of the deaf. Marcus's parents want him to learn ASL and spoken English.

Currently Marcus is enrolled at his local public school in a self-contained classroom for students who are deaf and hard of hearing. The teacher of the deaf provides instruction in both sign and spoken language. Marcus is in this classroom for most of the school day but attends physical education, art, and lunch with his hearing peers. Speech and language evaluations and academic progress reports indicate that Marcus has age-appropriate sign language skills. His listening and spoken language skills are 2 standard deviations below average.

Marcus's parents want him to receive a cochlear implant so he can improve listening and spoken language skills and interact independently with people who do not know sign language. Marcus has met the cochlear implant candidacy requirements and surgery is scheduled for next month.

Rehabilitation Recommendations

- Rehabilitation services
  - Work with a teacher of the deaf or speech-language pathologist to develop listening skills using the new implant and to develop spoken language, in addition to sign language.
- Educational placement and support
  - Review Marcus's IEP
    - Add new objectives related to listening and spoken language.
    - Update placement and services to maximize meaningful interaction with hearing peers.
    - Continue services with a teacher of the deaf to develop age-appropriate language and academic skills.
    - Increase services with the speech-language pathologist to develop age-appropriate listening and language skills.

Children with Multiple Disabilities

Approximately 40% of children with hearing loss have a sensory, cognitive, or neurologic disability in addition to hearing loss.[12] Today, the presence of a concomitant disability rarely precludes a child from receiving a cochlear implant. Studies indicate that children who have additional disabilities show progress in speech perception and language skills after implantation, but the rate of progress is slower than typically developing children with hearing loss.[20,27,28] The presence of multiple disabilities requires the rehabilitation team to address these additional needs:

- Inform parents about the potential impact of the additional disability on outcomes.
- Include professionals who are experts in the other disability/disabilities as part of the child's rehabilitation team.
- Establish realistic but high expectations for the child, noting that these might be different than those for children without additional disabilities who have similar audiological profiles.

An important point to consider is that additional disabilities are often diagnosed after implantation and may warrant a reevaluation of the child's educational plan.

Children from Bilingual Families

The number of bilingual families in the United States is steadily increasing. According to the 2005 to 2009 American Community Survey, nearly 20% of the population speaks more than 1 language at home.[29] Similarly, 20% of children with hearing loss live in a home where English is not the primary language.[12] Two issues commonly seen with bilingual families are (1) parents and caregivers have limited English proficiency, and (2) parents are bilingual and want the child to be bilingual as well. There is a dearth of research related to effective practices for intervention for families who do not speak English. Furthermore, there are a limited number of professionals who are bilingual and can provide services in the home language.[30]

Retrospective studies of children who have hearing loss and are reported to be bilingual suggest that it is possible for children who receive a cochlear implant at a young age and participate in auditory therapy to develop spoken language skills in 2 languages.[31,32] Some characteristics that were observed in children who were successful in developing 2 spoken languages were early age of implantation, consistent use of cochlear implant following implantation, focused therapy to develop listening and spoken language skills, parents fluent in the second language, consistent second language exposure at home, no additional disabilities, and better-than-average speech perception skills.[32] However, rehabilitation strategies that facilitate development of 2 spoken languages for children with cochlear implants are not well established and need further investigation.

SUMMARY

Cochlear implants have greatly expanded opportunities for children with profound hearing loss. The successful outcomes for children who receive cochlear implants are predicated largely by mindful collaboration between professionals and families. Professionals working with children who have a hearing loss must be aware that the definition of success with a cochlear implant is different for each child and each family. The goal should be to support children and help families achieve their desired outcomes through the development, implementation, and continuous evaluation of strong and realistic rehabilitation plans.

REFERENCES

1. Brown C. Early intervention: strategies for public and private sector collaboration. Presented at the 2006 Convention of the Alexander Graham Bell Association for the Deaf and Hard of Hearing. Pittsburgh(PA), June 23–27, 2006.

2. Svirsky M, Teoh S, Neuburger H. Development of language and speech perception in congenitally, profoundly deaf children as a function of age at cochlear implantation. Audiol Neurootol 2004;9(4):224–33.

3. Spencer L, Oleson J. Early listening and speaking skills predict later reading proficiency in pediatric cochlear implant users. Ear Hear 2008;29(2):270–80.

4. Cole E, Flexer C. Children with hearing loss developing listening and talking birth to six. San Diego (CA): Plural Publishing; 2007.

5. Geers A. Predictors of reading skill development in children with early cochlear implantation. Ear Hear 2003;24(1):S59–68.

6. Francis H, Koch M, Wyatt J, et al. Trends in educational placement and cost-benefit considerations in children with cochlear implants. Arch Otolaryngol Head Neck Surg 1999;125(5):499–505.

7. Wilkins M, Ertmer D. Introducing young children who are deaf or hard of hearing to spoken language: child's voice, an oral school. Lang Speech Hear Serv Sch 2002;33(3):196–204.

8. Hauser P, Marschark M. What we know and what we don't know about cognition and deaf learners. In: Marschark M, Hauser P, editors. Deaf cognition: foundations and outcomes. New York: Oxford University Press; 2008. p. 439–57.

9. Mitchell R, Karchmer M. Chasing the mythical ten percent: parental hearing status of deaf and hard of hearing students in the United States. Sign Language Studies 2004;4(2):138–63.

10. White K. Early intervention for children with permanent hearing loss: finishing the EHDI revolution. The Volta Review 2006;106(3):237–58.

11. Gallaudet Research Institute. Regional and national summary report of data from the 2007-2008 annual survey of deaf and hard of hearing children & youth. Available at: http://research.gallaudet.edu/Demographics. Updated January, 2001. Accessed January 4, 2011.

12. Gallaudet Research Institute. Regional and national summary report of data from the 2000-2001 annual survey of deaf and hard of hearing children & youth. Available at: http://research.gallaudet.edu/Demographics. Updated November, 2008. Accessed January 4, 2011.

13. Marvelli A. Highlights in the history of oral teacher preparation in America. The Volta Review 2010;110(2):89–116.

14. US Department of Education. The Individuals with Disabilities Education Act. 2004. Available at: http://frwebgate.access.gpo.gov/cgi-bin/getdoc.cgi?dbname=108_cong_public_laws&docid=f:publ446.108. Accessed April 1, 2011.

15. Pisoni D, Conway C, Kronenberger W, et al. Efficacy and effectiveness of cochlear implants in deaf children. In: Hauser P, Marschark M, editors. Deaf cognition: foundations and outcomes. New York: Oxford University Press; 2008. p. 52–101.

16. Zeng F. Trends in cochlear implants. Trends Amplif 2004;8(1):1–34.

17. Svirsky M, Robbins A, Kirk K, et al. Language development in profoundly deaf children with cochlear implants. Psychol Sci 2000;11(2):153–8.

18. Nicholas J, Geers A. Will they catch up? The role of age at cochlear implantation in the spoken language development of children with severe to profound hearing loss. J Speech Lang Hear Res 2007;50(4):1048–62.

19. Yoshinaga-Itano C. From screening to early identification and intervention: discovering predictors to successful outcomes for children with significant hearing loss. J Deaf Stud Deaf Educ 2003;8(1):11–30.

20. Waltzman S, Scalchunes V, Cohen N. Performance of multiply handicapped children using cochlear implants. Otol Neurotol 2000;21(3):329–35.

21. Pisoni D, Kronenberger W, Roman A, et al. Measures of digit span and verbal rehearsal speed in deaf children after more than 10 years of cochlear implantation. Ear Hear 2011;32:60S–74S.
22. Reed S, Antia S, Kreimeyer K. Academic status of deaf and hard-of-hearing students in public schools: student, home, and service facilitators and detractors. J Deaf Stud Deaf Educ 2008;13(4):485–502.
23. Antia S, Jones P, Reed S, et al. Academic status and progress of deaf and hard-of-hearing students in general education classrooms. J Deaf Stud Deaf Educ 2009;14(3):293–311.
24. Hyde M, Punch R, Komesaroff L. Coming to a decision about cochlear implantation: parents making choices for their deaf children. J Deaf Stud Deaf Educ 2010; 15(2):162–78.
25. Punch R, Hyde M. Children with cochlear implants in Australia: educational settings, supports, and outcomes. J Deaf Stud Deaf Educ 2010;15(4):405–21.
26. Houston T, Perigoe C. Speech-language pathologists: vital listening and spoken language professionals. The Volta Review 2010;110(2):219–30.
27. Daneshi A, Hassanzadeh S. Cochlear implantation in prelingually deaf persons with additional disability. J Laryngol Otol 2007;121(07):635–8.
28. Wiley S, Jahnke M, Meinzen-Derr J, et al. Perceived qualitative benefits of cochlear implants in children with multi-handicaps. Int J Pediatr Otorhinolaryngol 2005;69(6):791–8.
29. U.S. census bureau, 2005-2009 American community survey. Available at: http://factfinder.census.gov/servlet/STTable?_bm=y&-geo_id=01000US&-qr_name=ACS_2009_5YR_G00_S1601&-ds_name=ACS_2009_5YR_G00_. Updated September 22, 2009. Accessed April 1, 2011.
30. American Speech-Language-Hearing Association. Demographic profile of ASHA members providing bilingual and Spanish-language services. Available at: http://www.asha.org/uploadedFiles/Demographic-Profile-Bilingual-Spanish-Service-Members.pdf. Updated May, 2010. Accessed April, 2011.
31. Waltzman S, Robbins A, Green J, et al. Second oral language capabilities in children with cochlear implants. Otol Neurotol 2003;24:757–63.
32. Robbins A, Green J, Waltzman S. Bilingual oral language proficiency in children with cochlear implants. Arch Otolaryngol Head Neck Surg 2004;130:644–7.

Outcomes in Cochlear Implantation: Variables Affecting Performance in Adults and Children

Maura K. Cosetti, MD[a], Susan B. Waltzman, PhD[b],*

KEYWORDS

• Cochlear implants • Performance • Variables

COCHLEAR IMPLANTS AND POSTIMPLANTATION PERFORMANCE

Cochlear implantation allows most average, postlinguistically deafened pediatric and adult cochlear implant (CI) recipients to achieve meaningful auditory sensation and speech understanding. In the past 25 years, data on the postoperative outcomes following cochlear implantation have identified a wide spectrum of variables known to affect postimplantation performance (**Box 1**). These variables relate to the device itself, including electrode design, speech processing strategies, and device reliability, as well as individual patient characteristics such as cochleovestibular anatomy, presence of associated disabilities, or the cause of deafness. On a cellular level, factors believed to affect spiral ganglion cell survival and function have been shown to influence postoperative performance, including auditory deprivation, duration of deafness, and age at implantation. Social and educational factors, such as mode of communication, parent/family expectations, postimplantation rehabilitation, and socioeconomic status, are additional variables shown to affect postoperative performance. Novel variables capable of affecting performance, such as auditory training and focused attention, continue to emerge with increased understanding of auditory pathway development and neural plasticity. Despite extensive research examining

This work was supported by the Rienzi Foundation for Cochlear Implant Research.
The authors have nothing to disclose.
[a] Department of Otolaryngology, New York University School of Medicine, 550 First Avenue, Suite 7Q, New York, NY 10016, USA
[b] Department of Otolaryngology, New York University Cochlear Implant Center, New York University School of Medicine, 660 First Avenue, 7th Floor, New York, NY 10016, USA
* Corresponding author.
E-mail address: susan.waltzman@nyumc.org

Otolaryngol Clin N Am 45 (2012) 155–171
doi:10.1016/j.otc.2011.08.023
0030-6665/12/$ – see front matter © 2012 Elsevier Inc. All rights reserved.

Box 1
Variables affecting CI performance

1. CI technology
   a. Processing strategy
   b. Electrode design
   c. *Device reliability*
2. Neuronal cell physiology and function
   a. Age at implantation
   b. Duration of deafness/auditory deprivation
   c. Auditory neuroplasticity
   d. Auditory pathway development
3. Binaural hearing
4. Multiple disabilities
   a. Autism
   b. Auditory neuropathy/auditory dyssynchrony
5. Medical/surgical issues
   a. Anatomic abnormalities
   b. Meningitis
   c. CHARGE (coloboma, central nervous system anomalies, heart defects, atresia of the choanae, retardation of growth and/or development, ear anomalies and/or deafness) syndrome
6. Preoperative function: hearing level and speech performance
7. Education/rehabilitative environment
   a. Mode of communication
   b. *Multilingual or bilingual environment*
   c. Education and postimplantation rehabilitation services
8. Auditory training
9. Social factors
   a. Socioeconomic status
   b. Parent/family expectations and motivation

Items in italics are variables that research suggests do not affect performance.

---

both adult and pediatric postimplantation outcomes, the considerable variably in postoperative performance remains incompletely understood. Predictions of postimplantation benefit should be individualized and based on comprehensive preoperative assessment, with attention to the complex interplay of the aforementioned patient and device characteristics. Detailed knowledge of these variables not only improves clinician's predictive accuracy but may also reveal factors that can be manipulated to achieve optimal performance.

As initially narrow candidacy criteria have broadened to include many patients affected by sensorineural hearing loss (SNHL), including those at the extremes of age, such as infants and the elderly, patients with multiple handicaps, auditory neuropathy (AN)/auditory dyssynchrony (AD), abnormal cochlear anatomy, residual hearing, and even patients with unilateral deafness, variables affecting performance have become increasingly more complex. However, these interconnected variables can be examined in related groups, making understanding of the increasing list more manageable and less intimidating. This article highlights well-recognized variables known to affect CI performance, newly emerging factors warranting consideration, and certain key variables shown not to affect performance. Overall, the discussion focuses on data published from 2005 onward.

IMPLANT TECHNOLOGY

Since the introduction of cochlear implantation, advances in hardware, software, and speech processing technology have directly affected performance, successively improving postimplantation speech understanding with each significant technologic advance. Of these, the most significant factor affecting performance thus far is processing strategy. In time, changes in rate of electrode stimulation, mode (sequential or simultaneous, analog or pulsatile), number of channels, waveform or speech feature extraction of the auditory signal have led to increasingly advanced and sophisticated paradigms for electrode stimulation.

Speech Perception

Upgrades to spectral peak (SPEAK) from multipeak (MPEAK), and from SPEAK to continuous interleaved sampling (CIS) saw concomitant improvement in postoperative speech understanding. Multifactorial data obtained following each transition support the direct impact of superior processing strategy on outcome. Research on novel processing strategies continues to support this trend, especially regarding the newer goals of improved word understanding in noise and music appreciation. Use of virtual channels (VCs) in speech processing software has been recently incorporated in HiRes Fidelity 120 (HiRes 120), the commercial processing strategy developed by Advanced Bionics, LLC (Sylmar, CA) and available with the HiRes 90K CI. By varying the proportion of current delivered to each electrode of an electrode pair, current steering can increase the number of spectral channels beyond the number of physical electrodes provided by the CI array. In the HiRes 90K device, 16 active electrodes (and 15 electrode pairs) are used to create 8 additional stimulation sites, resulting in up to 120 virtual channels.[1–5]

Tonal Language Perception and Music Appreciation

Recent research by Firszt and colleagues[4] (2009) showed significant clinical benefit in both speech perception and music appreciation with the HiRes 120 current steering technology compared with traditional processing strategies. Subjective ratings of music pleasantness, sound quality, and instrument distinctness were also higher with the HiRes120 speech processing. Improved pitch resolution afforded by VC may be especially clinically relevant for speech perception of tonal languages, such as Mandarin or Cantonese, in which pitch may be the only auditory clue signaling a difference in word meaning. Recent research by Chang and colleagues[6] (2009) suggested that, compared with HiRes, HiRes 120 offered significant benefit to Mandarin-speaking pediatric CI recipients in areas of tone discrimination and speech perception. Additional research on native language is necessary, specifically the use of tonal language, as an independent variable affecting performance.

Neural Elements and Residual Hearing

Since the introduction of multi-electrode CI, advances in electrode design have focused on the development of smaller, less traumatic arrays that allow preservation of residual hearing and more selective activation of neural elements. Specific neuronal subpopulation stimulation depends on several factors, including the geometric arrangement of the electrodes, individual cochlear anatomy, and the proximity of the implanted array to the auditory neurons. Introduction of modiolar-hugging electrodes, such as used by the Nucleus CI512 (Sydney, Australia) by Cochlear, are designed to self-coil during or after insertion to reside close to the spiral ganglion cells in the modiolus. Perimodiolar arrays are intended to reduce the distance, and thereby the energy required, to stimulate neuronal cells as well as reduce insertion trauma. Unlike processing strategy modifications, introduction of modiolar-hugging electrodes has not been shown to definitively affect performance, although additional research is this area is ongoing. In contrast, ability to preserve residual hearing is intimately related to electrode configuration and size, as well as other factors such as atraumatic cochleostomy and insertion techniques. Preservation and use of residual hearing, as afforded by advances in all aspects of implant technology, including electrode design, seems to affect performance. This benefit has been attributed to improved frequency resolution and pitch discrimination afforded by preserved low-frequency residual hearing. The Nucleus Hybrid L24 is a 16-mm long 22-contact electrode array designed to preserve residual low-frequency hearing in the cochlear apex while providing a greater number of electrodes to the high-frequency and midfrequency regions. Lenarz and colleagues[7,8] (2006, 2009) reported initial and longer-term preservation of residual hearing with the Hybrid L24 using a round-window insertion approach. Patients with preserved residual hearing show improved speech understanding in noise and enhanced spatial hearing.[9] Similar results have been shown in the ongoing Nucleus Hybrid L24 Food and Drug Administration (FDA) clinical trial in the United States, which uses an atraumatic cochleostomy technique.[10]

Pediatric Residual Hearing

Limited data exist on the preservation of residual hearing in the pediatric population. Skarzynski and Lorens[11] (2010) reported their results of cochlear implantation on partial deafness in 15 children. Rates of speech perception in quiet improved from 34% before surgery to 67% after surgery and from 7% to 47% for hearing in noise.[11] Although promising, additional research on hearing preservation in the pediatric population, including long-term follow-up, is necessary.

Intraoperative Technology

Additional advances in implant technology include the capability for intraoperative objective, electrophysiologic measurements of the electrical compound action potential. Termed neural response telemetry (NRT) in the Nucleus implant by Cochlear (Sydney, Australia), neural response imaging (NRI) in CIs by Advanced Bionics, LLC (Symlar, CA, USA), and auditory nerve response telemetry (ART) for MED-EL (Innsbruck, Austria), these objective measures are used during surgery to assess the response of a patient's auditory system to electrical stimulation immediately following intracochlear insertion of the CI electrode. At the time of surgery, intraoperative NRT provides valuable information regarding the electrical output of the implant, the response of the auditory system to electrical stimulation, and preliminary device programming data; however, recent data suggest that it is not a valuable predictor of postoperative performance.[12] Furthermore, the absence of NRT does not necessarily indicate a lack of stimulation and, in itself, is not an important variable in postoperative outcome.

Device Reliability

A review of implant technology and its effect on performance is not complete without a discussion of CI device reliability. Although device failure remains an important concern for both patients and clinicians, increased reliability has been achieved in all devices over time. Although uncommon, implant failure requires device removal and reimplantation. The most common cause is a hard failure with sudden and complete loss of function.[13–17] Evidence by Carlson and colleagues[18] (2010) and Zeitler and colleagues[16] (2009) suggests that deactivation of 3 or 5 electrodes, respectively, can suggest impending device failure and warrant close monitoring and/or device removal. Overall, evidence to date suggests that reimplantation does not affect performance. Using careful surgical technique, revision surgery can lead to preservation or improvement in preoperative performance in most pediatric and adult patients.[13–17]

NEURONAL CELL PHYSIOLOGY AND FUNCTION: AGE AT IMPLANTATION, DURATION OF DEAFNESS/AUDITORY DEPRIVATION, AUDITORY PLASTICITY, AUDITORY PATHWAY DEVELOPMENT

These grouped variables relate to the survival, physiology, and function of spiral ganglion cells and the effects of the lack of auditory input over time. Positive effects of chronic electrical stimulation on spiral ganglion cells have been well shown in animal models. However, a critical period for auditory pathway development in humans has not been definitively established, although research in this area is ongoing and is described later. Effects of deprivation and plasticity on performance can be interpreted via their related clinical correlates: age at implantation and duration of deafness. Widespread newborn hearing screening has led to an increase in early diagnosis and greater opportunities for early intervention, including children younger than 1 year. Cochlear implantation in children less than age 12 months has shown both short-term and long-term safety and efficacy. Performance testing in very young children presents unique challenges because most tests are language based and not appropriate for children less than 1 year old. However, using methodology designed for age-appropriate abilities, a growing body of literature supports improved auditory and linguistic outcomes in children implanted before 12 months of age.[19–27]

Using the Infant-Toddler Meaningful Auditory Integration Scale (IT-MAIS) to assess speech perception, Waltzman and Roland[19] (2005) and Roland and colleagues[25] (2009) suggested that implantation before age 1 year may allow deaf children to reach their full hearing potential, which may approach that of normal-hearing peers in some cases. Colletti and colleagues[20] (2005) used the Category of Auditory Performance (CAP; a global measure of auditory receptive abilities) in their study of 10 children less than 12 months old. They found that outcomes in children less than 1 year old exceeded those of children implanted later. In an initial report involving 6 CI recipients less than 1 year old, Holt and Svirsky[23] (2008) did not find a difference between children implanted before 12 months of age and those implanted between 1 and 2 years old. However, recent data by these investigators including CI recipients less than 1 year old (N = 35) suggest a significant advantage in areas of speech perception compared with later-implanted groups.[26] Tajudeen and colleagues[26] (2010) found a benefit of early implantation when comparing children of the same age, but not when comparing children the same time after implantation. For this reason, they postulated that the sensitive period for word identification likely extends to at least 3 years old.

Evidence for a sensitive period for language development within the first 2 years of life is accumulating. Connor and colleagues[28] (2006) and Miyamoto and colleagues[24] (2008) provided data for improved speech perception and oral linguistic skills in children implanted before their second birthday compared with children implanted when older than 2 years of age. As mentioned earlier, postimplantation outcome assessment in children less than 1 year old requires unique methodology geared toward age-appropriate abilities. Using the Rosetti Infant-Toddler Language Scale (RI-TLS), Dettman and colleagues[21] (2007) examined communication abilities of 19 children implanted before 12 months of age. These children achieved rates of both receptive and expressive language growth comparable with their normally hearing peers and significantly greater than rates achieved by children implanted between 12 and 24 months of age. Nott and colleagues[29] (2009) compared lexical acquisition in CI recipients and normal-hearing children and found that those implanted earlier, before 12 months of age, were closest to their hearing peers in time to acquisition of their first and 100th word. Unlike Dettman and colleagues[21] (2007) Holt and Svirsky[23] (2008) found improved receptive language skills in children implanted before 1 year of age, but negligible differences in expressive ability between CI recipients less than 1 year old and those implanted between 12 and 24 months of age.[23] In a prospective study of pediatric CI recipients, Niparko and colleagues[27] (2010) showed improved rates of both speech and language performance in children implanted before 18 months of age, most of which paralleled the performance of normal-hearing controls. Although evidence regarding critical periods for auditory and linguistic development continues to emerge, the variables of age at implantation and length of deafness have a clear impact on CI performance in children.

In adolescent CI recipients, data suggest that performance is also affected by age at implantation and length of deafness. A study of 45 prelingually deafened adolescents with a mean age at implantation of 13.5 years (range 11–18 years) found age at implantation, duration of deafness, and preoperative hearing threshold to affect speech perception outcomes. All patients showed significant improvement from preoperative scores.[30]

At the other end of the age spectrum, cochlear implantation in elderly patients has raised issues of age-related degeneration of both peripheral and central auditory systems as well as overall cognitive deterioration and decreased neural plasticity associated with aging.[31] Successful cochlear implantation requires an intact and functional auditory processing pathway, from spiral ganglion cells to the auditory cortex. Research suggests that multiple areas along this pathway may be affected by the aging process, thereby influencing CI outcomes in the elderly.[32] Although histologic studies show that older individuals have lower spiral ganglion cell counts than younger individuals, the relationship between absolute number of remaining spiral ganglion cells and speech performance with a CI in the elderly is complex. Multiple studies show significant improvement in speech perception scores following implantation in elderly patients.[33–35] Budenz and colleagues[34] (2010) showed that, although younger patients out-performed elderly subjects, between-group differences correlated with duration of deafness rather than age. For quality-of-life outcomes, multiple studies support improvements in self-esteem, independence, and functional status, including a return to part-time or full-time employment, following cochlear implantation. Overall, evidence supports significant and widespread benefit of CIs in the elderly population and sheds light on the complex relationship between duration of auditory deprivation, age at implantation, neuronal plasticity, and outcome.

BINAURAL HEARING

Although a full discussion of the benefits of binaural hearing is beyond the scope of this article, improved performance is seen in bilateral CI recipients and bimodal users (individuals with a unilateral CI and contralateral hearing aid) compared with patients with a unilateral CI. In the last decade, research has shown improved accuracy in sound localization, spatial acuity, and speech understanding, especially in challenging listening environments, in patients with bilateral CIs.[36–45] These results have been shown for both simultaneous and sequential implantation in both children and adult recipients. Recent data for sound localization and spatial hearing following bilateral implantation suggest that these skills develop during the early stages of binaural hearing and improve over time with increasing experience.[41–43] In sequentially implanted children, localization abilities were greatest in children who received their first implant before age 2 years and those who attended a mainstream school (vs a school for the deaf).[46] In general, sound localization skills correlate positively with speech intelligibility in noise in that patients who are better able to localize a sound source perform better on tests of speech perception.[40,46] In a specific study of speech perception in noise, Dunn and colleagues[47] (2010) found that recipients of bilateral CIs showed significantly better performance than matched patients with unilateral CIs. In addition to objective measures, subjective data also support the binaural advantage with both adult bilateral recipients and parents of children with bilateral CIs reporting improved communication in daily life, including complex listening situations and spatial hearing.[37,48–50] Although multifactorial, the most significant determinant of postoperative speech performance following sequential bilateral implantation is performance after the first implantation. Data suggest that auditory perception benefits in children with sequentially implanted bilateral CIs are attained over time and, although related to age at initial implantation and chronologic age, seem unaffected by the length of time between implantations.[36,42,43]

Data comparing speech perception and localization skills of bimodal patients with bilateral CI recipients are less clear. Although some studies suggest that a greater binaural advantage is attained with a second CI compared with a hearing aid, others fail to show significant differences between the 2 groups.[51,52] Overall, the bimodal literature shows (1) a binaural advantage compared with unilateral CI, and (2) support for central integration of electric and acoustic hearing. Evidence for effective cortical integration of differing binaural auditory stimuli is also provided by Budenz and colleagues[53] (2009). In their study, benefits of bilateral implantation were unaffected by differing and/or newer technology in the second implanted ear, suggesting successful central or cortical integration of differing peripheral auditory input.

Performance data on simultaneously implanted patients parallel those of sequential bilateral CI recipients. Improved word recognition and sound localization abilities show stability in the long term with the greatest gains shown in the 12 months following implantation.[38,54,55] In adult simultaneous bilateral patients followed over time, localization abilities continued to improve up to 6 years following CI, suggesting that certain binaural advantages may develop in a longer time period. Whether using bimodal technology or bilateral CIs, evidence to date clearly shows a performance advantage with binaural hearing.

MULTIPLE DISABILITIES, INCLUDING AUTISM, AN/AD

Between 30% and 40% of children with SNHL show additional disabilities, including cognitive impairment, motor disorders, visual impairment, and behavioral/emotional spectrum disorders.[56] Each of these handicaps has the potential to affect performance with a CI. Additional disabilities may be congenital or acquired, diagnosed before, concurrent with, or after the diagnosis of hearing loss, and may range in severity across multiple dimensions. The significant heterogeneity of this population, combined with unique challenges in diagnosis and outcomes assessment, make generalized predictions of postimplantation success difficult. Despite this, evaluation of postimplantation outcomes, including speech perception, receptive and expressive language development, social interaction, environmental awareness, and quality of life suggest that cochlear implantation in patients with multiple disabilities can lead to substantial benefit across many dimensions. With respect to auditory speech perception skills, evidence supports improved word and speech recognition following implantation in those patients able to complete perception testing. Compared with children without additional disabilities, overall speech perception scores were lower and rates of skill acquisition slower in the multiply handicapped group.[57] Although some never received open-set speech recognition abilities, substantial benefit from implantation was shown in increased social interaction and environmental awareness. Berrettini and colleagues[57] (2008) reported on 23 pediatric CI recipients with additional diagnoses including cerebral palsy, mental retardation, autistic spectrum disorder, epilepsy, attention deficit and hyperactivity (ADHD), and learning disorders. Overall, most patients showed improved speech perception abilities compared with preoperative values, and 53% attained open-set speech recognition skills. Results of a parental questionnaire documented significant perceived postimplantation benefits: 100% of parents reported increased awareness of environmental sounds, 96% indicated improved interaction with peers, and 74% noted improvement in speaking skills. In addition, the percentage of patients using oral language increased from 28% (before surgery) to 67% after surgery.[57] Improved quality of life was also documented by Wiley and colleagues[58] (2005) with reported progress in communication skills, improved awareness of environmental sounds, and overall increased attentiveness and interaction with their environment.

Fewer studies have focused on language development in children with CIs and additional disabilities. Holt and Kirk[59] (2005) found substantial linguistic gains in 69 children with cognitive delay, although these achievements were significantly lower compared with patients with CIs and without cognitive delays. More recently, studies by Meinzen-Derr and colleagues[60,61] (2010) have shed light on preoperative predictors of language development using a metric adapted from the Gesell Developmental Schedule, the Nonverbal Cognitive Quotient (NVCQ.) In both studies, the NVCQ was found to be the strongest predictor of postimplantation language development. Well-known predictors in the general pediatric CI population (ie, patients without additional disabilities), such as age at hearing loss diagnosis, age at implantation, and implant duration, were not found to be significant predictors of postimplantation performance.[60] In their second study, the investigators compared 15 children with developmental disability and CIs with age-matched and NVCQ-matched controls to provide a novel control group based on assessments of cognitive function.[61] The CI group showed significantly lower rates of receptive and expressive language compared with age-matched and cognitively matched controls. They found their language delays to be disproportionate to their cognitive potential, meaning that children with CIs did not reach language levels commensurate with their cognitive potential.[61] This quantitative linguistic-cognitive discrepancy is a novel finding and may have implications for therapeutic strategy. Specifically, children with CIs and coexisting disabilities may need individualized augmentative and/or adaptive communication strategies to assist linguistic progress, such as speech-generating devices or visual aids. As in prior studies, benefits of CIs were recognized in many areas of quality of life and increased environmental awareness and social interaction.

On more traditional assessments of postimplantation success, multiply handicapped children generally score lower on tests of speech perception and language development than children without other disabilities. As in very young children, speech perception testing in this population is challenging because many tests are not appropriate for patients with multiple disabilities and/or cognitive impairment. For these patients, hearing impairment is not the only factor influencing response to sound. Neurologic deficits, visual impairments (including blindness), attention and hyperactivity disorders, AN, retardation and developmental delay, fine and gross motor impairments, and learning disabilities prohibit the use of, or complicate the information gained from, traditional assessments of speech and language development. Expansion of pediatric CI criteria to include increasingly younger children, as discussed earlier, has additional implications regarding predictions of postimplantation benefit because some disabilities are not detectable in infancy. Despite comprehensive CI evaluation and best diagnostic efforts, it may not be possible for clinicians to diagnose or predict unseen disabilities that do not become evident until the child is older. Even multidisciplinary developmental evaluations may be unable to predict future cognitive or developmental delay, such as autism. Preimplantation parent and family counseling in both very young children and the multiply handicapped should be based on individual assessment data, and expectations tailored to each child's specific set of disabilities.

Among the diverse group of patients with CI and multiple handicaps, 2 conditions deserve special discussion: autism and AN/AD. Research on pediatric CI recipients with autism shows significant variability in outcomes, with some studies suggesting minimal speech and language benefit in this population.[62] Daneshi and Hassanzadeh[63] (2007) reported quality-of-life improvements, such as increased responsiveness to sound, improved eye contact, greater attempt at vocalizations, and increased environmental awareness, but indicated that specific gains in communication skills were minimal. The investigators highlighted the need for intensive disease-specific rehabilitation to achieve minimal gains. This study and others emphasize the importance of appropriate preoperative parental counseling regarding expectations related to language acquisition in patients with autism spectrum disorder.

AN/AD describes a heterogeneous group of auditory processing abnormalities typically characterized by normal hair cell function with abnormal neural transmission. In older children and adults, a hallmark of diagnosis involves auditory perceptual deficits out of proportion with behavioral hearing levels. Presence of AN/AD affects postimplantation performance and prior research supports diverse outcomes in this group. For children (and adults) with AN/AD and minimal auditory capacity, multiple studies have confirmed CI outcomes commensurate with those of peers with other forms of SNHL.[64–66] However, recent evidence suggests that outcomes for a selected group of children with AN/AD treated with hearing aid amplification may equal or exceed those of children managed with CIs.[66,67] In addition, evidence exists for spontaneous recovery of AN/AD before 1 year of age.[64,68] Teagle and colleagues[67] (2010) examined 140 children with AN/AD of whom 52 (37%) received CIs. Although 50% of these children attained open-set speech perception skills after surgery, many were unable to participate in testing because of young age or developmental delay. Teagle and colleagues[67] (2010) and Rance and Barker[66] (2009) cautioned against CIs for all patients with AN/AD and instead suggested a stepwise management paradigm to better identify children who would benefit from amplification and those who are appropriate candidates for CIs.[66,67] Clearly a topic of ongoing debate, additional research is necessary to clarify issues of CI candidacy and performance in this population.

MEDICAL/SURGICAL ISSUES, INCLUDING ANATOMIC ABNORMALITIES, MENINGITIS, AND CHARGE SYNDROME

Optimal electrode placement is a prerequisite for maximizing CI success. Although numerous modifications to the cochlear implantation procedure exist, full atraumatic scala tympani electrode insertion is the goal of each surgery. Incorrect or suboptimal placement, or damaged or kinked electrodes can lead to suboptimal CI function or poor postoperative outcomes and may subject the patient to additional or revision surgery. A multitude of variables affect insertion, including anatomic abnormalities, characteristics of the electrode array itself, and surgical experience. Especially in patients with congenital cochlear malformations, such as common cavity, Mondini deformity, or hypoplastic cochlea, surgical experience can affect optimal electrode insertion and minimize complications. In anatomically challenging cases, familiarity and competence with fluoroscopic guidance is beneficial by allowing real-time visualization of electrode insertion.[69] Bending, kinking, roll-over, overinsertion, and placement in the internal auditory canal can be identified and addressed immediately. Because neural elements are likely located on the outer wall or septations with the cochlea, delicate electrode advancement helps reduce injury to these crucial structures. Experience and facility with a variety of electrode arrays, such as a straight electrode or double array, as well as surgical techniques such as fluoroscopy, are crucial for maximizing electrode insertion and, in turn, postoperative outcome in anatomically challenging cochleae.[69]

Most commonly caused by meningitis, cochlear ossification or labyrinthitis ossificans can result from otosclerosis, chronic otitis media, ototoxic agents, trauma (including iatrogenic), labyrinthine artery occlusion, ototoxic medications, leukemia, temporal bone tumors, viral infection, Wegener granulomatosis, and autoimmune and idiopathic processes. In these patients, degree of ossification is an important variable affecting performance. Up to 80% of patients with ossification have radiographic evidence of partial or complete obstruction of the proximal basal turn, thus preoperative imaging is important in surgical planning and electrode choice.[70] Postoperative performance of patients with significant intracochlear obstruction can be guarded and appropriate expectations should be discussed with both patients and their families before surgery. Although significant, long-term benefit from implantation has been documented, early intervention is encouraged to maximize electrode insertion and hearing outcomes.[71] In patients with meningitis, many of the previously mentioned variables may also affect their CI performance. Because of the frequent complexity of their health, medically necessary care can delay identification and treatment of hearing disorders, thereby increasing the age at implantation and length of auditory deprivation. In addition, neurologic compromise resulting from meningitic infection may introduce variables related to cognitive function.

As with some meningitic patients, patients with CHARGE syndrome exemplify the challenges presented by anatomic abnormalities combined with other disabilities. Characterized by coloboma of the eye (C), congenital heart defects (H), atresia or stenosis of the nasal choanae (A), retardation of growth or development and/or central nervous system anomalies (R), genital hypoplasia (G), and anomalies of the ear and/or deafness (E), children with CHARGE manifest a range of auditory impairments and frequent cochleovestibular abnormalities. Lanson and colleagues[72] (2007) showed varying, although consistently limited, auditory benefit from cochlear implantation, as shown by routine audiometry and the IT-MAIS in 10 patients with CHARGE syndrome.

PREOPERATIVE FUNCTION: HEARING LEVEL AND AUDITORY SPEECH PERFORMANCE

Preoperative hearing levels and measures of speech perception seem to have an effect on postoperative performance. In postlinguistically deafened adults and children, patients with high levels of preoperative hearing and speech understanding seem to perform better, although other variables, including those mentioned earlier such as device technology and age at implantation, may impart a greater effect on performance. Niparko and colleagues[27] (2010) and Arisi and colleagues[30] (2010) found preoperative hearing level to be one of several variables affecting CI performance in prelingually deafened children and adolescents, respectively. Adunka and colleagues[73] (2008) compared performance of 29 adult recipients of a standard, full-length CI with substantial preoperative residual hearing with age-matched controls without preoperative hearing. On measures of postoperative speech perception, they found no advantage of preoperative hearing level. As mentioned earlier, advances in electroacoustic stimulation (EAS) and hybrid electrode design have changed the parameters of CI candidacy to incorporate individuals with significant residual hearing in the low frequencies. Although a full discussion of EAS is beyond the scope of this article, the preservation of residual hearing seems to be an important determinant of postoperative performance, especially in challenging listening environments such as significant background noise and music appreciation. Extensive research in this area is ongoing and future studies are necessary to clarify the impact of hearing preservation on speech and hearing outcomes.

MODE OF COMMUNICATION, EDUCATION/REHABILITATIVE ENVIRONMENT

Regardless of preoperative mode of communication, both adult and pediatric CI recipients obtain speech perception benefit following cochlear implantation. Evidence suggests that individuals who, either primarily or exclusively, use oral communication (OC) before surgery perform better on tests of speech understanding following cochlear implantation. Because most deaf children are born to hearing parents, deaf children are commonly exposed to an early home life of oral communication. When OC and, to a lesser degree, total communication (TC) predominate in their educational environment, potentially by placement in a mainstream classroom setting, improved performance is seen on measures of speech perception and receptive and expressive language. As mentioned earlier, type and frequency of postimplantation rehabilitative services can greatly affect performance, and individualized education plans (IEPs) are a well-recognized tool to assist CI recipients to reach their full potential.

Exposure to a multilingual or bilingual environment has been investigated as a variable affecting language acquisition. Early research showed that successful acquisition of bilingual language proficiency in pediatric CI recipients and did not suggest a negative impact on CI performance.[74] Thomas and colleagues[75] (2008) found that exposure to a second language does not impair primary language (English) acquisition in unilaterally implanted children. Among German children implanted before 6 years old, Teschendorf and colleagues[76] (2010) suggested that speech and language performance in patients exposed to additional spoken languages were related to other factors such as compliance with the rehabilitation/educational program and parental/family support. Overall, data do not support exposure to a second language as a negative variable affecting CI performance.

AUDITORY TRAINING

An emerging area of CI research, studies suggest targeted auditory training and perceptual learning may positively affect CI performance in both adults and children.

Postoperative adaptation to electrically stimulated speech patterns produced by CIs seems to occur with passive, daily listening experiences. Evidence suggests that active auditory rehabilitation may accelerate or improve this adaptation and lead to improved speech recognition and music perception.[77–79] Initial testing in normal-hearing individuals showed that auditory training with spectrally shifted speech (an acoustic simulation of CI processing) improved speech recognition regardless of length of training period (ranging from 1 to 5 weeks).[80,81] Fu and Galvin[77] (2007) showed the effectiveness of a computer-assisted speech-training program used by adult, postlingually deafened patients with CIs at home on varying schedules. In prelingually deafened pediatric CI recipients, Chen and colleagues[79] (2010) found that use of a structured music training program improved pitch perception, with the degree of improvement related to duration of auditory training. Effects of auditory training can also be seen on neurophysiologic measures of cortical neural activity, specifically the N1-P2 complex.[82,83] Stimulus-specific auditory training increased left hemisphere P2 amplitudes in 13 normal-hearing subjects, and enhanced N1 pretraining amplitude seemed to predict above-average performance on posttraining testing.[83] Although preliminary, both clinical and neurophysiologic evidence supports auditory training–induced neural plasticity. Additional research is necessary to determine the full impact of auditory training on postimplantation performance.

SOCIAL FACTORS, INCLUDING SOCIOECONOMIC STATUS, PARENT/FAMILY EXPECTATIONS, AND MOTIVATION

Investigation into the relationship between socioeconomic status (SES) and CI performance stems from research in children with normal hearing for whom SES is a consistent and robust predictor of reading skills.[84] Epidemiology of pediatric cochlear implantation in the United States suggests a disparity among children with different ethnicity and SES in which minority children in lower SES groups have higher rates of SNHL but disproportionate rates of cochlear implantation.[85,86] In their prospective study of language development following cochlear implantation, Niparko and colleagues[27] (2010) found a relationship between SES and performance: children with higher SES showed greater rates of improvement in spoken language and comprehension. Higher family income predicted better baseline language performance as well as gains over time. However, multivariate analysis attenuated the influence of income and revealed bidirectional associations between SES, level of maternal education, and degree of maternal engagement in communication. In their comparison of patients with Medicaid versus private insurance, Chang and colleagues[87] (2010) found lower SES to be associated with higher rates of postoperative complications, decreased follow-up compliance, and lower rates of sequential bilateral implantation. However, they found that lower SES was not a barrier to access to cochlear implantation. A complex and multifactorial issue, data suggest that an impact of SES on performance must be carefully interpreted in the greater context of variables known to influence outcome.

Parental and family motivation and expectations are crucial variables affecting cochlear implantation outcomes and cannot be underestimated. As mentioned earlier, Niparko and colleagues[27] (2010) examined variables of maternal engagement in early communication, parental/caregiver mentoring, and early oral language exposure and found positive relationships with language performance in pediatric CI recipients. The importance of parental or caregiver involvement in postoperative rehabilitation is easy to identify, but direct effects on outcome are difficult to quantify. In practical terms, compliance with the demanding schedules of postoperative programming appointments and postimplantation rehabilitation requires significant parental and family commitment. Similarly essential are appropriate familial expectations regarding postoperative speech and language acquisition. Flexibility and understanding of the potential range of outcomes and variable rates of improvement are key to maximizing individual CI performance.

SUMMARY

Variables affecting performance with a CI are diverse, symbiotic, and continually evolving with advances in implant technology and ever-expanding candidacy criteria. Research into the factors discussed in this article, as well as their complex interrelationships, affords both clinicians and patients a greater understanding of postimplantation performance. The variables that are dominant in their effect on CI performance evolve with advances in implant technology, expanding candidacy groups, and a multitude of other factors. Even within an individual CI recipient, the significance of certain variables may change with time, with increasing patient age, new technology, or increased experience with the implant.

Despite remarkable auditory perception in most traditional CI recipients, considerable variability in performance remains incompletely understood. Attempts to characterize this significant variability, especially as it pertains to patients with unexpectedly poor performance, have focused on the multiplicity of variables discussed earlier. In the coming years, greater focus on issues of neural plasticity, cognition, auditory training, and sensitive periods for speech and language development will likely contribute to a greater understanding of variables affecting cochlear implantation outcome as well as clinical interventions for those with poor performance.

REFERENCES

1. Koch DB, Downing M, Osberger MJ, et al. Using current steering to increase spectral resolution in CII and HiRes 90K users. Ear Hear 2007;28(Suppl 2): 38S–41S.
2. Brendel M, Buechner A, Krueger B, et al. Evaluation of the Harmony soundprocessor in combination with the speech coding strategy HiRes 120. Otol Neurotol 2008;29(2):199–202.
3. Buechner A, Brendel M, Krueger B, et al. Current steering and results from novel speech coding strategies. Otol Neurotol 2008;29(2):203–7.
4. Firszt JB, Holden LK, Reeder RM, et al. Speech recognition in cochlear implant recipients: comparison of standard HiRes and HiRes 120 sound processing. Otol Neurotol 2009;30(2):146–52.
5. Landsberger DM, Srinivasan AG. Virtual channel discrimination is improved by current focusing in cochlear implant recipients. Hear Res 2009;254(1–2):34–41.
6. Chang YT, Yang HM, Lin YH, et al. Tone discrimination and speech perception benefit in Mandarin-speaking children fit with HiRes Fidelity 120 sound processing. Otol Neurotol 2009;30(6):750–7.
7. Lenarz T, Stover T, Buechner A, et al. Temporal bone results and hearing preservation with a new straight electrode. Audiol Neurootol 2006;11(Suppl 1):34–41.
8. Lenarz T, Stover T, Buechner A, et al. Hearing conservation surgery using the Hybrid-L electrode. Results from the first clinical trial at the Medical University of Hannover. Audiol Neurootol 2009;14(Suppl 1):22–31.
9. Buchner A, Schussler M, Battmer RD, et al. Impact of low-frequency hearing. Audiol Neurootol 2009;14(Suppl 1):8–13.

10. Roland JT, Shapiro WS, Waltzman SB. Preliminary results of Nucleus L24 in the United States. International Conference on Cochlear Implants and Other Auditory Implantable Technologies. Stockholm (Sweden), June 30–July 3, 2011.
11. Skarzynski H, Lorens A. Electric acoustic stimulation in children. Adv Otorhinolaryngol 2010;67:135–43.
12. Cosetti MK, Shapiro WH, Green JE, et al. Intraoperative neural response telemetry as a predictor of performance. Otol Neurotol 2010;31(7):1095–9.
13. Venail F, Sicard M, Piron JP, et al. Reliability and complications of 500 consecutive cochlear implantations. Arch Otolaryngol Head Neck Surg 2008;134(12):1276–81.
14. Trotter MI, Backhouse S, Wagstaff S, et al. Classification of cochlear implant failures and explantation: the Melbourne experience, 1982-2006. Cochlear Implants Int 2009;10(Suppl 1):105–10.
15. Zeitler DM, Budenz CL, Roland JT Jr. Revision cochlear implantation. Curr Opin Otolaryngol Head Neck Surg 2009;17(5):334–8.
16. Zeitler DM, Lalwani AK, Roland JT Jr, et al. The effects of cochlear implant electrode deactivation on speech perception and in predicting device failure. Otol Neurotol 2009;30(1):7–13.
17. Gosepath J, Lippert K, Keilmann A, et al. Analysis of fifty-six cochlear implant device failures. ORL J Otorhinolaryngol Relat Spec 2009;71(3):142–7.
18. Carlson ML, Archibald DJ, Dabade TS, et al. Prevalence and timing of individual cochlear implant electrode failures. Otol Neurotol 2010;31(6):893–8.
19. Waltzman SB, Roland JT Jr. Cochlear implantation in children younger than 12 months. Pediatrics 2005;116(4):e487–93.
20. Colletti V, Carner M, Miorelli V, et al. Cochlear implantation at under 12 months: report on 10 patients. Laryngoscope 2005;115(3):445–9.
21. Dettman SJ, Pinder D, Briggs RJ, et al. Communication development in children who receive the cochlear implant younger than 12 months: risks versus benefits. Ear Hear 2007;28(Suppl 2):11S–8S.
22. Tait M, De Raeve L, Nikolopoulos TP. Deaf children with cochlear implants before the age of 1 year: comparison of preverbal communication with normally hearing children. Int J Pediatr Otorhinolaryngol 2007;71(10):1605–11.
23. Holt RF, Svirsky MA. An exploratory look at pediatric cochlear implantation: is earliest always best? Ear Hear 2008;29(4):492–511.
24. Miyamoto RT, Hay-McCutcheon MJ, Kirk KI, et al. Language skills of profoundly deaf children who received cochlear implants under 12 months of age: a preliminary study. Acta Otolaryngol 2008;128(4):373–7.
25. Roland JT Jr, Cosetti M, Wang KH, et al. Cochlear implantation in the very young child: long-term safety and efficacy. Laryngoscope 2009;119(11):2205–10.
26. Tajudeen BA, Waltzman SB, Jethanamest D, et al. Speech perception in congenitally deaf children receiving cochlear implants in the first year of life. Otol Neurotol 2010;31(8):1254–60.
27. Niparko JK, Tobey EA, Thal DJ, et al. Spoken language development in children following cochlear implantation. JAMA 2010;303(15):1498–506.
28. Connor CM, Craig HK, Raudenbush SW, et al. The age at which young deaf children receive cochlear implants and their vocabulary and speech-production growth: is there an added value for early implantation? Ear Hear 2006;27(6):628–44.
29. Nott P, Cowan R, Brown PM, et al. Early language development in children with profound hearing loss fitted with a device at a young age: part I–the time period taken to acquire first words and first word combinations. Ear Hear 2009;30(5):526–40.

30. Arisi E, Forti S, Pagani D, et al. Cochlear implantation in adolescents with prelinguistic deafness. Otolaryngol Head Neck Surg 2010;142(6):804–8.
31. Mahncke HW, Bronstone A, Merzenich MM. Brain plasticity and functional losses in the aged: scientific bases for a novel intervention. Prog Brain Res 2006;157: 81–109.
32. Dickstein DL, Kabaso D, Rocher AB, et al. Changes in the structural complexity of the aged brain. Aging Cell 2007;6(3):275–84.
33. Eshraghi AA, Rodriguez M, Balkany TJ, et al. Cochlear implant surgery in patients more than seventy-nine years old. Laryngoscope 2009;119(6): 1180–3.
34. Budenz CL, Cosetti MK, Coelho DH, et al. The effects of cochlear implantation on speech perception in older adults. J Am Geriatr Soc 2010;59(3):446–53.
35. Carlson ML, Breen JT, Gifford RH, et al. Cochlear implantation in the octogenarian and nonagenarian. Otol Neurotol 2010;31(8):1343–9.
36. Zeitler DM, Kessler MA, Terushkin V, et al. Speech perception benefits of sequential bilateral cochlear implantation in children and adults: a retrospective analysis. Otol Neurotol 2008;29(3):314–25.
37. Laske RD, Veraguth D, Dillier N, et al. Subjective and objective results after bilateral cochlear implantation in adults. Otol Neurotol 2009;30(3):313–8.
38. Litovsky RY, Parkinson A, Arcaroli J. Spatial hearing and speech intelligibility in bilateral cochlear implant users. Ear Hear 2009;30(4):419–31.
39. Koch DB, Soli SD, Downing M, et al. Simultaneous bilateral cochlear implantation: prospective study in adults. Cochlear Implants Int 2010;11(2):84–99.
40. Litovsky R, Harris S, Born M. Acquisition of spatial hearing abilities in two-year-old children: role of auditory experience and bilateral cochlear implantation. J Acoust Soc Am 2010;128(4):2425.
41. Litovsky R, Misurelli S, Godar S. Source segregation in noisy environments by children with normal hearing and bilateral cochlear implants. J Acoust Soc Am 2010;128(4):2425.
42. Grieco-Calub TM, Litovsky RY. Sound localization skills in children who use bilateral cochlear implants and in children with normal acoustic hearing. Ear Hear 2010;31(5):645–56.
43. Godar SP, Litovsky RY. Experience with bilateral cochlear implants improves sound localization acuity in children. Otol Neurotol 2010;31(8):1287–92.
44. Sparreboom M, van Schoonhoven J, van Zanten BG, et al. The effectiveness of bilateral cochlear implants for severe-to-profound deafness in children: a systematic review. Otol Neurotol 2010;31(7):1062–71.
45. Mok M, Galvin KL, Dowell RC, et al. Speech perception benefit for children with a cochlear implant and a hearing aid in opposite ears and children with bilateral cochlear implants. Audiol Neurootol 2010;15(1):44–56.
46. Van Deun L, van Wieringen A, Scherf F, et al. Earlier intervention leads to better sound localization in children with bilateral cochlear implants. Audiol Neurootol 2010;15(1):7–17.
47. Dunn CC, Noble W, Tyler RS, et al. Bilateral and unilateral cochlear implant users compared on speech perception in noise. Ear Hear 2010;31(2):296–8.
48. Galvin KL, Mok M, Dowell RC, et al. Speech detection and localization results and clinical outcomes for children receiving sequential bilateral cochlear implants before four years of age. Int J Audiol 2008;47(10):636–46.
49. Scherf F, Van Deun L, van Wieringen A, et al. Subjective benefits of sequential bilateral cochlear implantation in young children after 18 months of implant use. ORL J Otorhinolaryngol Relat Spec 2009;71(2):112–21.

50. Summerfield AQ, Lovett RE, Bellenger H, et al. Estimates of the cost-effectiveness of pediatric bilateral cochlear implantation. Ear Hear 2010;31(5): 611–24.
51. Mok M, Galvin KL, Dowell RC, et al. Spatial unmasking and binaural advantage for children with normal hearing, a cochlear implant and a hearing aid, and bilateral implants. Audiol Neurootol 2007;12(5):295–306.
52. Bond M, Mealing S, Anderson R, et al. The effectiveness and cost-effectiveness of cochlear implants for severe to profound deafness in children and adults: a systematic review and economic model. Health Technol Assess 2009;13(44): 1–330.
53. Budenz CL, Roland JT Jr, Babb J, et al. Effect of cochlear implant technology in sequentially bilaterally implanted adults. Otol Neurotol 2009;30(6):731–5.
54. Eapen RJ, Buss E, Adunka MC, et al. Hearing-in-noise benefits after bilateral simultaneous cochlear implantation continue to improve 4 years after implantation. Otol Neurotol 2009;30(2):153–9.
55. Chang SA, Tyler RS, Dunn CC, et al. Performance over time on adults with simultaneous bilateral cochlear implants. J Am Acad Audiol 2010;21(1):35–43.
56. Chilosi AM, Comparini A, Scusa MF, et al. Neurodevelopmental disorders in children with severe to profound sensorineural hearing loss: a clinical study. Dev Med Child Neurol 2010;52(9):856–62.
57. Berrettini S, Forli F, Genovese E, et al. Cochlear implantation in deaf children with associated disabilities: challenges and outcomes. Int J Audiol 2008;47(4): 199–208.
58. Wiley S, Jahnke M, Meinzen-Derr J, et al. Perceived qualitative benefits of cochlear implants in children with multi-handicaps. Int J Pediatr Otorhinolaryngol 2005;69(6):791–8.
59. Holt RF, Kirk KI. Speech and language development in cognitively delayed children with cochlear implants. Ear Hear 2005;26(2):132–48.
60. Meinzen-Derr J, Wiley S, Grether S, et al. Language performance in children with cochlear implants and additional disabilities. Laryngoscope 2010;120(2):405–13.
61. Meinzen-Derr J, Wiley S, Grether S, et al. Children with cochlear implants and developmental disabilities: a language skills study with developmentally matched hearing peers. Res Dev Disabil 2011;32(2):757–67.
62. Donaldson AI, Heavner KS, Zwolan TA. Measuring progress in children with autism spectrum disorder who have cochlear implants. Arch Otolaryngol Head Neck Surg 2004;130(5):666–71.
63. Daneshi A, Hassanzadeh S. Cochlear implantation in prelingually deaf persons with additional disability. J Laryngol Otol 2007;121(7):635–8.
64. Rance G. Auditory neuropathy/dys-synchrony and its perceptual consequences. Trends Amplif 2005;9(1):1–43.
65. Gibson WP, Sanli H. Auditory neuropathy: an update. Ear Hear 2007;28(Suppl 2): 102S–6S.
66. Rance G, Barker EJ. Speech and language outcomes in children with auditory neuropathy/dys-synchrony managed with either cochlear implants or hearing aids. Int J Audiol 2009;48(6):313–20.
67. Teagle HF, Roush PA, Woodard JS, et al. Cochlear implantation in children with auditory neuropathy spectrum disorder. Ear Hear 2010;31(3):325–35.
68. Raveh E, Buller N, Badrana O, et al. Auditory neuropathy: clinical characteristics and therapeutic approach. Am J Otolaryngol 2007;28(5):302–8.
69. Coelho DH, Waltzman SB, Roland JT Jr. Implanting common cavity malformations using intraoperative fluoroscopy. Otol Neurotol 2008;29(7):914–9.

70. Jackler RK, Luxford WM, Schindler RA, et al. Cochlear patency problems in cochlear implantation. Laryngoscope 1987;97(7 Pt 1):801–5.
71. Philippon D, Bergeron F, Ferron P, et al. Cochlear implantation in postmeningitic deafness. Otol Neurotol 2010;31(1):83–7.
72. Lanson BG, Green JE, Roland JT Jr, et al. Cochlear implantation in children with CHARGE syndrome: therapeutic decisions and outcomes. Laryngoscope 2007; 117(7):1260–6.
73. Adunka OF, Buss E, Clark MS, et al. Effect of preoperative residual hearing on speech perception after cochlear implantation. Laryngoscope 2008;118(11): 2044–9.
74. Waltzman SB, Robbins AM, Green JE, et al. Second oral language capabilities in children with cochlear implants. Otol Neurotol 2003;24(5):757–63.
75. Thomas E, El-Kashlan H, Zwolan TA. Children with cochlear implants who live in monolingual and bilingual homes. Otol Neurotol 2008;29(2):230–4.
76. Teschendorf M, Janeschik S, Bagus H, et al. Speech development after cochlear implantation in children from bilingual homes. Otol Neurotol 2011;32(2):229–35.
77. Fu QJ, Galvin JJ 3rd. Perceptual learning and auditory training in cochlear implant recipients. Trends Amplif 2007;11(3):193–205.
78. Fu QJ, Galvin JJ 3rd. Maximizing cochlear implant patients' performance with advanced speech training procedures. Hear Res 2008;242(1–2):198–208.
79. Chen JK, Chuang AY, McMahon C, et al. Music training improves pitch perception in prelingually deafened children with cochlear implants. Pediatrics 2010; 125(4):e793–800.
80. Fu QJ, Nogaki G. Noise susceptibility of cochlear implant users: the role of spectral resolution and smearing. J Assoc Res Otolaryngol 2005;6(1):19–27.
81. Nogaki G, Fu QJ, Galvin JJ 3rd. Effect of training rate on recognition of spectrally shifted speech. Ear Hear 2007;28(2):132–40.
82. Tremblay KL, Kraus N. Auditory training induces asymmetrical changes in cortical neural activity. J Speech Lang Hear Res 2002;45(3):564–72.
83. Tremblay KL, Shahin AJ, Picton T, et al. Auditory training alters the physiological detection of stimulus-specific cues in humans. Clin Neurophysiol 2009;120(1): 128–35.
84. Connor CM, Zwolan TA. Examining multiple sources of influence on the reading comprehension skills of children who use cochlear implants. J Speech Lang Hear Res 2004;47(3):509–26.
85. Stern RE, Yueh B, Lewis C, et al. Recent epidemiology of pediatric cochlear implantation in the United States: disparity among children of different ethnicity and socioeconomic status. Laryngoscope 2005;115(1):125–31.
86. Mehra S, Eavey RD, Keamy DG Jr. The epidemiology of hearing impairment in the United States: newborns, children, and adolescents. Otolaryngol Head Neck Surg 2009;140(4):461–72.
87. Chang DT, Ko AB, Murray GS, et al. Lack of financial barriers to pediatric cochlear implantation: impact of socioeconomic status on access and outcomes. Arch Otolaryngol Head Neck Surg 2010;136(7):648–57.

Language Outcomes After Cochlear Implantation

Hillary Ganek, MA, CCC-SLP, LSLS Cert. AVT[a],*,
Amy McConkey Robbins, MS, CCC-SLP[b], John K. Niparko, MD[a]

KEYWORDS

- Family-centered intervention
- Sound and symbol correspondence • Auditory training
- Incidental learning • Total communication
- Oral communication

Whereas the impact of hearing loss in an adult varies considerably, the impact of a sensorineural hearing loss in infancy and early childhood can be pervasive. Virtually every aspect of communication and spoken language learning is supported by early access to the phonology of speech.[1]

For more than 2 decades, the proportion of cochlear implants (CIs) provided to young children with hearing loss has increased. Auditory thresholds of children with CIs provide improved access to auditory information beyond that available to deaf children using conventional amplification (hearing aids), offering a critical substrate for auditory learning.[2] To the extent that a CI can encode the sounds of speech with precision, the device can provide opportunities for learning spoken language.

LANGUAGE ACQUISITION IN CHILDREN WITH CIs

The primary goal of implantation in children is to facilitate communication in the modality that is native to the families of the vast majority of deaf children: spoken language. Language is defined as a vehicle for shaping and relating abstractions for communication[3] in which meaning is independent of the immediate situation. Practical use of speech is based on the assignment of a single name to various appearances and situations under varying conditions. Spoken language involves a conversion of thought into speech, and relies on mental representations of phonological (sound) structure and syntactic (phrase) structure.[3] The CI, because it provides improved access to sound and phrase structure, may improve spoken language outcomes.

[a] Department of Otolaryngology–Head and Neck Surgery, The Listening Center at Johns Hopkins, The Johns Hopkins University, 601 North Caroline Street, Baltimore, MD 21287, USA
[b] Communication Consulting Services, 8512 Spring Mill Road, Indianapolis, IN 46260, USA
* Corresponding author.
E-mail address: hganek1@jhmi.edu

Otolaryngol Clin N Am 45 (2012) 173–185
doi:10.1016/j.otc.2011.08.024
0030-6665/12/$ – see front matter © 2012 Elsevier Inc. All rights reserved.

oto.theclinics.com

Published studies now provide substantial evidence regarding the effects of CIs on language development in children. Robbins[4] has identified trends that have emerged from those studies:

Earlier Age at CI is Associated with Better Communication Development

This finding is robust and has been verified in multiple studies by researchers using different assessment tools. The research literature suggests a substantial advantage for language acquisition in children receiving their CIs at young ages in comparison with older ages.[5–7] Niparko and colleagues[8] used a controlled prospective, longitudinal, multisite design to evaluate age at implantation in relation to spoken language development as part of the Childhood Development after Cochlear Implantation (CDaCI) study. Children implanted prior to18 months of age followed language development trajectories similar to hearing peers. Implantation after 18 months created less favorable trajectories.

These findings should compel us to examine just how early deaf children may need to receive a CI if language-learning gaps relative to hearing children are to be avoided. Even for children whose language-learning rate after implantation does not match that of normal-hearing (NH) peers, rates postimplantation have been shown to be consistently faster than those established preimplantation. In addition, higher increases in comprehension and expression were associated with greater residual hearing before implantation, higher parent-child interaction scores, and higher socioeconomic status.[8]

Nicholas and Geers[9] used spontaneous language samples and the Preschool Language Scale to evaluate 76 children whose age at cochlear implantation ranged from 12 to 36 months and who had used oral-only communication since implantation. Children implanted at the youngest ages, between 12 and 16 months, were more likely to achieve age-appropriate spoken language. By contrast, children implanted after 24 months of age did not catch up with NH peers when tested at age 4.5 years. The investigators concluded that children who receive a CI as late as age 3 years may experience great difficulty catching up with NH age mates.

Manrique and colleagues[10] studied 130 CI children using the Peabody Picture Vocabulary Test and the Reynell Scales. Their findings suggested that children implanted before 2 years of age exhibited better language development than those implanted after age 2.

The effect of age at cochlear implantation was studied using scores from the Infant-Toddler Meaningful Auditory Integration Scale (IT-MAIS) in 3 groups of children who had received a CI at the age of 12 to 18 months, 19 to 23 months, or 24 to 36 months, respectively.[11] Scores from each age group, obtained at pre-CI, then at 3, 6, and 12 months post-CI, were compared with IT-MAIS scores obtained from a large group of children with normal hearing.[12] The results were consistent with those cited above: The most impressive scores were obtained from children in the youngest-implanted group, in which more than half of the subjects achieved scores after 6 months of CI use that matched the scores of NH peers. Although substantial gains in scores associated with CI use were also obtained from the two groups implanted at older ages, the trend was less dramatic for those implanted between ages 19 and 23 months, and still less dramatic for those implanted between ages 24 and 36 months. In addition, the scatter in scores was much wider for the oldest than the youngest group, indicating that it became harder to predict post-CI performance as children's age at implantation increased.

The basis for improving the language-learning trajectory with young age at CI relates to sensitive periods and neural plasticity. Using the latency of the P1 cortical auditory evoked potential as a measure of central auditory pathway maturity, Sharma and colleagues[13] found that children implanted at 3.5 years or younger showed age-appropriate latency responses by 6 months post-CI. These investigators concluded that in the absence of normal stimulation, a sensitive period persists for about 3.5 years during which the human central auditory system remains maximally plastic.[13]

Other central nervous system factors play a role in language outcomes. For example, there is superior potential for younger children to learn language incidentally. Although children who are older at the time of CI may still benefit from incidental learning, it is likely that their rehabilitation and environment will need to address greater deficits.

Improved speech processing strategies provide more communication enhancement. The amount and quality of information provided by the speech processor has a measurable effect on language. Data from Geers and colleagues[14] have shown that children whose CIs were upgraded on a regular basis with state-of-the-art speech-processing improvements outperformed children using older speech-processing technologies. A wide dynamic range and optimal growth of loudness characteristics contribute substantially to a child's ability to hear speech. Accordingly, outdated processors should be revised in favor of technology that can enhance the child's listening experience.

Children with CIs Outperform their Profoundly Deaf Peers Who Use Hearing Aids

Faster rates of language learning and higher overall language achievement levels are consistently documented in CI children relative to their unimplanted, deaf peers.[6,15] The average profoundly deaf child with hearing aids learns language at about half the rate of NH children, acquiring 6 months of language in 1 year's time.[6,16,17] This trend for deaf children to acquire language, on average, at only about half the level of NH peers is found repeatedly in the literature, going back to such studies as those by Osberger.[18] If the thresholds of hearing for a profoundly deaf child are improved to a level those similar to those experienced by a hard-of-hearing child,[19,20] this conversion represents an enormous improvement in auditory learning potential, given the differences in performance that have been documented between children with profound versus aidable sensorineural hearing loss.

CIs Enable Some Children to Acquire Language at a Rate Similar to that of Normal-Hearing Children

The CI changes the trajectory of spoken language learning in most recipients, elevating the rate of learning relative to the pre-CI period. Several studies demonstrated that the average child who received a CI learned approximately 1 year of language in 1 year's time.[6,21,22] Blamey and colleagues[23] documented a rate of language learning in a group of CI children that was considerably slower than that reported in other studies.[6,8,23,24] However, some children in the Blamey and colleagues[23] study had not received their CI until as late as age 8 years, a factor that likely contributed to the more modest improvements in language. As more data have been analyzed, especially from large-scale studies,[8] it is clear that language outcomes are substantially more favorable if implantation occurs before a wide and persistent gap develops between chronologic and language age. In addition, it is estimated that 40% of deaf children have additional disabilities.[25,26] An increasing number of children from that group, which makes up a substantial percentage of all deaf children, are receiving CIs. Among that group, a language-learning rate comparable to that of children with normal hearing would be the exception rather than the rule. This finding underscores the need to consider that certain conditions should prompt a thorough consideration.

Many Children Remain Delayed in their Language Skills Even After Implantation

In a nationwide sample of 8- to 9-year-olds who received a CI between 24 and 35 months of age, only 43% achieved combined speech and language skills within the average range, relative to NH peers.[27] Recall that significant delays in language development already exist in most children by the time they receive their CI, even in those who are implanted early. As Tyszkiewicz and Stokes[28] note, a 2-year-old hearing child has a highly tuned auditory system used since birth, generating a large auditory repertoire. The 2-year-old who is implanted has a very different starting position, with little of this knowledge in place. To prevent a continued delay, children must either learn language at a rate faster than normal after CI, or receive their CIs early enough to prevent an insurmountable chronologic language gap from forming in the first place. Unfortunately, language-learning rates that exceed those of hearing children are rare.

A Wide Range of Language Benefit is Observed Across Children

Studies of language ability in CI children consistently yield a wide range of performance outcomes. This wide range is found in virtually every study of CI users and requires that data be interpreted with caution, particularly when these data are presented as average performance. Large standard deviations in data limit the usefulness of looking at "average" scores. Regardless of the specific device used, some children do extremely well with their implants, performing at the upper end of the continuum, whereas a small number of children receive limited benefit from their implants. The attempt to identify the factors that might account for this variability requires a multivariate use.

Children Using both Oral and Total Communication Improve in their Language Skills After CI; but as a Group, Oral Communication Users Outperform Those Using Total Communication

This trend is robust, having been reported in a variety of observational studies[7,22,29] using different assessment procedures. However, these studies are without controls, thus preventing analyses of covariates and confounders (eg, those related to specifics of the hearing history and the family environment). Underlying language skills are the domain in which total communication (TC) children with CIs have competed most favorably with oral communication (OC) children, when each group of children is tested in its preferred modality—that is, TC children tested in sign plus speech, OC children tested in oral-only mode. Under these conditions, Geers and colleagues[22] found no significant differences in language comprehension or verbal reasoning between OC and TC children with CIs who were implanted by age 5 years. However, better performance of the OC children emerged when other aspects of language were assessed, including expressive vocabulary, morphosyntactic use, utterance length, and narrative form—all measured via spontaneous language samples. This advantage of the OC over the TC group was apparent even when the TC children were credited with signed as well as oral productions.

As mentioned, methodological challenges persist in this research related to confounding influences. TC and OC children may not be equal at the start of their intervention. It is not clear whether the mechanisms by which language is enhanced via a CI are the same for children using OC and TC. These studies almost all used subjects implanted before the age of 5 years. If children with long-standing profound deafness are implanted when they are older than 4 years, the likelihood that they will require sign to augment language learning is very high.[30] This is especially true for language presented in academic settings where the pace of presentation is rapid and the amount of material introduced is voluminous. The advantages of the OC over the TC group have been even more striking in studies assessing speech perception and speech production in children with CIs.[31,32]

Grammatical Development, Including Syntax and Morphology, is Mastered More Slowly than Other Language Skills in Children with CIs

Even in CI children who demonstrate language comprehension within the average range, expressive use of morphologic markers is often delayed.[5,15,16,22,29] Deficits in this domain also persist longer than deficits in other language areas in NH children with specific language impairment,[33,34] suggesting that morphosyntactic skills are a fragile aspect of language, vulnerable to delays. This vulnerability is compounded for children with hearing loss because morphologic markers are almost always in word-final position in English, and consist of high-frequency consonants such as s, z, and t that are often poorly audible, especially in conversation.[35]

Cochlear implantation also affects the development of early communication skills such as eye contact and turn-taking. Tait and Lutman[36] found that these skills begin to develop within 6 months of implantation.

LITERACY SKILLS IN CHILDREN WITH CIs

The nature of a child's language development, whether manual or oral, will depend on the quantity and quality of exposure to a complete language system. Early and appropriate language stimulation appears to be an important factor in the acquisition of visual language as manifest in comprehension (reading) and expression (writing), as well as in acquisition of spoken language. For example, reading comprehension ability among deaf 15-year-old students who use American Sign Language as their primary mode of communication is at the third-grade level, whereas the average 15-year-old hearing student reads at a tenth-grade level.[37]

Reading requires a combination of abilities including sound and symbol correspondence, strong vocabulary skills, and an extensive world knowledge. Sound symbol is the ability to decode a word by associating written letters with the reader's phonologic system. Historically, children who are deaf have not been able to access the entire phonologic system. Therefore they have relied more on whole-word recognition than on sound and symbol correspondence. Strong vocabulary skills allow readers to apply more cognitive analysis to processing complex syntax and become more successful readers.[38,39] Children who are deaf typically have vocabulary deficits likely rooted in limitations in phonological processing, particularly those referencing abstract concepts.[40] Such deficits can prevent the full processing capacity needed to understand higher-level texts.

Early readers bring their world knowledge to their first literacy experiences. Children who are deaf often face a parent-child communication barrier that prevents exposure to the kinds of conversation about higher-level abstract concepts that provides hearing peers with a foundation for reading comprehension.[41] Without these preliteracy skills, children without access to sound struggle to develop age-appropriate reading skills.[42]

Data reported by Tomblin and colleagues[15] indicate that reading levels among schoolchildren with CIs, however, approaches that of their hearing peers with extended CI experience. Geers[43] notes that whereas many children with CIs achieve literacy skills within the average range for their hearing peers, others do not do as well. High nonverbal IQ scores, good CI function, an oral mode of communication, and overall language competence including comprehension, production, and the use of narrative forms are all associated with better literacy outcomes.[44,45]

Pisoni and Geers[46] investigated the impact of working memory on measures of speech perception, speech intelligibility, language processing, and reading in implanted children with prelingual deafness. The investigators evaluated correlations between children's ability to recall lists of digits presented in the auditory-only modality and their performance on these measures. Moderate to high correlations were found between auditory memory and performance in each outcome area, suggesting that working memory plays an important role in mediating performance across these higher communication tasks. Pisoni and Geers postulate that there is commonality in the perceptual processes used in these tasks. The ability to formally register speech sounds, coupled with rehearsal, can be used to encode and retrieve the representations of spoken words from lexical memory.

AUDITORY REHABILITATION AFTER COCHLEAR IMPLANTATION

The uniqueness of the listening experience enabled by a CI is underscored by qualitative differences in how sound perception is elicited in comparison with other strategies of auditory rehabilitation. For example, a hearing aid filters, amplifies, and compresses the acoustic signal, thereby delivering a processed signal to the cochlea for transduction. By contrast, a CI receives, processes, and transmits acoustic information by generating electrical fields. Electrical stimulation bypasses nonfunctional cochlear transducers and directly depolarizes auditory nerve fibers. Implant systems convey an electrical code based in those selected features of speech that are critical to phoneme and word understanding in normal listeners, without the advantages of signal preparation provided by cochlear mechanisms of sound processing that render complex sounds listenable and discriminable. As noted, the CI listening experience also differs from normal audition in the timing of when that experience begins. These factors directly affect CI rehabilitation.

Rehabilitation needs should be considered in the context of prelingual versus postlingual onset of deafness. The postlingually deafened child, having experienced profound hearing loss after the acquisition of language, typically shows more rapid improvements in speech recognition with the device.[47] From an auditory training perspective, postlingually deafened children are often characterized as more like the postlingually deafened adult than like the prelingually deaf child. Rehabilitation with the postlingually deafened child is often short term, with emphasis on communication strategies and on mapping the new percepts from the implant onto an existing linguistic code. By contrast, the prelingually deaf child with a CI must use information from the implant to develop such a code de novo, with early auditory training necessarily emphasizing early constructs of spoken language.

Robbins[4] described 12 guiding premises, reiterated here, that underlie the rehabilitation for prelingually deaf children with CIs. These premises are the synthesis of research findings and clinical experience with a broad range of implanted children. The reader will note that much of what enhances learning in CI children is consistent with developmental learning in all children. Because the sensory deficit in the case of deaf children with CIs interferes with spoken language acquisition, developmental approaches, while still allowing a child to gain insights into comprehension and production, need to be taken to their fullest extent over a protracted period of time.

PREMISES 1 AND 2: OVERARCHING GOALS
Premise 1. The Child Must Learn to Attach Meaning to What is Heard Through the CI

To learn a spoken language via a CI, two conditions must be met. First, the listener must have sufficient (not necessarily perfect) auditory access to the language code—the vowels, consonants, and suprasegmental patterns that make up that language. In other words, one must be able to hear a language to learn it. Auditory access is essential, but not sufficient, for language acquisition. A second, critical condition must also be met: The sounds must gradually be attached to meaning. Attaching meaning to the sounds transmitted by a CI is a critical task, whether it is a postlingual child who must remap the new signal onto an existing linguistic code or a child with prelingual deafness who must develop the code de novo. The CI and its technology provide access, but rehabilitation, parental follow-up, a nurturing listening- and spoken-language environment at home and at school, and the child's emergent cognitive ability is necessary to allow him or her to create the opportunities for meaning to be established. The older the child at the time of implantation, the more specific and intensive the training must be to ensure that sound is rendered meaningful.

Premise 2. The Ultimate Goal for All Children with Hearing Loss, Including Those with CIs, is Communicative Competence

This premise means that the child can adequately express and understand human communication at a level commensurate with his or her age and/or cognitive ability. Modes of communication for children with hearing loss are on a spectrum from mostly oral to mostly visual (**Fig. 1**). Some children with CIs will learn to rely heavily on their listening abilities. For others, communicative competence will include the use of sign language or cued speech, either full-time or only in academic settings, or only for receptive clarification. There is an assumption, though, that if parents have sought a CI, they value their child's auditory and spoken language skills and intend to devote energy to improving them. Not all families of children with hearing loss share these values, and parent choice should always be respected. Parents should be encouraged to select the options for their child that reflect the values they hold as parents, consistent with their goals for their child's future.

PREMISES 3, 4, 5: THE LEARNING ENVIRONMENT
Premise 3. Skills Learned in a Therapy Setting Must be Transferred Out of the Therapy Room and into the Classroom, Home, and Other Aspects of the Child's Everyday World

Clinicians must develop and practice skills within the therapy room but always with the greater goal that those skills will generalize out of the therapy room, into the child's classroom, home setting, and other everyday environments.

Studies and clinical experience support the notion that the parents are primary agents in their child's communicative competence and overall development.[48,49] Clinicians should view their role largely as one of helping parents facilitate their child's communication progress all day, every day, within the typical range of activities and interactions that comprise family life. For older children whose parents are not at school every day, it is especially important to convey the message that parents are

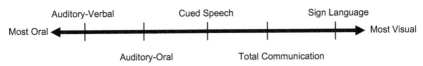

Fig. 1. Communication methods for children with hearing impairment are found on a spectrum ranging from completely oral to completely visual. Each family must choose what place on the spectrum best fits their needs.

essential to their child's success. Sharing of information between home and school has great benefit for all involved and can be accomplished in a variety of ways, including through a communication notebook that travels from home to school and back. Parents can also be encouraged to complete an interview such as the Children's Home Inventory for Listening Difficulties (CHILD) that reflects the child's auditory behaviors in the home. Clinical experience suggests that strong parental involvement can sometimes negate the effects of a weak educational setting, whereas the reverse is far less likely.

Premise 4. Rehabilitation Sessions Should Integrate Goals of Speech, Language, Perception, and Pragmatics Within an Environment that has Appropriate Social/Emotional Context

Compelled by law and school policy, clinicians typically write rehabilitation plans that compartmentalize the various domains of communication, writing separate goals for the child in each of these domains. In essence, as clinicians we break apart the complex, unified phenomenon of communication into artificially separate pieces. Our challenge in rehabilitation is to address those goals but to do so in a way that integrates or reunifies the pieces into a whole. This goal is one that is not always achievable in every rehabilitation session. Sometimes we must practice and over-learn a particular skill through a traditional drill method that is unlike natural communication. This practice is acceptable, as long as the clinician seeks to put that skill back into purposeful communication as soon as the child is capable. We seek to use what Fey[24] has termed a "hybrid" approach to intervention, balancing structured practice with naturalistic interactions.

Premise 5. Parents are the Most Potent Influence on the Child's Progress

Due to the identification of hearing loss in babies via universal newborn hearing screening (UNHS) in the United States and other countries, and the growing number of children with hearing loss implanted as infants and toddlers, an increasing number of clinicians are serving this population. Some clinicians are not trained to work with babies or to provide services within a model of family-centered intervention. Such intervention focuses on the parents and the family as a whole, rather than on therapizing the child with a CI (**Fig. 2**). Moeller[48] cites statistics from Dunst[49] that 2 hours per week, perhaps spent in therapy, make up only 2% of a toddler's waking hours,

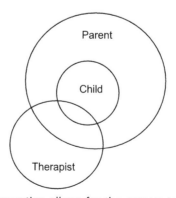

Fig. 2. Family-centered intervention allows for the parents to be the primary language models for their children just as they are for hearing children. The therapist guides and coaches the parents rather than focusing solely on the child with a cochlear implant.

whereas everyday activities such as diapering and feeding occur at least 2000 times before the child's first birthday. This statistic is a convincing statement about the power of families, rather than clinicians, to be the change agents in their child's communication after cochlear implantation. Parents who take advantage of only 10 interactions each waking hour of a child's day will have provided more than 36,000 teachable moments between ages 1 and 2 years.[48]

PREMISES 6 TO 10: CONTENT AND EXPERIENCE
Premise 6. Almost All Children with CIs Require a Combination of Didactic Instruction and Incidental Learning to Acquire Spoken Language

Auditory development in children with profound deafness has been traditionally viewed as requiring rote training. This viewpoint implied that the child required didactic instruction to achieve each of the listening skills along a hierarchy of auditory development, and virtually hundreds of such skills were required to achieve mastery. The assumption was that the child learned only what was directly taught.

This approach was not unreasonable, given limitations in conveying the highly nuanced information contained in speech to deaf children before the advent of multichannel CIs. That is, many profoundly deaf children with hearing aids were pattern perceivers, able to recognize only patterns of auditory information rather than discriminate the fine temporal and spectral structure of speech.

In fact, CIs provide the potential for deaf children to make use of incidental learning to an unprecedented degree. Incidental spontaneous learning provides the means by which NH children acquire spoken language and, theoretically, provides the most efficient, socially motivated, and naturalistic way to learn a native language. Nevertheless, the signal provided by the implant is not complete; even CI recipients using state-of-the-art speech-processing technology receive a degraded auditory signal. In addition, many children receive a CI after a period of auditory deprivation during which they have learned to process information visually. Even with the improved auditory signal provided by the CI, these youngsters may need systematic and intensive training to reach their full auditory potential. Thus, both didactic instruction and incidental learning have advantages for the CI child. In general, the older the child is at the time of cochlear implantation, the more structured, didactic instruction is generally required in rehabilitation.

Premise 7. A Diagnostic Teaching Approach to CI Therapy Yields the Most Benefit, Both to Children and to Parents and Teachers

Such an approach seeks to identify what the child can do and to adjust the level of difficulty of tasks. Here, the child is always challenged to achieve greater communication autonomy while the conditions that can either enhance or impede learning are always under assessment. This approach stands in contrast to a traditional therapy approach in which goals are set for a child and in each session similar activities are used. The underlying assumption of a traditional approach is that, with continued practice over multiple sessions, a child will increase the accuracy of the skill—a "practice makes perfect" philosophy. This approach is reinforced by the way individualized education programs are usually written, often using a format such as "Johnny will demonstrate x skill x number of times using a set of x alternative responses with x% accuracy."

In a diagnostic teaching approach the setting of appropriate individual goals is still critical, but the clinician uses the child's performance during each session to determine directions needed for subsequent sessions. If a child is successful with an activity under quiet conditions in a session, the child practices it during the next session to reach a level of automaticity, then the activity is made more challenging in the following session. The clinician continually monitors which factors are favorable or unfavorable to the child's learning, focusing prominently on the positive aspect of the question: "What are the things that help this child learn most efficiently?" A diagnostic teaching approach works well for a flexible and creative clinician who is willing to try new things, knowing that even if a technique fails with a child, something valuable has been learned—that is, what approach *not* to use. Clinicians can team up with the classroom teacher to share factors identified in therapy that may be useful or challenging to the child in the classroom setting, and vice versa.

Premise 8. Content from a Child's Educational Program Should be Used as Material in Rehabilitation for Maximum Reinforcement and Most Efficient Use of Instructional Time

Rather than using stimuli unrelated to the child's other goals, clinicians are encouraged to use concepts, vocabulary, music, and other current classroom materials within therapy activities. Clinicians who assure teachers that their goal is to make the teacher's job easier, not harder, will often build alliances with regular education staff that promote goodwill throughout the child's years at the school. These alliances become all the more important as a greater number of children with CIs are fully included in regular education settings.

Premise 9. Music is a Complex Auditory Experience that Dovetails with Auditory and Spoken Language Development and, Thus, Should be Integrated Within Intervention

An increasing number of research and observational reports suggest that CI children seek out and appreciate music to a degree that is qualitatively different from that of adults who receive CIs.[50–53] Clinical experience strongly supports the use of music as an integral component, rather than a separate domain, of rehabilitation with CI children. There are multiple beneficial effects of integrating music into a therapy session and encouraging its use at home, including articulation suprasegmental accuracy, language development, listening development, social skills and turn taking, and cultural assimilation.

Premise 10. Infants and Toddlers with Implants Require an Approach that is Quite Different from that for Children Implanted After this Age. Therapy with CI Babies is Not Just About Developing Words or Auditory Skills

Early communication skills are seen to flow from experiences in which an infant and caregiver share affective states, joint attention, and intentions to communicate.[54] Communicative abilities that develop during infancy form the foundation for emerging language. Clinicians should emphasize the importance of parents providing stimulating communication to infants as a key step in their development.

PREMISES 11 AND 12: MONITORING PROGRESS
Premise 11. Auditory Milestones that have been Established May be Used to "Red Flag" Children who are Progressing at a Slower than Expected Rate

Research and clinical findings have documented the auditory milestones achieved by the average child with a CI during the first year of device use.[11,30,55,56] Three different groups of CI children reflect different preimplant characteristics and show different patterns of skill achievement. When a child is identified as progressing at a slower rate than expected, red flags are raised and specific steps taken, allowing clinicians to intervene as early as possible and identify the source of the problem.[57]

Premise 12. Formal Assessment Tools, Although Important for Monitoring Progress, May Paint an Inadequate Picture of a CI Child's Overall Competence with Spoken Language

Formal assessments conducted with CI children are necessary to support a format of progress in the child's communication.[21] However, careful analysis of results is warranted. The problem lies in the interpretation of the tests, not in the tests themselves. Because tests other than spontaneous language samples are artificial measures of language that use probes such as picture pointing of 4 pictured choices, they may bear little resemblance to real-life communication demands. Children with hearing loss often have extensive experience with this type of format, and may perform well on structured tests that have a repetitive nature. Therefore, interpretations should be cautious when children with CIs score within the average range on test instruments, because these instruments may not be sensitive to the more subtle and higher-level demands of inference, problem solving, and topic shifts that characterize real-world conversation.[58]

REFERENCES

1. Berliner K, Eisenberg L. Methods and issues in the cochlear implantation of children: an overview. Ear Hear 1985;6(Suppl 3):6S–13S.
2. Ling D. Foundations of spoken language for hearing impaired children. Washington, DC: Alexander Graham Bell Assoc for the Deaf; 1989.
3. Jackendoff R. Phonological structure. In: Jackendoff R, editor. Patterns in the mind: language and human nature. New York: Basic Books; 1994. p. 53–65.
4. Robbins AM. Rehabilitation after cochlear implantation. In: Niparko J, editor. Cochlear implants: principles & practices. 2nd edition. Philadelphia: WoltersKluwer/Lippincott, Williams & Wilkins; 2009. p. 269–312.
5. Nikolopolous T, Dyar D, Archbold S, et al. Development of spoken language grammar following cochlear implantation in prelingually deaf children. Arch Otolaryngol Head Neck Surg 2004;130(5):629–33.
6. Svirsky M, Robbins AM, Kirk KI, et al. Language development in profoundly deaf children with cochlear implants. Psychol Sci 2000;11(2):153–8.
7. Hammes D, Novak M, Rotz LA, et al. Early identification and cochlear implantation: critical factors for spoken language development. Ann Otol Rhinol Laryngol Suppl 2002;189:74–8.
8. Niparko J, Tobey E, Thal D, et al. Spoken language development in children following cochlear implantation. JAMA 2010;303(15):1498–506.
9. Nicholas JG, Geers A. Will they catch up? The role of age at cochlear implantation in the spoken language development of children with severe to profound hearing loss. J Speech Lang Hear Res 2007;50:1048–62.
10. Manrique M, Cervera-Paz F, Huarte A, et al. Advantages of cochlear implantation in prelingual deaf children before 2 years of age when compared with later implantation. Laryngoscope 2004;114:1462–9.
11. Robbins AM, Koch DB, Osberger MJ, et al. Effect of age at cochlear implantation on auditory skill development in infants and toddlers. Arch Otolaryngol Head Neck Surg 2004;130:570–4.
12. Kishon-Rabin L, Taitelbaum R, Elichai O, et al. Developmental aspects of the IT-MAIS in normal-hearing babies. Isr J Speech Hear 2001;23:12–22.
13. Sharma A, Dorman M, Spahr A. A sensitive period for the development of the central auditory system in children with cochlear implants: implications for age of implantation. Ear Hear 2002;23:532–9.

14. Geers A, Brenner C, Davidson L. Factors associated with development of speech perception skills in children implanted by age five. Ear Hear 2003;24(1):25S–35S.
15. Tomblin JB, Spencer L, Flock S, et al. A comparison of language achievement in children with cochlear implants and children using hearing aids. J Speech Lang Hear Res 1999;442:497–511.
16. Robbins AM, Svirsky MA, Miyamoto RT. Aspects of linguistic development affected by cochlear implants. In: Waltzman SB, Cohen NL, editors. Cochlear implants. New York: Thieme Medical Publishers; 2000. p. 269–92.
17. Boothroyd A, Geers A, Moog J. Practical implications of CIs in children. Ear Hear 1991;12:81S–9S.
18. Osberger MJ. Language and learning skills of hearing-impaired students. ASHA Monogr 1986;(23):41–53.
19. Boothroyd A, Eran O. Auditory speech perception capacity of child implant users expressed as equivalent hearing loss. Volta Rev 1994;96:151–68.
20. Eisenberg K, Kirk KI, Martinez AS, et al. Communication abilities of children with aided residual hearing: comparison with cochlear implant users. Arch Otolaryngol Head Neck Surg 2004;130(5):563–9.
21. Robbins AM. Language development in children with cochlear implants. In: Waltzman SB, Roland JT, editors. Cochlear implants. 2nd edition. New York: Thieme Medical Publishers; 2006. p. 153–66.
22. Geers A, Nicholas J, Sedey A. Language skills of children with early cochlear implantation. Ear Hear 2003;24(1):46S–58S.
23. Blamey PJ, Sarant J, Paatsch L, et al. Relationships among speech perception, production, language, hearing loss and age in children with impaired hearing. J Speech Lang Hear Res 2001;44(2):264–85.
24. Fey M. Language intervention with young children. San Diego (CA): College-Hill; 1986.
25. Parrish R, Roush J. When hearing loss occurs with other disabilities. Volta Voices 2004;11(7):20–1.
26. Yoshinaga-Itano C, Sedey AL, Coulter D, et al. Language of early- and later-identified children with hearing loss. Pediatrics 1998;102:1161–71.
27. Geers A. Speech, language and reading skills after early cochlear implantation. Arch Otolaryngol Head Neck Surg 2004;130:634–8.
28. Tyszkiewicz E, Stokes J. Paediatric rehabilitation. In: Cooper H, Craddock L, editors. Cochlear implants—a practical guide. 2nd edition. London: Whurr Publishers; 2006. p. 322–37.
29. Kirk KI, Firszt J, Hood L, et al. New directions in pediatric cochlear implantation: effects on candidacy. ASHA Leader 2006;11(16):6–7, 14–5.
30. McClatchie A, Therres MK. Auditory speech & language (AuSpLan). Washington, DC: AG Bell; 2003.
31. Toby E, Geers A, Brenner C, et al. Factors associated with development of speech production skills in children implanted by age five. Ear Hear 2003; 24(1):36S–45S.
32. Osberger MJ, Fisher L, Phillips SZ, et al. Speech recognition performance of older children with cochlear implants. Am J Otol 1998;2(19):152–7.
33. Goffman L, Leonard J. Growth of language skills in preschool children with specific language impairment: implications for assessment and intervention. Am J Speech Lang Pathol 2000;9:151–61.
34. Rice M, Wexler K, Hershberger S. Tense over time: the longitudinal course of tense acquisition in children with specific language impairment. J Speech Lang Hear Res 1998;41:1412–30.

35. Rudmin F. The why and how of hearing/s/. Volta Rev 1983;263–9.
36. Tait M, Lutman M. Comparison of early communicative behavior in young children with cochlear implants and with hearing aids. Ear Hear 1994;15:352–62.
37. Holt J. Stanford achievement test—8th edition. Am Ann Deaf 1993;138:172–5.
38. Yurkowski P, Ewoldt C. A case for the semantic processing of the deaf reader. Am Ann Deaf 1986;131:243–7.
39. Geers A, Moog J. Factors predictive of the development of literacy in profoundly hearing impaired adolescents. Volta Rev 1989;91:69–86.
40. Hayes H, Geers AE, Treiman R, et al. Receptive vocabulary development in deaf children with cochlear implants: achievement in an intensive auditory-oral educational setting. Ear Hear 2009;30(1):128–35.
41. Maxwell MM. Beginning reading and deaf children. Am Ann Deaf 1986;91:69–86.
42. Schopmeyer B. Reading and deafness. In: Niparko J, editor. Cochlear implants: principles and practices. Philadelphia: Lippincott, Williams, Wilkins; 2000. p. 263–6.
43. Geers A. Predictors of reading skills development in children with early cochlear implantation. Ear Hear 2003;24:59S–68S.
44. Geers A. Factors affecting the development of speech, language, and literacy in children with early cochlear implantation. Lang Speech Hear Serv Sch 2002;33:172–83.
45. Geers A, Brenner C, Nicholas J, et al. Rehabilitation factors contributing to implant benefit in children. Ann Otol Rhinol Laryngol 2002;111:127–30.
46. Pisoni DB, Geers AE. Working memory in deaf children with cochlear implants: correlations between digit span and measures of spoken language processing. Ann Otol Rhinol Laryngol Suppl 2000;185:92–3.
47. Cheng A, Grant G, Niparko J. A meta-analysis of the pediatric cochlear implantation. Ann Otol Rhinol Laryngol 1999;177:124–8.
48. Moeller MP. Early intervention and language development in children who are deaf and hard of hearing. Pediatrics 2000;106(3):e43. Available at: www.pediatrics.org/cgi/content/full/106/3/e43. Accessed September 24, 2011.
49. Dunst CJ. Parent and community assets as sources of young children's learning opportunities. Asheville (NC): Winterverry Press; 2001.
50. Gfeller K. Accommodating children who use cochlear implants in music therapy or educational setting. Music Ther Perspect 2000;18:122–30.
51. Gfeller K, Witt S, Spencer L, et al. Musical involvement and enjoyment of children who use cochlear implants. Volta Rev 1998;100(4):213–33.
52. Stordhal J. Song recognition and appraisal: a comparison of children who use cochlear implants and normally hearing children. J Music Ther 2002;39(1):2–19.
53. Barton C. Bringing music to their bionic ears: nurturing music development in children with cochlear implants. Issue 1. In: Loud and clear. Valencia (Spain): Boston Scientific; 2006. p. 1–8.
54. Wetherby A. Communication and language intervention for preschool children. Buffalo (NY): United Educational Services, Inc; 1992.
55. Waltzman SB, Cohen N. Implantation of patients with prelingual long-term deafness. Ann Otol Rhinol Laryngol Suppl 1999 177;108(4):84–87.
56. Osberger MJ, Zimmerman-Phillips S, Barker MJ, et al. Clinical trial of the Clarion cochlear implant in children. Ann Otol Rhinol Laryngol Suppl 1999 17;108(4):88–92.
57. Robbins AM. Clinical red flags for slow progress in children with cochlear implants. Issue 1. In: Loud and clear. Valencia (CA): Advanced Bionics; 2005. p. 1–8.
58. Dorman D, Hickson L, Murdoch B, et al. Outcomes of an auditory-verbal program for children with hearing loss: a comparative study with a matched group of children with normal hearing. Volta Rev 2007;107(1):37–54.

New Frontiers in Cochlear Implantation: Acoustic Plus Electric Hearing, Hearing Preservation, and More

Sarah E. Mowry, MD[a], Erika Woodson, MD[b], Bruce J. Gantz, MD[a],*

KEYWORDS

- Hearing preservation • Cochlear implantation
- Electric and acoustic processing • Hybrid

 ▶ Video of Surgical Technique for Hearing Preservation accompanies this article at http://www.oto.theclinics.com/.

In the past 30 years, cochlear implantation has changed from being an experimental procedure to representing the standard of care. Advances in processing strategies, implant design, and patient selection criteria have improved implant users' performance significantly. The current frontiers in implantation involve strategies to preserve residual acoustic hearing and the development of algorithms to combine electrical and acoustic hearing. It is also important to consider preserving apical Organ of Corti structures to take advantage of new developments that might lead to regeneration of the inner ear in the future.

Cochlear implantation with a standard-length electrode has become a routine treatment for profound deafness; however, interest is mounting to expand electrical speech-processing capabilities to those individuals with more residual acoustic hearing, as those with implants demonstrate significantly better speech understanding than severely hearing–impaired individuals using hearing aids. Over the past 10 years,

This work was sponsored in part by grant numbers RO1DC00037 and 2P50DC00242 from the NIDCD and by GCRC/NCRR grant number RR00059.

Disclosures: Dr Gantz is a consultant for Cochlear Corporation and Advanced Bionics Corporation. Drs Mowry and Woodson have no disclosures.

[a] Department of Otolaryngology, University of Iowa Hospital and Clinics, 200 Hawkins Drive, PFP 21212, Iowa City, IA 52249, USA

[b] Head and Neck Institute, Cleveland Clinic Foundation, A71, 9500 Euclid Avenue, Cleveland, OH 44195, USA

* Corresponding author.

E-mail address: Bruce-gantz@uiowa.edu

Otolaryngol Clin N Am 45 (2012) 187–203

doi:10.1016/j.otc.2011.09.001

individuals with substantial low-frequency acoustic hearing below 1500 Hz have received varying electrode designs, including shortened cochlear implants, in an attempt to preserve this remaining inner ear function. These patients have not been considered candidates for implantation using standard criteria, due to their residual low-frequency hearing. However, patients with severe to profound high-frequency hearing loss above 1500 Hz and relative preservation of low-frequency hearing do poorly, even with bilateral amplification. This loss of fidelity occurs because different qualities of sound are encoded in various frequencies of sound energy. In the low frequencies, information about vocal fold vibration is relayed (ie, the ability to distinguish between "s" and "z"), whereas frequencies above 1000 Hz encode information regarding the vocal formants and spectral patterns (such as the difference between "b" and "g").[1] The information provided by the low frequencies requires only that the patient be able to distinguish differences in loudness and speech patterns, whereas the information provided in the high frequencies requires the listener to distinguish between various spectral patterns. Patients with high-frequency losses are able to use loudness and speech pattern cues, but they lack the ability to distinguish differences in spectral patterns. This particular hearing-loss pattern results in significant reductions in word discrimination scores as the ability to distinguish between the different consonant sounds erodes. Amplification of these frequencies is insufficient to improve speech recognition scores when thresholds exceed 55 dB.[2]

ELECTRIC AND ACOUSTIC HEARING
Shortened Electrodes

In many patients with some residual hearing, cochlear implantation with a standard-length electrode and standard surgical technique results in complete loss of the remaining acoustic hearing.[3,4] However, in 1997 Hodges and colleagues[5] reported on a series of patients who had preserved residual hearing after implantation. Since that time, multiple studies have demonstrated the ability to retain residual low-frequency hearing following standard-length electrode implantation.[6,7] However, it is difficult to maintain speech discrimination in addition to pure tones when electrodes are passed beyond the basal turn.[6] Passing a standard-length electrode beyond the basal turn of the cochlea can result in damage to the organ of Corti, due to migration of the electrode through the basilar membrane.

The development of acoustic plus electric hearing has evolved from the work of two independent groups of researchers from the Iowa Cochlear Implant Clinical Research Center in Iowa City, Iowa, USA, and the Johann-Wolfgang-Goethe-University in Frankfurt, Germany.

In 1995, the University of Iowa CI research team began the development of a shortened electrode array, or Hybrid S, in collaboration with the Cochlear Corporation (Lane Cove, Australia). The goals and theories behind development of the short electrode are fundamentally different than merely inserting a standard-length electrode into the cochlea under modified technique. The Hybrid project stemmed from work by Shepherd and colleagues[8,9] that showed that preservation of the apical regions of the feline cochlea could be spared anatomically and functionally following limited electrode insertion. The Hybrid electrode was thus intentionally designed to only insert into the lower basal turn of the cochlea and stimulate the missing areas of high frequency in subjects with steeply descending audiograms. The design was predicated on the concept that once the electrode was advanced beyond the upper basal turn it could not be controlled, and could migrate through the basilar membrane as it was advanced against the lateral wall. Limiting the length of the electrode prevents this type of damage. The electrode is specifically intended for patients with good to excellent low-frequency thresholds but severe to profound loss in the higher frequencies. The concept of hearing preservation and cochlear implantation was first presented at the National Institutes of Health-National Institute on Deafness and other Communication Disorders Tenth Anniversary celebration meeting in late 1998. The first volunteer was implanted under the initial US Food and Drug Administration (FDA) trial in 1999.

The Hybrid-S electrode is smaller in diameter than the standard electrode, measuring 0.2 mm × 0.4 mm (**Fig. 1**). Other modifications include a Dacron washer positioned to prevent the electrode from insertion past the 10-mm mark, and a titanium marker to orient the electrodes toward the modiolus.[10] The initial electrode was 6 mm in length and contained 6 electrodes. The most important finding in the original 3 volunteers receiving the 6-mm device was the ability to preserve residual acoustic hearing close to their preoperative levels. Two of the subjects complained that the sound was very high-pitched and not very useful.[11] The initial electrode design was then lengthened to 10 mm, with 6 electrodes within the distal 6 mm. The ideal insertion depth is approximately 195° of the basal turn of the cochlea.[12]

Candidates for implantation with this shorter electrode must have less than 60 dB hearing loss between 125 and 500 Hz and less than 80 dB hearing loss above 2000 Hz. Further, they may have substantial consonant nucleus consonant (CNC) word scores in the best aided situation between 10% and 60% correct in the worse hearing ear and up to 80% correct in the better hearing ear (**Fig. 2**).

In 2003, Gantz and Turner[11] reported on the first 6 patients implanted with the Hybrid electrode. Three volunteers received the 6-mm electrode and 3 received the 10-mm electrode. All patients had normal to mild hearing loss up to 750 Hz. All patients had preservation of their residual hearing. Patients receiving the 6-mm electrode saw a benefit of 10% in the consonant recognition scores, whereas those who received the 10-mm electrode improved by 40% on average within the first year following implantation. The final results of the initial feasibility study included the original 6 patients plus 3 more who received the 10-mm device. All 9 patients had preserved low-frequency hearing within 15 dB of their preoperative levels. Patients who received the 10-mm electrode did considerably better in the combined mode (cochlear implant + hearing aids in bilateral ears) than those who received the 6-mm electrode. Of the 4 patients implanted with the 10-mm electrode after 12 months or more of follow-up, 3 scored more than 80% on CNC words in the combined mode.[13]

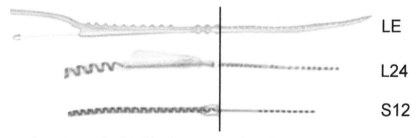

LE

L24

S12

Fig. 1. Photomicrograph of Cochlear Corporation electrodes. The Hybrid S electrode is inserted through 195° of the basal turn while the Hybrid L is inserted through 270°. The standard-length Contour Advanced electrode (LE) with 24 channels is antimodular, and full insertion extends through 450° of the cochlea. The Contour Advance is 19 mm in length, the L24 is 16 mm in length, and the S10 is 10 mm in length. The vertical line indicates the optimal insertion depth at the cochleostomy. (Photo provided *courtesy of* Cochlear™ Americas, © 2009 Cochlear Americas.)

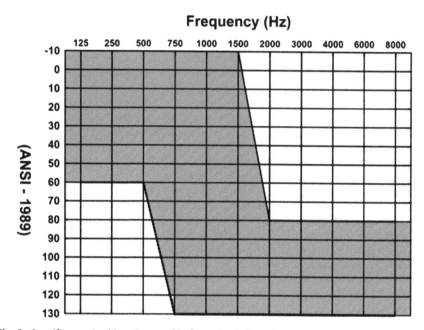

Fig. 2. Specific required hearing profile for Hybrid clinical trial candidates. The shaded area represents hearing loss appropriate for acoustic plus electric hearing clinical trials. ANSI, American National Standards Institute.

Following the feasibility study, a larger multicenter phase 1 FDA trial was conducted for the Hybrid S 10-mm electrode. Eighty-seven patients were recruited at 13 medical centers. Preliminary data on long-term hearing outcomes was published in 2009.[14] Two patients lost all residual hearing within 1 month of implantation for an initial hearing preservation rate of 98%. Over the course of the study (between 3 and 24 months after activation), 6 more patients lost residual hearing for a long-term hearing preservation rate of 91%. Over time, 30% of patients experienced low-frequency threshold changes of greater than 30 dB (between 3 and 36 months post activation).

In the Hybrid S trial, 16 patients (18% of the subjects) did not improve or worsened on performance measures. A multivariate analysis was performed to determine which factors negatively influenced the outcomes for the poor-performer group. A long duration of deafness (longer than 40 years) and low preoperative CNC word scores were found to negatively impact on functional outcomes (**Table 1**).[14]

Another short electrode has been developed in conjunction with the Cochlear Corporation, the Hybrid L24, which is 16 mm in length and contains 22 electrodes (see **Fig. 1**). The optimal insertion is through 250° of the basal turn of the cochlea. This longer electrode would still preserve residual hearing in the apical portions of the cochlea, but if the low-frequency hearing is lost the Hybrid L can be used as a traditional electric-processing only device as it has 22 electrodes, similar to a standard electrode. The FDA trial for the Hybrid L is closed and is now accruing data. Preliminary results from the European clinical trial with this electrode have been published recently, and demonstrate the ability to preserve residual hearing (see **Table 1**).[15] The European trial included 32 patients, 24 of whom were hybrid candidates and 8 long-electrode candidates. Hearing was preserved within 30 dB of preoperative

Table 1
Clinical trials of cochlear implants

	Cochlear Hybrid S10[14]	Cochlear Hybrid L24[15]	Med-El Flex[EAS,21]
Number of patients	87	32 total 24 implanted with L24	18
Average length of follow-up, months (range)	9–12 (3–36)	Not stated 16 patients completed testing at 12 mo 22 patients had reached 6 mo	15 (range not given)
Average change in threshold	13.5 dB (n = 80)	10 dB	Not given
% within 30 dB of preoperative thresholds	70%	94%	66%
Number with complete loss of residual hearing	2 immediate; 6 delayed	None	3 delayed
Average word scores	73% on CNC words	45.1% on FMT	44% on FMT 71% on open-set sentences

Abbreviations: CNC, Consonant Nucleus Consonant test; FMT, Freiberg Monosyllable Test.

thresholds in 96% of patients, and 68% were within 15 dB. These results were stable over time. Of the 16 patients with 12 months of experience, 94% retained hearing within 30 dB of preoperative thresholds. The ongoing US trial of the L24 electrode is demonstrating similar hearing preservation rates to the S8 US trial. This study also noted a negative impact from prolonged duration of hearing loss. It additionally confirmed the findings from the Hybrid S trial that there is a significant learning period for patients with short electrodes.[16] Those in the European trial showed significant improvement on word scores between the 6-month and 12-month marks.

The Med-El Corporation (Innsbruck, Austria) has also developed a shortened electrode for electric and acoustic hearing. Their standard-length electrode, the Combi40+, has a goal insertion length of 31 mm. The shortened electrode, the M, is 22 mm in length and its goal insertion is 360° through the basal turn of the cochlea. Recent adaptations of the electrode include a significantly reduced diameter of the distal portion of the electrode and a very flexible tip. This Flex[EAS] electrode can be used for both cochleostomy and round window insertion techniques.[17] Much of the data regarding the Med-El system involves mixed cohorts of patients.

Before the development of the shortened electrode, surgeons in Europe were using a standard-length electrode but limiting the depth of insertion. Therefore, results regarding the shortened electrode from several studies are difficult to interpret.[18–20] However, results related to the M electrode specifically were reported in 2008 (see **Table 1**).[21] In this series, 18 patients were implanted with the M device. Twelve of the 18 (66%) had low-frequency hearing preservation that could be usefully amplified. Three other patients had some residual low-frequency hearing but did not find amplification useful. Three patients (16%) lost all residual hearing. Of interest, the loss of residual hearing was not immediate, but delayed by 3 to 6 months after hybrid activation. Of the 18 patients implanted, 6 used the hybrid mode on a regular basis.

Standard-Length Electrodes

The ability to preserve residual acoustic function rests in both the type of electrode used and the techniques with which it is inserted. An alternative strategy for hearing preservation has been developed with standard-length electrodes. Kiefer and colleagues[4] reported on 14 patients implanted with the Med-El Combi 40+ electrode. Depth of insertion was intentionally limited to less than 24 mm (full insertion is 31.5 mm) and a "soft insertion" technique was used. Useful low-frequency hearing (less than 20 dB change in thresholds) was maintained in 12 of 14 patients, with 2 patients losing all residual hearing. Fraysse and colleagues[22] reported on a multicenter prospective trial using the Nucleus 24 Contour Advance electrode. The optimal insertion depth was 450° from the cochleostomy. Twenty-seven patients were implanted during the study, but only 12 had no deviations from the reported surgical protocol. Approximately 40% of patients lost the residual hearing completely, and only 19% to 33% (depending on frequency tested) of patients retained hearing thresholds within 20 dB of preoperative scores. Using modified surgical techniques and standard-length electrodes, other investigators have reported preserved hearing within 20 dB of preoperative thresholds in 67% to 89% of patients.[4,22–25] However, not all of these patients retain the ability to discriminate. Balkany and colleagues[6] reported that although patients experienced an average of only 15 dB change in the low frequencies, the average acoustic CNC word score postoperatively was 0%. This result was statistically significant ($P<.001$). In all of the previously mentioned studies, the electrodes were inserted through the entire basal turn of the cochlea. The optimal depth of insertion for the Nucleus 24, a perinodular 19-mm electrode, is between 450° and 540° (see **Fig. 1**). The Med-El Combi 40+ has a goal insertion of 31 mm. Prentiss and colleagues[26] have reported on their experience with deep electrode insertion with the goal of acoustic hearing preservation. Eighteen patients were implanted with the Med-El Pulsar100 to depths of 24 to 28 mm. All patients retained some acoustic hearing, with 16 of 18 patients within 30 dB of their preoperative thresholds.

Discussion

There is controversy in the literature about which electrode length is preferred. There is a higher rate of reduced thresholds and anacusis with the long electrodes. Some investigators argue that the long electrodes should be used for this reason, so that if residual hearing is lost the patient can have the full-length electrode to use in an electric-only listening mode.

The short electrode, at 10 mm in length, accesses only the 2800- to 4700-Hz range according to the Greenwood frequency-place map of the basilar membrane. Thus, using the electrode in the electric-only listening mode should cause significant tonotopic place mismatch. While this mismatch causes decreased word discrimination in normal-hearing listeners, Hybrid S electrode users in the electric-only mode performed similarly to long-electrode users on consonant recognition tasks.[27] Improved performance with the shorter 10-mm Hybrid electrode does require a longer adaptive time. Patients continue to improve even after the first 12 months of use.[16,27] Long-electrode users frequently require between 6 and 12 months to adapt to electric hearing.

Another argument in favor of implanting patients with a longer electrode is the likelihood of progressive low-frequency hearing loss. Yao and colleagues[28] retrospectively reviewed the audiometric records of 28 patients who met the criteria for implantation with a Hybrid electrode. Linear regression analysis of each patient's thresholds over time at each frequency from 250, 500, 750, 1000, and 2000 Hz was performed. The average for several groups was then calculated: more than 10 years of data, less than 10 years of data, age greater than 45 years at initial audiogram, and age less than 45 years at initial audiogram.

This study demonstrated no difference in the rate of change between the two groups based on age. Patients with less than 10 years of data had very wide standard deviations as a result of having fewer data to analyze. However, the rate of change was similar between all groups. The average rate of change for all frequencies was 1.05 dB per year. These data suggest that low-frequency hearing is relatively stable over time despite severe/profound loss in the high frequencies. If low-frequency hearing can be preserved at the time of operation, it is likely that the patient will experience minimal further hearing loss in the long term.[28]

Another concern in regard of the Hybrid or electrode acoustic stimulation (EAS) studies is the progression of hearing loss after activation of the electrical processing. At the time of implantation, very few patients lose all of their residual acoustic hearing. Only 2 of 87 (2%) lost all hearing with implantation in the phase 1 Hybrid S10 trial.[14] Between activation and 3 months, 9 of 87 (10%) subjects experienced a 30 dB drop in their pure-tone average at 125, 250, and 500 Hz. The cause of this loss is not known. Originally it was thought that this could be an immune reaction to the electrode; however, that now seems unlikely. Another possibility is loss of afferent spiral ganglion neuron synapse at the hair cell related to the combination of acoustic amplification and electrical stimulation. Puel and colleagues[29] and Wang and colleagues[30] have reported this finding as the initial injury in noise-induced hearing loss. This mechanism of delayed hearing loss is presently under investigation at the authors' center. The authors are also adapting programming strategies to protect the residual structures by reducing the stimulating current at initial activation and widening pulse rates.

BENEFITS OF ACOUSTIC AND ELECTRIC PROCESSING

The full benefits of acoustic and electrical stimulation of the ipsilateral cochlea are still being investigated. However, the available literature suggests several discrete advantages to the use of both modalities. There is a significant body of literature that reports on the benefits of "bimodal" hearing. In this situation, the user receives electrical stimulation in the implanted ear and uses a hearing aid in the contralateral ear. A full review of this listening condition is beyond the scope of this article. The reader is referred to a review on the subject by Firszt and colleagues[31] for more detailed information.

The benefits of "combined" hearing are discussed here. In this situation, the user receives electric stimulation in the implanted ear as well as acoustic information through the use of bilateral hearing aids. Improvements in speech discrimination, signal-to-noise ratio (SNR), and music perception are discussed.

Speech Discrimination

As discussed previously, patients with preserved low-frequency hearing have significant improvements in their discrimination scores. Those implanted with shorter electrode arrays, such as the Hybrid S/L or Med-El M/Flex[EAS] electrodes, are achieving significant improvements in discrimination tasks as well. Patients implanted with the Hybrid S electrode continue to demonstrate improvement in CNC scores beyond 1 to 2 years after activation in the combined mode.[16] At the time of publication of the Hybrid 10 clinical trial, 68 of 87 patients in the multicenter trial had follow-up lengths of greater than 9 months. Improvements in speech reception threshold (SRT) or CNC word score occurred in 74% of patients. Nearly half of patients (48%) had improvement in both SRT and CNC scores. Improvement on CNC testing ranged from 10% to 70% better than preoperative scores for 45 of 61 patients with long-term follow-up.[14] For those implanted with the Hybrid L24, word recognition scores improved by 21% on average; one patient demonstrated improvement from 5% to 95% on the Freiburg Monosyllabic word test (FMT).[15]

Some patients score more than 90% on the CNC monosyllabic word test in the combined mode with all electrodes. Patients implanted with the Flex[EAS] electrode also scored well. Preoperative open-set sentence recognition was 24% and after 12 months of use, scores averaged 71% (P<.05). Monosyllable recognition also improved; preoperative scores averaged 16% on the FMT and postoperative scores averaged 44% (P<.05). One patient in this cohort achieved scores above 90% discrimination postoperatively.[21] As demonstrated in multiple studies, exceptional improvement in speech understanding is possible for patients in the combined mode with all electrodes activated.

Patients receiving long electrodes with preserved low-frequency cochlear function also routinely improved on discrimination tasks. Patients receiving the Med-El Combi40 with 19 to 24 mm of insertion scored 75% on monosyllabic words at 1 year; preoperative scores averaged 9%.[4] Fraysse and colleagues[22] reported on those receiving a Nucleus 24 Contour Advance. Preoperative word scores averaged 15%. At 3 months, patients in the combined condition had improved to 55%. Long-term data for this patient group are not available, but patients may continue to improve in the combined condition as is seen in other studies.

Hearing in Noise

Although cochlear implants significantly improve speech understanding in quiet, traditional cochlear implant users have difficulty in noisy environments. Distinguishing the correct words in a background of competing talkers is an even more difficult task. Normal-hearing listeners are able to understand 50% of the presented words when the background noise is 30 dB louder; thus normal-hearing listeners have an SNR of −30 dB (lower numbers are better). For competing talkers, the average SNR in normal-hearing listeners is −15 dB.[32] The average long-electrode user requires an SNR of +3 dB for unmodulated background noise and +8 for multitalker babble (MTB), meaning that the talker has to be 3 dB louder than competing noise or 8 dB louder than MTB.[32–34]

Hybrid S recipients do better than traditional cochlear implant patients but not as well as normal-hearing listeners in background noise. SNRs varied from −12 to +17 dB in a subgroup of 27 Hybrid S patients with 12 months or greater experience. The average SNR for the Hybrid S group was −9 dB.[14] Elevated SNRs occurred in those patients who experienced greater than 30 dB changes to their low-frequency hearing. The results for Hybrid S patients in MTB are similar to hearing-impaired patients with SRTs between 81 and 100 dB (severe/profound) (**Fig. 3**).

Patients receiving the Hybrid L electrode also improved their SNR when tested in the combined mode. The average SNR preoperatively was 12.1 dB, and postoperatively the SNR dropped to 2.1 dB.[15]

Those with the Flex[EAS] electrode also improved speech understanding in noise. Preoperative open-set sentence scores in SNR of +10 were 14% and after 1 year in the EAS mode scores averaged 60% (P<.05).[21]

Patients receiving a long electrode with hearing preservation also benefit when listening in noise. Patients with the Med-El Combi40+ and low-frequency thresholds of <80 dB scored better than patients with a cochlear implant and no residual hearing at an SNR of +5 dB (P<.01).[22] Others have reported a similar improvement with sentence recognition in noise.[23]

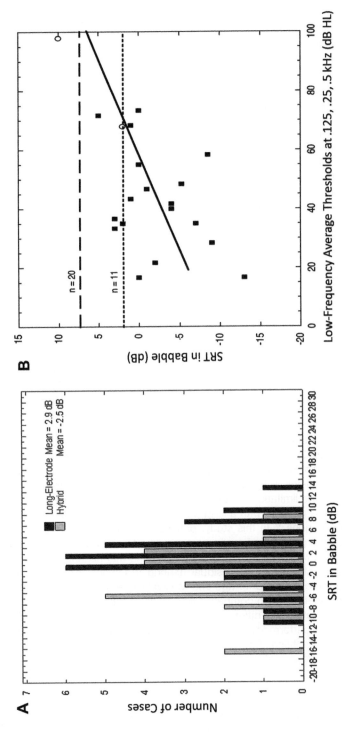

Fig. 3. Benefit of low frequency hearing in noise. (A) Preservation of low frequency hearing in multitalker babble. Hybrid S and long electrode users were matched based on CNC scores in quiet. The 2 groups were then compared in multitalker babble. On average, long electrode users required a SNR of +2.9 dB to achieve 50% correct. Hybrid S users were able to correctly respond with a SNR of −2.5 dB. (B) Better SNRs are correlated with the amount of LF hearing preserved. Users with mild to moderate LF hearing loss have improved SNRs. This correlation was significant (P<.05) (Turner et al., 2008).

Music Appreciation

Identification and enjoyment of music have been areas where traditional cochlear implant users have had significant difficulty. The extremely complex spectral information that is encoded in music is very difficult for traditional cochlear implant users to appreciate. Extensive work by the Iowa CI Research team has identified several components of music for which cochlear implant users perform well, and other areas where they struggle. Patients with long electrodes and no residual hearing (traditional cochlear implant users) can distinguish lyrics to a certain degree but have significant trouble with pitch, timbre, and melody recognition.[32,35]

Music appreciation has been a part of the research protocol for the Hybrid S/L trials. Subjects with preserved low-frequency hearing have a distinct advantage over traditional cochlear implant recipients in several music-processing functions. Pitch perception is one of the most basic functions of the auditory system with respect to music appreciation. Hybrid users perform better on these types of tasks when compared with long-electrode users, but are still significantly poorer-performing than normal-hearing listeners.[36] When provided with lyrics to easily recognizable American songs, Hybrid users were able to identify the songs correctly 65% to 100% of the time, similar to normal-hearing listeners. When the lyrics were removed and only the melody was presented, Hybrid patients did less well (50% correct) but still much better than traditional long-electrode users (fewer than 10% correct).[35]

Instrument recognition is also an important part of music appreciation. These tests determine the ability to distinguish a piano from an oboe, for example. The difference in sound quality produced by these different instruments is referred to as timbre. Gfeller and colleagues[35] tested 3 subject groups: normal-hearing individuals, hybrid patients in combined mode, and long-electrode recipients. Instruments were grouped into 3 categories based on the "most characteristic" frequency of the instrument (low, medium, high tones). Normal-hearing listeners were able to distinguish among these instruments between 80% and 100% of the time, depending on the frequency. Hybrid users did less well than normal-hearing individuals ($P<.001$) on instruments with medium-frequency and high-frequency characteristics. Long-electrode users did significantly worse than both the normal-hearing and hybrid users ($P<.001$ and $P<.005$ respectively) for low- and high-frequency instruments. There was no statistical difference between the Hybrid and long-electrode group for medium-frequency instruments. These findings likely represent the benefits of acoustic hearing in the low frequencies, and the limitations of the electric hearing in high frequencies.

Music testing in EAS patients with a long-electrode insertion has been studied by Brockmeier and colleagues.[37] In this study, patients received a Med-El Combi40+ inserted with a soft surgery technique to preserve low-frequency residual hearing. Thirteen EAS patients were then compared with both normal-hearing listeners and those with a long electrode but no residual hearing (traditional cochlear implant patients). Subjects were matched for age and musical experience. EAS patients did well on pitch discrimination when compared with traditional cochlear implant candidates, and were not statistically different from normal-hearing listeners on this task. However, EAS patients performed poorly on melody discrimination, instrument detection, and instrument identification; on these tests, EAS patients' scores were not significantly different to those of traditional cochlear implant users.

Pitch-Place Perception

Perhaps the most interesting finding of the Hybrid clinical trial is the concept of place-pitch shifts that take place within the auditory system. Before the development of the short electrode and expansion of implantation criteria, this type of analysis could not be made because the severity of hearing loss in the contralateral ear precluded objective comparative acoustical testing. In general, early studies in this area suggested the perceived pitch could be as much as 3 octaves different from that expected according to the Greenwood pitch-place map, but that patients adapt to this information.[38,39]

In 2007, Reiss and colleagues[16] described a series of 10-mm Hybrid users who underwent testing to compare the perceived pitch of electrical stimulus to acoustic stimulation in the contralateral ear. A series of 18 patients were provided with an electrical stimulus to the most apical electrode (number 6), a short time delay, and then an acoustic stimulus to the contralateral ear. Subjects were asked to rate whether the acoustic stimulus was higher, lower, or similar in pitch to the electric stimulus. The acoustic tone was then varied to match the electric stimulus perception. Patients also underwent speech discrimination testing to determine if pitch perception affected implant performance. Five of the 18 patients underwent serial testing over a period of up to 5 years from activation. For 3 of these patients, the perceived pitch decreased significantly over time (as much as 2 octaves). The change in pitch-place perception could not be explained by progressive hearing loss in the contralateral ear or changes in word recognition, as these remained constant over time. Nor could these changes be attributed to alteration in hardware performance, as all integrity testing and impedances remained stable. Patients with short follow-up time (up to 13 months) also demonstrated little change. It is interesting that in these hybrid patients the speech perception testing was correlated with pitch perception soon after implantation. However, in long-term users this correlation was abolished.

Further data were published in 2008 regarding the changes in pitch perception over time in Hybrid users. Early and late measures of pitch-place perception were compared with the most apical electrode preferred MAPs. Early measurements were commonly one octave or more different from the preferred MAP. Late measurements were much closer to the preferred MAP.[27]

Taken together, the results of pitch matching and correlation of speech recognition imply significant plasticity within the auditory system. The correlation between these variables early in Hybrid use suggests a stimulation pattern according to the tonotopic organization of the afferent pathways. However, late data imply pitch perception is heavily modulated by central processes. A recent review of the concept of neural plasticity with regard to cochlear implantation was recently published by Fallon and colleagues.[40] The mechanism for this shift is not entirely clear, but may be driven by the severe spectral mismatch between the electric stimulation and the residual acoustic hearing within the auditory cortex.

SURGICAL TECHNIQUE FOR HEARING PRESERVATION

A "soft surgery" technique was first described by Lehnhardt in the early 1990s.[41] Modifications of the original technique have been described by other investigators.[4,12,13,42] The technique used at the University of Iowa for implantation of the Cochlear Hybrid S and L devices is described here. A video of this technique is available online in conjunction with this *Clinics* publication (Video).

A standard 3-dimensional mastoidectomy is performed through a postauricular incision positioned in the hairline. A portion of the superior margin of the mastoid cortex is left in place to create a ledge of bone in the area of the anterior tegmen mastoideum for securing the electrode. A suture is passed through the cortex to anchor the electrode before placing it in the cochlea. This suture reduces the spring of the electrode and helps prevent movement of the electrode during placement in the scala tympani (ST) (**Fig. 4**). A bony well for the internal processor is also created in the same manner as for a standard Cochlear Corporation receiver/stimulator. A ridge of bone between the mastoid cavity and the well is left to prevent the implant from sliding anteriorly. A subperiosteal pocket is created deep to the temporalis muscle and pericranium. The facial recess is opened widely. Removal of the bone overlying and anterior to the facial nerve is important to provide full exposure of the round window niche. The bone anterior to the nerve should be removed down to the level of the stapedius muscles. This wide exposure cannot be overemphasized. The bony overhang of the round window niche is drilled away to expose the entire round window membrane using a 1-mm diamond burr.

In the United States a cochleostomy is the preferred strategy for placing the electrode, whereas surgeons in Europe favor placement through the round window membrane. There are proponents of both approaches.[10,12,43–45]

If a cochleostomy is to be used, it must be performed in the appropriate position with special care. Cochleostomy is the preferred method of the senior author (B.J.G.) to enter the ST. Meticulous anatomic and histologic analysis of the ST and osseous spiral lamina (OSL) has detailed a precarious curvature to the OSL at the terminal end (hook region) of the ST. The unique relationship of the OSL and round window predisposes to fracture of the OSL when using the round window technique.[45,46] Furthermore, insertion through the round window may result in a conductive hearing loss, as was revealed in the recently published data for the Hybrid-L European trial.[15]

The opening of the cochlea should be treated in a similar way to a "drill-out" stapedotomy procedure. Before creating the cochleostomy, the surgical field is irrigated to remove as much bone chip and blood debris. Meticulous hemostasis is important to prevent entry of any blood into the cochlea on opening. Suctioning of perilymph must be avoided as well.

The cochleostomy is created 1 to 2 mm anterior and inferior to the anterior floor of the round window membrane (**Fig. 5**). Entry into the ST in this location prevents damage to the basilar membrane and facilitates insertion in the correct trajectory to avoid injury to cochlear structures. The bone of the promontory is quite thick in this area, and as much as 1 to 2 mm of bone must be removed to reach the endosteum of the ST. The bone of the promontory should be widely saucerized with a 1.5-mm diamond burr anterior to the annulus of the round window membrane. The bone over the cochleostomy is thinned with a 0.5-mm diamond burr.

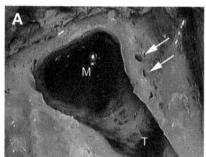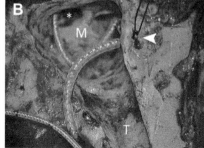

Fig. 4. Location of the electrode sling stitch. (*A*) The sling stitch is placed through holes (*arrows*) drilled in the tegmen mastoideum using a 1.5-mm diamond drill. (*B*) The stitch (*arrowhead*) provides stabilization of the Hybrid S electrode to prevent recoil or movement of the electrode during and following insertion. *Asterisk*, facial recess; M, mastoid cavity; T, trough to the receiver/stimulator well.

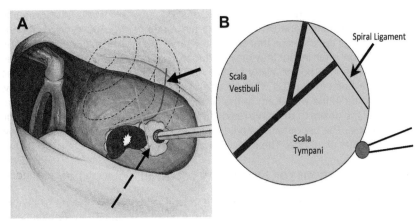

Fig. 5. Appropriate cochleostomy placement. (*A*) Position of cochleostomy in the inferior-posterior quadrant of a box created by drawing a line at the superior margin of the round window and a perpendicular line at the inferior margin of the round window (*dashed arrow*). Basilar membrane position (*solid arrow*), round window membrane (*star*). (*B*) The cochlea is oriented in the temporal bone such that the basal turn is tipped anterior-superior with the helicotrema deep to the tensor tympani muscle. The black line indicates the approximate position of the spiral ligament. The cochleostomy should be placed inferior to the spiral ligament to prevent damage to the basilar membrane. (*From* Gantz BJ, Turner CW, Gfeller KE, et al. Preservation of hearing in cochlear implant surgery: advantages of combined electrical and acoustic speech processing. Laryngoscope 2005;115(5):798; with permission.)

Before opening the endosteum of the cochleostomy, the electrode and processor should be seated in position. The electrode array (not the ground electrode) for the Hybrid S and L is secured within the mastoid. To do this, 2 holes are drilled into the tegmen tympani that allow a 2-0 nylon suture to be passed through the bone. Once the processor and electrode are seated and secured, a "washer" of temporalis fascia 1.5 mm × 1.5 mm in diameter is harvested and flattened in a fascial tissue press. This fascia is then punctured with a straight needle, and the electrode is inserted through the fascia up to the Dacron collar. This fascia "washer" is used to seal the ST at the cochleostomy. Opening the endosteum into the ST should be the final act of the procedure to minimize the time the cochlea is open to the middle ear. The ST is entered with a 0.2-mm footplate hook. The electrode is advanced into the ST with a fine-tip smooth forceps (such as a jeweler's forceps) positioned at the Dacron collar and the claw-type instrument distally. The trajectory of insertion is parallel to the posterior auditory canal wall (see **Fig. 5**). The electrode is advanced slowly into the ST over 1 to 2 minutes. This slow insertion allows displacement of perilymph and minimizes insertional trauma. The electrode is advanced to the fascia "washer" to ensure a tight seal.

Currently intraoperative ABR is being evaluated as a strategy to monitor the residual hearing during electrode insertion. To do this, a preoperative ABR is obtained to confirm the patient has a well-formed response to click stimuli and to establish the stimulus level for monitoring. The intensity of stimulus is chosen to be the lowest level above threshold that results in a relatively stable amplitude with repeated measures. Due to the extent of the high-frequency hearing loss, wave V of the ABR has increased latency. The amplitude of the response is a more reliable measure in these patients. A click is used to generate the response, and is believed to represent activation of the most basal functioning hair cells. Presumably this will be the area of the cochlea first affected adversely by the insertion process, and intervention at this point may preserve cochlear function in more apical regions. Because amplitude measures in the ABR are typically quite variable, recordings are made in two 500-sweep sets. This approach reduces the chances that changes in amplitude will be ascribed to changing cochlear function when in fact they may be due to normal variability. The surgeon must pause during the insertion to allow for the ABR data to be collected. More than 10 subjects have been implanted with the use of intraoperative ABR, and no changes have been noted in the waveform at the time of surgery in any subject.

Because of the desire to preserve residual hearing, the middle ear is not packed with muscle or fascia. The periosteum should then be closed completely over the receiver/stimulator and the electrode. The soft tissues are then closed in the standard fashion.

CANDIDACY/INDICATIONS FOR HYBRID-TYPE COCHLEAR IMPLANTATION

Implanting an electrode into the cochlea of a patient with residual hearing would have been unthinkable 15 years ago. However, the evidence suggests that patients who meet the current criteria for hybrid implantation gain tremendous benefit from these devices. Other patient populations may also benefit from these devices.

Apical cochlear preservation may become a significant issue in the future. It is entirely possible that treatments will emerge that require naïve cochlear tissue (hair cell generation, tissue transfer, and so forth). This aspect is particularly relevant for families weighing the risks and benefits of bilateral cochlear implantation for deaf children. The University of Iowa CI research team has recently implanted 9 children with bilateral cochlear implants: one ear with a standard long electrode and the other with the Hybrid S12 research electrode.[47] The goal of the feasibility study was to determine whether these children would perform as well as children who receive bilateral long electrodes. Preliminary data are available from these children using the Preschool Language Scale-3 (PLS-3), a standardized and normalized tool to assess children from age 2 weeks to 7 years. Children in the study scored an average of 80 (range 73–87). The average score for children with bilateral long electrodes is 83. These data suggest that use of a unilateral short electrode provides adequate auditory information in the situations tested. The children in this small study were only 12 to 24 months of age at implantation, so long-term follow-up is necessary to determine whether the trends seen in this study are long lasting. A larger-scale study is currently under way.

SUMMARY

Preservation of residual low-frequency hearing during implant surgery is both achievable and desirable.

- The act of inserting an electrode into the inner ear while maintaining residual cochlear function is technically challenging.
- Use of shorter electrode arrays is currently under investigation in the United States.
- Patients undergoing hearing preservation surgery can expect a long-term low-frequency hearing preservation rate of 50% to 70%.
- Preservation of low-frequency hearing allows for improved speech discrimination in quiet. Patients demonstrate average improvements on CNC words of 20% to 40% over preoperative scores, with some patients scoring well above 80% correct.
- Implant recipients with preserved low-frequency hearing can expect improved hearing in noise. SNRs are similar to those with moderate to severe hearing loss rather than the SNRs of traditional long-electrode users.

- Music appreciation is still difficult for EAS patients. The residual low-frequency hearing improves some quantitative measures of music discrimination, but subjective music appreciation continues to be as difficult for a majority of EAS patients as their standard electrode counterparts.

Few would have imagined the progress that has been made in the past 30 years regarding cochlear implantation. The future promises to be equally exciting. Developments in both hardware (electrode design) and software (speech-processing strategies) have provided significant improvement in the lives of many patients. The burgeoning practice and technology behind hearing-preservation cochlear implant surgery promises to expand these benefits to a much larger hearing-impaired population.

ACKNOWLEDGMENTS

The authors would like to thank Dr Chris Turner and Christine Etler for their assistance with the article.

REFERENCES

1. Turner CW, Gantz BJ, Karsten S, et al. Impact of hair cell preservation in cochlear implantation: combined electric and acoustic hearing. Otol Neurotol 2010;31(8):1227–32.
2. Hogan CA, Turner CW. High frequency audiability: benefits for hearing impaired listeners. J Acoust Soc Am 1998;104(1):432–41.
3. Rizer FM. Post operative audiometric evaluation of cochlear implant patients. J Otolaryngol 1988;98:203–6.
4. Kiefer J, Gstoettner W, Baumgartner W, et al. Conservation of low-frequency hearing in cochlear implantation. Acta Otolaryngol 2004;124(3):272–80.
5. Hodges AV, Schloffman J, Balkany T. Conservation of residual hearing with cochlear implantation. Am J Otol 1997;18(2):179–83.
6. Balkany TJ, Connell SS, Hodges AV, et al. Conservation of residual acoustic hearing after cochlear implantation. Otol Neurotol 2006;27(8):1083–8.
7. von Ilberg C, Kiefer J, Tillein J, et al. Electric-acoustic stimulation of the auditory system. New technology for severe hearing loss. ORL J Otorhinolaryngol Relat Spec 1999;61(6):334–40.
8. Ni D, Shepherd RK, Seldon HL, et al. Cochlear pathology following chronic electrical stimulation of the auditory nerve. I: normal hearing kittens. Hear Res 1992;62(1):63–81.
9. Xu J, Shepherd RK, Millard RE, et al. Chronic electrical stimulation of the auditory nerve at high stimulus rates: a physiological and histopathological study. Hear Res 1997;105(1–2):1–29.
10. Gantz BJ, Turner CW, Gfeller KE, et al. Preservation of hearing in cochlear implant surgery: advantages of combined electrical and acoustic speech processing. Laryngoscope 2005;115(5):796–802.
11. Gantz BJ, Turner CW. Combining acoustic and electrical hearing. Laryngoscope 2003;113(10):1726–30.
12. Roland JT Jr, Zeitler DM, Jethanamest D, et al. Evaluation of the short hybrid electrode in human temporal bones. Otol Neurotol 2008;29(4):482–8.
13. Gantz BJ, Turner CW. Combining acoustic and electric speech processing: Iowa/nucleus hybrid implant. Acta Otolaryngol 2004;24:344–7.
14. Gantz BJ, Hansen MR, Turner CW, et al. Hybrid 10 clinical trial. Audiol Neurootol 2009;14(Suppl 1):32–8.

15. Lenarz TA, Stover T, Buechner A, et al. Hearing conservation surgery using the Hybrid-L electrode. Audiol Neurootol 2009;14(Suppl 1):22–31.
16. Reiss LA, Turner CW, Erenberg SR, et al. Changes in pitch with a cochlear implant over time. J Assoc Res Otolaryngol 2007;8:241–57.
17. Hochmair I, Nopp P, Jolly C, et al. Med-El cochlear implants: state of the art and a glimpse into the future. Trends Amplif 2006;10(4):201–20.
18. Helbig S, Baumann U. Acceptance and fitting of the DUET device—a combined speech processor for electric acoustic stimulation. Adv Otorhinolaryngol 2010; 67:81–7.
19. Gstoettner WK, Kiefer J, Baumgartner WD, et al. Hearing preservation in cochlear implantation for electric acoustic stimulation. Acta Otolaryngol 2004;124(4):348–52.
20. Kiefer J, Pok M, Adunka O, et al. Combined electric and acoustic stimulation of the auditory system: results of a clinical study. Audiol Neurootol 2005;10(3):134–44.
21. Gstoettner WK, van de Heyning P, O'Connor AF, et al. Electric acoustic stimulation of the auditory system: results of a multi-centre investigation. Acta Otolaryngol 2008;128(9):968–75.
22. Fraysse B, Macias AR, Sterkers O, et al. Residual hearing conservation and electroacoustic stimulation with the Nucleus 24 Contour Advance cochlear implant. Otol Neurotol 2006;27(5):624–33.
23. Gstoettner WK, Helbig S, Maier N, et al. Ipsilateral electric acoustic stimulation of the auditory system: results of long-term hearing preservation. Audiol Neurootol 2006;11(Suppl 1):49–56.
24. Di Nardo W, Cantore I, Melilo P, et al. Residual hearing in cochlear implant patients. Eur Arch Otorhinolaryngol 2007;264(8):855–60.
25. Garcia-Ibanez L, Macias AR, Morera C, et al. An evaluation of the preservation of residual hearing with the Nucleus Contour Advance electrode. Acta Otolaryngol 2009;129(6):651–64.
26. Prentiss S, Sykes K, Staecker H. Partial deafness cochlear implantation at the University of Kansas: techniques and outcomes. J Am Acad Audiol 2010;21:197–203.
27. Reiss LAJ, Gantz BJ, Turner CW. Cochlear implant speech processor frequency allocations may influence pitch perception. Otol Neurotol 2008;29:160–7.
28. Yao WN, Turner CW, Gantz BJ. Stability of low-frequency residual hearing in patients who are candidates for combined acoustic plus electric hearing. J Speech Lang Hear Res 2006;49(5):1085–90.
29. Puel JL, Ruel J, Gervais d'Aldin C, et al. Excitotoxicity and repair of cochlear synapses after noise-trauma induced hearing loss. Neuroreport 1998;22(9): 2109–14.
30. Wang Y, Hirose K, Liberman MC. Dynamics of noise-induced cellular injury and repair in the mouse cochlea. J Assoc Res Otolaryngol 2002;3(3):248–68.
31. Firszt JB, Reeder RM, Skinner MW. Restoring hearing and symmetry with two cochlear implants or one cochlear implant and one hearing aid. J Rehabil Res Dev 2008;45(5):749–67.
32. Turner CW, Gantz BJ, Vidal C, et al. Speech recognition in noise for cochlear implant listeners: benefits of residual acoustic hearing. J Acoust Soc Am 2004; 115(4):1729–35.
33. Nelson P, Jin SH, Carney AE, et al. Understanding speech in modulated interference: cochlear implant uses and normal-hearing listeners. J Acoust Soc Am 2003;113(2):961–8.
34. Gantz BJ, Turner CW, Gfeller KE. Acoustic plus electric speech processing: preliminary results of a multicenter clinical trial of the Iowa/Nucleus Hybrid implant. Audiol Neurootol 2006;11(Suppl 1):63–8.

35. Gfeller KE, Olszewski C, Turner CW, et al. Music perception with cochlear implants and residual hearing. Audiol Neurootol 2006;11(Suppl 1):12–5.
36. Gfeller KE, Turner CW, Oleson J, et al. Accuracy of cochlear implant recipients on pitch perception, melody recognition, and speech reception in noise. Ear Hear 2007;28(3):412–23.
37. Brockmeier SJ, Peterreins M, Lorens A, et al. Music perception in electric acoustic stimulation users as assessed by the Mu.S.I.C. test. Adv Otorhinolaryngol 2010; 67:70–80.
38. Boex C, Baud L, Cosendai G, et al. Acoustic to electric pitch comparisons in cochlear implant subjects with residual hearing. J Assoc Res Otolaryngol 2006; 7(2):110–24.
39. Fu QJ, Nogaki G, Galvin JJ 3rd. Auditory training with spectrally shifted speech: implications for cochlear implant patient auditory rehabilitation. J Assoc Res Otolaryngol 2005;6(2):180–90.
40. Fallon JB, Irvine DR, Shepherd RK. Neural prostheses and brain plasticity. J Neural Eng 2009;6(6):065008.
41. Lehnhardt E. Intracochlear placement of cochlear implant electrodes in a soft surgery technique. HNO 1993;41(7):356–9.
42. James C, Albegger K, Battmer R, et al. Preservation of residual hearing: how and why. Acta Otolaryngol 2005;125(5):481–91.
43. Skarzynski H, Lorens A, Piotrowska A, et al. Preservation of low frequency hearing in partial deafness cochlear implantation (PDCI) using the round window surgical approach. Acta Otolaryngol 2007;127(1):41–8.
44. Adunka O, Unkelbach MH, Mack M, et al. Cochlear implantation via the round window membrane minimizes trauma to cochlear structures: a histologically controlled insertion study. Acta Otolaryngol 2004;124(7):807–12.
45. Wright CG, Roland PS. Temporal bone microdissection for anatomic study of cochlear implant electrodes. Cochlear Implants Int 2005;6(4):159–68.
46. Briggs RF, Tykocinski M, Stidham K, et al. Cochleostomy site: implications for electrode placement and hearing preservation. Acta Otolaryngol 2008;125(8):870–6.
47. Gantz BJ, Dunn CC, Walker EA, et al. Bilateral cochlear implants in infants: a new approach-Nucleus Hybrid S12 project. Otol Neurotol 2010;31:1300–9.

Revision Cochlear Implantation in Children

Alejandro Rivas, MD[a],*, George B. Wanna, MD[a],
David S. Haynes, MD[b]

KEYWORDS

- Revision cochlear implantation • Hard failure • Soft failure
- Device defect • Electrode extrusion • Infection • Children
- Retained electrode

Since the first intrascalar cochlear implant (CI) placement by House and Edgerton[1] in 1961, cochlear implantation has evolved to become an effective and widely performed procedure for the restoration of sound in severe and profound hearing impaired individuals. The number of patients benefiting from this technology continues to grow exponentially. Any threat to the functional gains evokes concern in all users, especially children and their families who fear the loss of newly found access to sound and communication. As the experience with CI grows, replacement or revision cochlear implant (RCI) surgery has become an important procedure. In 1985, Hochmair-Desoyer and Burian[2] reported the first RCI. Since then, multiple publications have addressed the safety of this procedure, including the preservation or enhancement of speech perception performance.[3–8] Initial reports encountered decrements in electrode activation,[9] diminished speech perception,[10] and intracochlear trauma,[11] suggesting that RCI could have a negative functional outcome. However, with the advances in technology, particularly the use of thinner electrodes, and the increased surgical experience of the otologic community, RCI is a safe procedure that, nonetheless, requires careful consideration of the indications and expected benefits.

No disclosures (A.R., G.B.W.); David S. Haynes is a consultant for Cochlear America, Zeiss.
[a] Department of Otolaryngology–Head and Neck Surgery, Division of Otology-Neurotology and Skull Base Surgery, Vanderbilt Bill Wilkerson Center, Vanderbilt University, 1215 21st Avenue South, 7209 Medical Center East, South Tower, Nashville, TN 37232, USA
[b] Otology Group of Vanderbilt, Department of Otolaryngology–Head and Neck Surgery, Vanderbilt Bill Wilkerson Center, Vanderbilt University, 1215 21st Avenue South, 7209 Medical Center East, South Tower, Nashville, TN 37232, USA
* Corresponding author.
E-mail address: alejandro.rivas@vanderbilt.edu

Otolaryngol Clin N Am 45 (2012) 205–219
doi:10.1016/j.otc.2011.09.005
0030-6665/12/$ – see front matter © 2012 Elsevier Inc. All rights reserved.

INDICATIONS

In general, the reported rate of revision surgery accounts for approximately 3% to 15%[12] of CI operations in different studies. This variability can be explained by differences between centers and different study characteristics. Moreover, some of those studies combined pediatrics and adult populations, which increases the incidence of revision surgery because children have a higher rate of device failure because of an increased association with head trauma.[13]

Although there is less data available regarding revision CI surgery in children alone, when compared with adults, the prevalence seems to double. In later studies whereby centers looked separately at their population, Arnoldner and colleagues[14] found an incidence of RCI of 7% in adults versus 14% for children, whereas Rivas and colleagues[8,15] encountered 4.8% versus 13.0%, in adults and children respectively, in a 10-year period.

To facilitate the approach for RCI and to guide required interventions, there are 2 main indications: non–device-related indications and device-related indications. The first one, although less common (26%), includes those patients who require RCI because of infections, allergic reactions, cholesteatomas, misplacements of the electrode, electrode extrusions, and, rarely, single-channel upgrades.

Non–Device-Related Indications

Infections

The incidence of infectious complications in patients with CI range from 1.7% to 8.2%.[16,17] Scalp flap infections can initially present as tenderness over the receiver/stimulator, progressing to edema, erythema, and eventually an underlying abscess. The initial treatment should be conservative, usually requiring close observation and intravenous (IV) antibiotics. In cases of persistence or recurrence of symptoms, the authors proceed with wound debridement, wash out, and cultured-guided antibiotics in an attempt to maintain the implant integrity. This practice, however, represents a real challenge because of the potential formation of biofilms.

Bacterial biofilms are composed of communities of bacteria enclosed in a self-produced polymeric matrix of mainly exopolysaccharides with a propensity to attach and persist on the surface of biomaterials.[18] The biofilm may develop defense mechanisms against both a host immune system and antimicrobial agents preventing them from treating the infection. In this circumstance, the removal of implanted devices is often inevitable to eradicate the disease. In cases whereby IV antibiotics and local wound care fail to resolve infection, the device should be removed leaving the electrode within the cochlea. The patients are treated with parenteral antibiotics for at least 6 weeks, followed by RCI.

The mechanisms responsible for intractable infection of CI are unclear. *Staphylococcus aureus* has been the most common pathogen identified in implant infections, which suggests a nonotologic source because this is not a common middle ear pathogen.[19] Moreover, the safety of implanting CI with a low rate of postoperative device infection in middle ears that are chronically contaminated[20] or intermittently, acutely infected[21–23] has been reported. However, the problem is more complex than simple exposure of the device to bacteria. In fact, Ruellan and colleagues[24] detected bacterial biofilm on 9 CI removed because of device failure, without evidence of infection, demonstrating the need for investigating the pathophysiology of CI-associated biofilms.

This finding may lead to the development of biomaterials that could limit the formation of biofilm or to the creation of implants with drug delivery systems that could treat such formation.[25] Aids in this process include hand hygiene, aseptic technique, and routine use of careful antibiotic irrigation during implantation.

Cholesteatoma

In the 1980s, CI was contraindicated in patients with otitis media[26] because it was hypothesized to be associated with a higher incidence of inner ear infections and intracranial complications. However, later studies of complications of CI in children did not show an increased incidence of otitis media.[21,27] Most of the time these children are treated conservatively with oral antibiotics.[21,28] Only a few reports of patients requiring explantation have been described.[16,29–31] Some of them, although rare, secondary to cholesteatoma.[32–34] Lin,[35] for example, identified 4 out of 186 children with a CI having cholesteatoma; all required surgery, and 3 of them eventually needing explantation to eradicate the disease. Although the overall incidence of cholesteatoma is similar to that of children with normal hearing,[36] the decision making and treatment options in managing cholesteatoma in children with CIs are challenging for clinicians.[35]

Different approaches are used in an attempt to maintain the implant survival, prevent complications, and eradicate the cholesteatoma. Intact canal wall tympanomastoidectomy and modified radical mastoidectomy with nonobliterative closure of the external auditory canal are the most-used techniques to clear the ear of disease.[37] The type of procedure performed depends on the extent of the cholesteatoma and the involvement of the disease with relation to the electrode array.

In cases whereby the electrode array is uninvolved and the cholesteatoma is small, a canal wall up cartilage tympanomastoidectomy is recommended in an attempt to maintain the ear canal and the existing CI (**Fig. 1**).[38] This technique provides postoperative visualization of the tympanic membrane to monitor recurrence. This visualization is the major advantage over canal overclosure techniques whereby entrapment of squamous epithelium is a risk and magnetic resonance imaging cannot be perform because of the magnet and the signal void around the CI.[39]

Regardless of the technique used, most surgeons prefer a staged procedure to confirm eradication of the disease or to excise any recurrence.[40–48] Moreover, when the cholesteatoma surrounds the electrode array, explantation is necessary to prevent tracking of the squamous epithelium into the cochleostomy. This decision is difficult to make because the removal of the CI imparts the loss of auditory input to a child who is

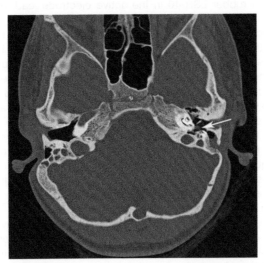

Fig. 1. Axial cut of temporal bone computed tomography demonstrating a small area of soft tissue density in the middle ear compatible with cholesteatoma (*arrow*), tracking along the electrode array.

already cognitively impaired, especially when reimplantation is often difficult because the soft-tissue tract that the electrode occupies can close. The use of a nonmetallic spacer has been proposed to keep this tract open during absence of the implant.[28] The replacement of the CI should be delayed 6 to 12 months if the disease is eradicated.

Despite repeated procedures, it may not be possible to completely and permanently eradicate all cholesteatoma. In these cases, because of the risk of meningitis, permanent explantation should be considered with implantation of the contralateral ear.[35,39]

In conclusion, although the treatment of cholesteatoma in children with CI is challenging, it is possible to preserve the CI in some cases. If the electrode array is involved, the CI must be removed and appropriate measures must be taken to prepare the ear for reimplantation and to minimize potential risks, such as the recurrence of entrapped epithelium, extrusion of the device, and meningitis. An appropriate procedure should be based on the individual clinical presentation at the initial evaluation and time of surgery.

Allergic reactions

Although wound infection is the most common cause of device extrusion, other rare causes must be suspected when recurrent extrusion is encountered. Silicone allergy should be considered, particularly in delayed-onset device extrusion with negative wound culture results or no response to antibiotics. Four cases of CI extrusion as a result of silicone allergy have been reported. Puri and colleagues[49] documented hypersensitivity to the silicone liquid silicone rubbers (LSR)-30 component of a Nucleus 24 Contour device (Cochlear Ltd, Sidney, Australia), whereas Kunda and colleagues[50] documented extrusion secondary to allergic reactions to the room temperature vulcanization (RTV) silicone adhesive from the CI casing. The silicone components used in CI differ in the 3 major CI manufacturers: Advanced Bionics, Cochlear, and Med-El. LSR-70 is used in the receiver-stimulator of Advanced Bionics devices, whereas cochlear devices are cased in liquid silicone rubber LSR-30 and RTV silicone adhesive. Med-El devices use RTV silicone adhesive, liquid silicone rubber LSR-40 in the active electrode lead, and silicone tube high consistency rubber 50 durometer in the reference electrode lead.[50]

All 3 CI manufacturers carry an allergy kit. These kits provide the samples of materials contained in the specific type of CI. The different tests that can be used in allergy testing of CI components include the patch test, prick test, and intradermal test. Patch testing is used in contact dermatitis and is appropriate for nonsoluble materials. In this test, a small amount of allergen is placed over the skin and covered with a watertight bandage for 48 to 96 hours.[51] Evidence of edema or erythema over at least half of the tested area is considered a positive result. This test has a sensitivity and specificity of 70%.[52] The prick test is used with soluble or crushed, diluted nonsoluble allergens. This test involves pricking or scratching the skin with a drop allergen. When a result is negative or equivocal, intradermal testing is a more sensitive option. This test includes a dilute sterile extract with diluting agent alone as a negative control and histamine as a positive control. A result is considered positive if a wheal forms and it is at least 5 mm larger than the control reaction after 15 minutes.[52]

On confirmation of silicon allergy and the specific component to avoid, explantation and reimplantation is warranted. There are different options for RCI, including a custom-made CI without the affecting allergen or the use of a ceramic receiver stimulator. Because only a few cases have been reported in the literature, there is no consensus on the time of reimplantation. However, all reported cases have been reimplanted in a delay fashion. The authors advocate the removal of the receiver stimulator, leaving the electrode within the cochlea to prevent ossification, followed by reimplantation at least 6 weeks later.

Extracochlear electrodes

Extracochlear electrodes are the most common cause of reimplantation after device-related indications in children.[8] In this group, there can be misplacement of the electrode array (**Fig. 2**) or, more commonly, electrode array extrusion.

Patients experiencing migration of the electrode array usually present with reduced speech perception and lack of progress in receptive and productive skills. Pain with audition, facial nerve stimulation, and vertigo has also been reported.[8,15] Audiologic evaluation usually shows an increase in clinical unit levels, a loss of neural response telemetry, and an increase in impedance levels. Programming changes alleviated some of these symptoms through the removal of basal channels from the map. However, all of these findings can also be encountered in device failures. Computed tomography scan makes the differentiation and reveals the displacement of electrodes in migration cases.

Extrusion occurs more frequently in patients who had only partial insertions initially and in patients with known cochlear ossification. This condition poses a particular challenge for RCI because of fibrosis and obliteration of the distal electrode tract, which often prevents the possibility to attain a full reinsertion.

Electrode extrusions tend to occur in younger-aged patients, potentially because of the decreased stability of the electrode lead in smaller mastoid cavities.[8] This condition can cause a springlike effect leading to progressive electrode withdrawal. The slow decline in speech perception found in these patients before RCI suggests that extrusion may be a dynamic process that can progress.[8]

The underlying cause of electrode extrusion is unknown, but several theories exist. In children, it is proposed that extrusion occurs as the skull grows, putting a strain on the electrode, although Roland and colleagues[53] have shown no electrode migration in the pediatric population over time. Ossification of the cochlea and the physical forces placed on the outer wall by the electrode have been associated with extrusion. The use of perimodiolar electrodes may decrease this occurrence.[54]

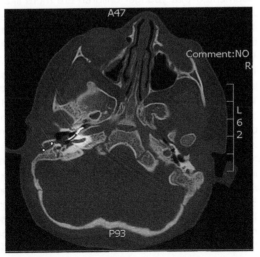

Fig. 2. Axial cut of temporal bone computed tomography showing an electrode array misplaced inside the eustachian tube.

To reduce the probability of electrode extrusion, some techniques have been proposed. Probably the most widely used is tightly packing the cochleostomy with tissue (fascia, muscle, or perichondrium) to hold the electrode in place. Cohen and Kuzma[55] have used a titanium clip to hold the electrode to the incus buttress. Balkany and Telischi[56] developed the split-bridge technique in an attempt to reduce the incidence of electrode migration.

Device-Related Indications

Device-related indications have been the most common cause of reimplantation in most centers (74%) and include those cases where there is facial nerve stimulation and confirmed or suspected device failures.[8]

Facial nerve stimulation

The facial nerve electric stimulation is a complication after CI with rates between 1% and 15%.[57–60] Possible explanation of this adverse effect is a leakage of currents caused by a change in the electric properties of the bone or close proximity of the facial nerve to the outer wall of the cochlea, together with the need for high electric current to stimulate the auditory nerve (ie, malformations or ossified cochleae).

In theory, the perimodiolar electrodes with contacts facing toward the modiolus have less current flow toward the outer wall of the cochlea and might reduce the problem of facial nerve stimulation. Reimplantation, therefore, seems a viable option when the new device is equipped with such a perimodiolar electrode.[61]

Confirmed or suspected device failures

It is important that clinicians are able to diagnose suboptimal or anomalous implant performance and counsel CI candidates, and their families, on prospects for improved performance with RCI. An important concern relates to the fact that device defects may be missed in children with limited language capabilities unless an observant parent, therapist, or teacher is able to detect a decline in speech perception or less-than-expected progress. This concern is particularly important because Marlow and colleagues[8] documented that younger children are more likely to achieve and exceed previous peak performance than their older counterparts. This observation emphasizes the detrimental effect of delayed RCI in children who are in crucial periods of speech recognition and language development.

When concerns with implant performance arise, 3 principal factors are considered. The audiologist will first exchange external equipment and adjust program settings. The medical status of patients and the placement of the electrode array are then assessed. Finally, internal-device integrity testing may be needed. In cases whereby patients report no sound, defective external equipment has been ruled out, and the telemetric locking capability of the system is lost, the device is confirmed to be defective (hard failure).

Confirmed device failure is defined as the absence of auditory input or electronic lock between external and internal components. These patients receive no auditory input from the device, which usually occurs as a sudden loss of sound perception. Approximately 30% of patients might experience preceding non–life-threatening head trauma or short-term (less than 4 months) signs and symptoms of atypical tinnitus, intermittent function, shocking sensation, fluctuating impedances, loss of electrodes, or open circuits before the loss of sound or telemetric lock.[8] The evaluation confirms that no connection can be made with the device by external means and the decision to revise is straightforward.

However, in patients who continue to perceive sound but experience diminished benefit, fail to progress, or develop aberrant symptoms, a device defect may be suspected.

Suspected device failure (soft failure) is considered a clinical malfunction of the CI whereby the device may still provide some auditory input but patients develop a decrement in performance (*lack of progress*) or unacceptable aversive symptoms. Those symptoms include intermittent CI function; programming difficulties; aberrant sounds; increased loudness; or nonauditory symptoms, like pain, vertigo, or headaches. Information about declining performance, particularly when accompanied by programming difficulties and open or short circuits, should prompt consideration of RCI.[62]

The clinical impression of suspected device malfunction must be investigated by clinical, audiologic, and radiographic criteria in an effort to exclude medical problems and hardware- or software-related causes of performance deterioration. However, clinical acuity is the cornerstone of the decision to proceed with revision surgery in these cases because most of these children present with normal integrity testing.[8,15] Furthermore, integrity tests done by the manufacturers before RCI have shown that approximately 50% of the suspected device-failure cases function within manufacturer specifications, and integrity tests do not correlate with ex vivo device analysis.[8,15] Therefore, the diagnosis is supported by the return of function with subsequent reimplantation.[28,63]

On completion of RCI surgery, all explanted failed devices must be sent to the manufacturer for ex vivo device analysis and identification of the source of the failure. The most common causes of device failure include case fracture or loss of hermetic seal.[15,64–66]

OUTCOMES OF REVISION COCHLEAR IMPLANTATION

Since the Hochmair-Desoyer and Burian report, others studies addressed the safety of RCI, including the preservation or enhancement of speech perception performance. RCI has been shown to be a safe procedure with postoperative hearing results comparable to the initial CI performance.

When comparing preoperative speech performance immediately before RCI and speech performance 6 or more months after reimplantation, most studies have demonstrated that revision surgery maintains or improves speech perception in 89% to 100% of the cases (**Table 1**).[4,5,8,15,67,68] This finding is particularly true for non–device-related indication and confirmed device failures. Those few cases whereby patients do not return to peak performance are usually suspected failures. Marlow and colleagues[8] found that depending on the definition of success, (1) a return to previous peak performance or (2) an increase in speech perception in cases of low performance and failure to progress, suspected device failure was deemed to be successful in 67% of the cases with low and stagnant performance versus 83% of the cases with previous decrements in performance. Importantly, aversive auditory symptoms, like intermittent/decline or poor performance, atypical tinnitus, increased loudness, or nonauditory symptoms, like pain or headache, were the most common clinic manifestations that usually resolve with RCI and were found to be positive prognostic factors of improvement in speech perception.

There are inherent risks to RCI, however. Poorer speech perception in 3% of children was associated with a 45% decline in activated electrodes after RCI,[8] which underlines the negative consequences resulting from incomplete electrode activation in children.[69,70] Reports of decrements in electrode activation,[9] diminished speech

Table 1
Revision cochlear implantation in children: review of the literature

Report	Incidence RCI[a]/Device Failure[b] (%)	Average Duration First Device (y)	Indication hf/sdf/other (n)	Postoperative Speech Perception Better/Same/Worse[c] (%)	Device Defect Found (%)
Chung et al,[86] 2010[d]	7.5	4.5	26/14/73	71/29/0[e]	26
Marlow et al,[8] 2010	13/-	3.4	26/18/18	87/10/3	84
Brown et al,[65] 2009[d]	5.5/4.2	—	24/10/10	—	86
Cullen et al,[66] 2008	11.2/-	2.6	49/16/42	—	88
Battmer et al,[92] 2007[d]	-/3.8	—	—	—	—
Cote et al,[68] 2007	8.0/6.2	6.4	19/2/6	26/63/11	68
Migirov et al,[93] 2007	12.5/6.9	—	21/1/16	—	—
Fayad et al,[87] 2006	5.6/3.2	—	17/1/9	—	—
Tambyraja et al,[88] 2005[d]	—	—	416/71/305	—	—
Lassig et al,[67] 2005	6.4/4.2	3.9	16/4/10	72/16/11	—
Beadle et al,[89] 2005	-/26.7[f]	3.4	—	—	—
Weise et al,[13] 2005	-/5.4	2.0	—	—	—
Arnoldner et al,[14] 2005	-/13.9	—	—	—	—
Maurer et al,[90] 2005	12.6/11.2	—	15/0/2	—	100
Parisier et al,[4] 2001	-/6.7	2.7	—	37/63/0	—
Alexiades et al,[5] 2001	4.7/4.3	2.7	17/1/2	53/47/0	—
Balkany et al,[3] 1999[d]	5.7/2.2	—	—	—	—
Miyamoto et al,[9] 1997	-/6.3	—	—	—	—
Parisier et al,[91] 1996	-/14.9	—	—	—	100

Abbreviations: hf, hard failure; other, other indications of RCI; sdf, suspected device failure.
[a] Revision for all indications/devices replaced for proven defect.
[b] Device-related indications only.
[c] Relative to immediate preoperative speech perception scores.
[d] Includes adults and children.
[e] Suspected device failures (soft failures) only.
[f] Cumulative rate for children with 10 to 14 years of implant experience.

perception,[10] and intracochlear trauma[11] should prompt careful consideration of the indications and expected benefits of RCI.

The potential benefit of RCI should be considered carefully, regardless of patient age, taking into account the magnitude and time course of observed changes of performance as well as clinical and device characteristics. After all other strategies for restoring functional deficits are ruled out, RCI surgery should be considered to restore previous performance and enhance the potential for future benefit.

SURGICAL CONSIDERATIONS

RCI requires thoughtful planning and special attention to several surgical considerations. The use of the same incision from the first operation is usually preferred and similar flaps are developed.

Monopolar cautery should be avoided to prevent current spread through the electrode lead to the neural elements of the cochlea as well as direct damage to the device itself.[5] The use of monopolar electrocautery, with appropriate precautions, has only been approved to be safely used below the neck in CI recipients.[71] Nonetheless, studies in pigs using 30 minutes of continuous electrocautery in the nasopharynx have shown to maintain the integrity of the CI.[72] Furthermore, Labadie and colleagues[73] reported one case whereby no subjective degradation of performance or malfunction on integrity testing was encountered after electroconvulsive therapy. Despite these observations, using monopolar cautery during RCI could pose a risk of getting in direct contact with the device and render an ear unsuitable for reimplantation. The bipolar cautery is preferred by the authors for RCI surgery and has allowed adequate hemostasis without adverse effects on the patients' speech perception outcomes or on ex vivo device analysis done by the manufacturers after explantation.

Roland and colleagues[5,54,74,75] have advocated the use of the Shaw heated scalpel (Hemostatix Medical Devices, Cherry Hill, NJ, USA), which is effective in controlling bleeding without affecting wound healing or flap viability. Others use the Ultracision harmonic scalpel (Ethicon, Cincinnati, OH, USA) that is capable of cutting tissue and establishes complete hemostasis with minimal thermic lesion by using mechanical vibrations to cause denaturation of proteins.[76,77]

During explantation, mechanical trauma to the device must be avoided. The electrode lead might be encased in soft tissue and the use of a 12-blade scalpel has been proven useful to cut the adhesions and follow the wire down to the facial recess at which point the array is cut. The intracochlear electrode is left in place until the new electrode, of similar or smaller size and diameter, is ready for reinsertion.[75] The removal of the electrode array should be done under direct visualization just before insertion of a new lead through the same intracochlear tract.[68,78] Improper technique may contribute to incomplete or traumatic electrode insertions, which may result in fewer active electrodes and declined performance.[8–10,15]

When premature removal of the electrode array occurs, Rivas and colleagues[15] described the use of laser to ablate the intrascalar fibrous tissue that obstructs the cochleostomy tract, which provides accessibility for easy insertion of a new array. Without these measures, the intracochlear pseudocapsule can be lost,[78] which may lead to intracochlear dissection insult,[11] electrode manipulation, decreased insertion depth, and even cerebrospinal fluid leak.[4,6,12,15,67,68]

Although most revision surgeries are performed without complications, occasionally the extraction of an indwelling CI electrode array may not be straightforward. A rare but potential complication is the incomplete electrode extraction during RCI surgery. Alexiades and colleagues[5] were the first to describe a retained ball tip of an Ineraid implant electrode (Symbion Corporation, Salt Lake City, Utah) inside the cochlea during explantation. In that case, a full electrode array insertion was achieved in the same cochlea with good speech performance.[5] Brown and colleagues[65] reported one case whereby the electrode array fractured and the distal portion of the electrode lead was retained within the cochlea precluding insertion and requiring implantation of the contralateral ear. Kang and colleagues[79] described a similar experience in 2 of 3 children with incomplete electrode extraction. The third child received a partial electrode insertion in the same cochlea but was unable to return to peak levels of speech recognition performance, requiring further implantation in the contralateral ear. Nadol and colleagues[80] performed histopathologic studies demonstrating the formation of dense fibrous and bony tissue response that extended from the cochleostomy into the intrascalar compartment. This finding provides a potential explanation regarding why electrode may fracture within the cochlea. This inflammatory response may be even more pronounced in cases whereby a positioner was used.[79] Anecdotally, the authors have encountered one case of incomplete electrode extraction during RCI surgery in one adult with a nonfunctioning single-channel electrode and history of meningitis (**Fig. 3**). The known increased inflammatory response in patients with history of meningitis helps support the argument of osteoneogenesis around the electrode lead as a potential cause for intracochlear electrode fixation. Although this complication is rare, it is prudent to discuss its implications with patients and their families before surgery, particularly in patients with known positioners in place and those with a history of meningitis.

After successful reinsertion of the electrode array, the cochleostomy is then packed in the usual manner with muscle, fascia, or periosteum to secure the electrode lead in place. As previously mentioned, the split-bridge technique,[56] or the use of a titanium clip against the incus buttress,[55] decreases the forces of migration and the incidence of electrode extrusion[81]; however, this technique is rarely required unless previous electrode extrusion was encountered.

Once a CI has been explanted, the internal CI device must be sent to the manufacturer for testing and reliability reporting. For the past 10 years, the reliability of CI has been similar between the 3 major manufacturers.[8,15,64,65] In the future, manufacturers must follow the 2010 international classification of reliability for implanted CI receiver stimulators to report device failures in a manner that is fair and consistent to all manufacturers.[82]

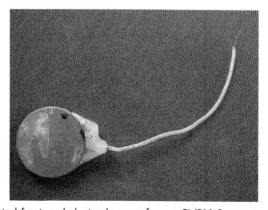

Fig. 3. The explanted fractured electrode array from a CI (3M Company, Maplewood, Minnesota) after incomplete electrode extraction from a patient with history of meningitis.

This practice will provide a standard way to generate cumulative survival curves for CI components and gives the necessary information to CI centers for patient counseling.

FUTURE CONSIDERATIONS

Electroacoustic stimulation (EAS) is a topic that has received considerable attention over the last 10 years. This promising technology targets individuals with severe to profound hearing loss who may still have some measurable hearing in the low frequencies preventing them from receiving a standard CI. Recent reports from Arnolder and colleagues[83] describe the use of a MED-EL Flex EAS (MED-EL, Innsbruck, Austria) electrode in adults and children, with a rate of complete or partial hearing preservation of 100% after a mean postoperative period of 7 months. Others have not achieved as encouraging results. Talbot and Hartley[84] completed a systematic review of 25 publications involving hearing-preservation CI surgery and encountered that 24% and 13%, out of 254 patients, developed a significant increase in acoustic hearing loss or total loss, respectively, using a short CI electrode. Under such conditions, a short electrode may be ineffective in providing enough speech understanding, and reimplantation with a standard electrode array may be warranted. Fitzgerald and colleagues[85] reported 2 users of hybrid CI who lost their residual hearing in the implanted ear after a few months with subsequent limited speech perception. Both patients were reimplanted with a full array and developed a steep improvement in word recognition and speech understanding. This report underscores a new indication for RCI in EAS users who loose their residual hearing and develop suboptimal speech acquisition.

SUMMARY

RCI surgery is an important tool in the armamentarium of CI programs. Early recognition of complications and suboptimal device performance is crucial for children who are in pivotal periods of speech understanding and language development. A discussion regarding RCI with patients and parents must be considered when the progressive clinical assessment reveals an unfavorable course in the acquisition of communication skills. A delay in reimplantation may carry negative consequences because benefits seem to decrease with age. The potential benefit of RCI must be reviewed with patients and parents, but they must recognize that, although rare, revision surgery does not always lead to successful outcomes. Integrity testing provides important but not definitive information when diagnosing device failure, thus, the decision for RCI surgery must be based on device and patient factors to obtain a positive result that impacts verbal development and communication.

REFERENCES

1. House W, Edgerton B. A multiple-electrode cochlear implant. Ann Otol Rhinol Laryngol 1982;91:104–16.
2. Hochmair-Desoyer I, Burian K. Reimplantation of a molded scala tympani electrode: impact on psychophysical and speech discrimination abilities. Ann Otol Rhinol Laryngol 1985;94:65–70.
3. Balkany T, Hodges A, Gomez-Marin O, et al. Cochlear reimplantation. Laryngoscope 1999;109:351–5.
4. Parisier S, Chute P, Popp A, et al. Outcome analysis of cochlear implant reimplantation in children. Laryngoscope 2001;111:26–32.
5. Alexiades G, Roland JJ, Fishman A, et al. Cochlear reimplantation: surgical techniques and functional results. Laryngoscope 2001;111:1608–13.

6. Buchman C, Higgins C, Cullen R, et al. Revision cochlear implant surgery in adult patients with suspected device malfunction. Otol Neurotol 2004;25: 504–10.

7. Gantz B, Lowder M, McCabe B. Audiologic results following reimplantation of cochlear implants. Ann Otol Rhinol Laryngol 1989;142:12–6.

8. Marlowe A, Chinnici J, Rivas A, et al. Revision cochlear implant surgery in children: the Johns Hopkins experience. Otol Neurotol 2010;31(1):74–82.

9. Miyamoto R, Svirsky M, Myres WA, et al. Cochlear implant reimplantation. Am J Otol 1997;18:S60–1.

10. Henson A, Slattery WI, Luxford W, et al. Cochlear implant performance after reimplantation: a multicenter study. Am J Otol 1999;20:56–64.

11. Shepherd R, Clark G, Xu SA, et al. Cochlear pathology following reimplantation of a multichannel scala tympani electrode array in the macaque. Am J Otol 1995;16: 186–99.

12. Fayad JN, Baino T, Parisier SC. Revision cochlear implant surgery: causes and outcome. Otolaryngol Head Neck Surg 2004;131:429–32.

13. Weise JB, Muller-Deile J, Brademann G, et al. Impact to the head increases cochlear implant reimplantation rate in children. Auris Nasus Larynx 2005;32:39–43.

14. Arnoldner C, Baumgartner WD, Gstoettner W, et al. Surgical considerations in cochlear implantation in children and adults: a review of 342 cases in Vienna. Acta Otolaryngol 2005;125:228–34.

15. Rivas A, Marlowe A, Chinnici J, et al. Revision cochlear implantation surgery in adults: indications and results. Otol Neurotol 2008;29:639–48.

16. Bhatia K, Gibbin KP, Nikolopoulos TP, et al. Surgical complications and their management in a series of 300 consecutive cochlear implantations. Otol Neurotol 2004;25:730–9.

17. Hopfenspirger MT, Levine SC, Rimell FL. Infectious complications in pediatric cochlear implants. Laryngoscope 2007;117:1825–9.

18. Hall-Stoodley L, Costerton JW, Stoodley P. Bacterial biofilms: from the natural environment to infectious diseases. Nat Rev Microbiol 2004;2:95–108.

19. Antonelli PJ, Lee JC, Burne RA. Bacterial biofilms may contribute to persistent cochlear implant infection. Otol Neurotol 2004;25:953–7.

20. El-Kashlan HK, Arts HA, Telian SA. Cochlear implantation in chronic suppurative otitis media. Otol Neurotol 2002;23:53–5.

21. Luntz M, Hodges AV, Balkany T, et al. Otitis media in children with cochlear implants. Laryngoscope 1996;106:1403–5.

22. Kempf HG, Johann K, Weber BP, et al. Complications of cochlear implant surgery in children. Am J Otol 1997;18:S62–3.

23. Luntz M, Teszler C, Shpak T, et al. Cochlear implantation in healthy and otitis-prone children: a prospective study. Laryngoscope 2001;111:1614–8.

24. Ruellan K, Frijns JH, Bloemberg GV, et al. Detection of bacterial biofilm on cochlear implants removed because of device failure, without evidence of infection. Otol Neurotol 2010;8(31):1320–4.

25. Johnson TA, Loeffler KA, Burne RA, et al. Biofilm formation in cochlear implants with cochlear drug delivery channels in an in vitro model. Otolaryngol Head Neck Surg 2007;136:577–82.

26. Belal A Jr. Contraindications to cochlear implantation. Am J Otol 1986;7:172–5.

27. Cohen NL, Hoffman RA. Complications of cochlear implant surgery in adults and children. Ann Otol Rhinol Laryngol 1991;100:708–11.

28. Kempf HG, Johann K, Lenarz T. Complications in pediatric cochlear implant surgery. Eur Arch Otorhinolaryngol 1999;256:128–32.

29. Yu KC, Hegarty JL, Gantz BJ, et al. Conservative management of infections in cochlear implant recipients. Otolaryngol Head Neck Surg 2001;125:66–70.
30. Donnelly MJ, Pyman BC, Clark GM. Chronic middle ear disease and cochlear implantation. Ann Otol Rhinol Laryngol Suppl 1995;166(Suppl):406–8.
31. Roehm PC, Gantz BJ. Cochlear implant explantation as a sequela of severe chronic otitis media: case report and review of the literature. Otol Neurotol 2006;27(3):332–6.
32. Fayad JN, Wanna GB, Micheletto JN, et al. Facial nerve paralysis following cochlear implant surgery. Laryngoscope 2003;113:1344–6.
33. Dutt SN, Ray J, Hadjihannas E, et al. Medical and surgical complications of the second 100 adult cochlear implant patients in Birmingham. J Laryngol Otol 2005;119:759–64.
34. Gysin C, Papsin BC, Daya H, et al. Surgical outcome after paediatric cochlear implantation: diminution of complications with the evolution of new surgical techniques. J Otolaryngol 2000;29:285–9.
35. Lin YS. Management of otitis media-related diseases in children with a cochlear implant. Acta Otolaryngol 2009;129(3):254–60.
36. House WF, Luxford WM, Courtney B. Otitis media in children following the cochlear implant. Ear Hear 1985;6(Suppl 3):24S–6S.
37. Hellingman CA, Dunnebier EA. Cochlear implantation in patients with acute or chronic middle ear infectious disease: a review of the literature. Eur Arch Otorhinolaryngol 2009;266(2):171–6.
38. Migirov L, Dagan E, Kronenberg J. Surgical and medical complications in different cochlear implant devices. Acta Otolaryngol 2009;129(7):741–4.
39. El-Kashlan HK, Telian SA. Cochlear implantation in the chronically diseased ear. Curr Opin Otolaryngol Head Neck Surg 2004;12(5):384–6.
40. Axon PR, Mawman DJ, Upile T, et al. Cochlear implantation in the presence of chronic suppurative otitis media. J Laryngol Otol 1997;111(3):228–32.
41. Bendet E, Cerenko D, Linder TE, et al. Cochlear implantation after subtotal petrosectomies. Eur Arch Otorhinolaryngol 1998;255(4):169–74.
42. Gray RF, Irving RM. Cochlear implants in chronic suppurative otitis media. Am J Otol 1995;16(5):682–6.
43. Gray RF, Ray J, McFerran DJ. Further experience with fat graft obliteration of mastoid cavities for cochlear implants. J Laryngol Otol 1999;113(10):881–4.
44. Himi T, Harabuchi Y, Shintani T, et al. Surgical strategy of cochlear implantation in patients with chronic middle ear disease. Audiol Neurootol 1997;2(6):410–7.
45. Incesulu A, Kocaturk S, Vural M. Cochlear implantation in chronic otitis media. J Laryngol Otol 2004;118(1):3–7.
46. Kim CS, Chang SO, Lee HJ, et al. Cochlear implantation in patients with a history of chronic otitis media. Acta Otolaryngol 2004;124(9):1033–8.
47. Marangos N, Laszig R. Cochlear implant surgery and radical cavities. Adv Otorhinolaryngol 1997;52:147–50.
48. Takahashi H, Naito Y, Fujiki N, et al. Cochlear implant surgery in ears with chronic otitis media. Adv Otorhinolaryngol 2000;57:93–5.
49. Puri S, Dornhoffer JL, North PE. Contact dermatitis to silicone after cochlear implantation. Laryngoscope 2005;115:1760–2.
50. Kunda LD, Stidham KR, Inserra MM, et al. Silicone allergy: a new cause for cochlear implant extrusion and its management. Otol Neurotol 2006;27: 1078–82.
51. Parslow TG, Stites DP, Terr AI, et al, editors. Medical immunology. 10th edition. New York: Lange Medical Books/McGraw-Hill; 2001. p. 394–7.

52. Adkinson NF Jr, Yunginger JW, Busse WW, et al, editors. Middleton's allergy: principles and practice. 6th edition. Philadelphia: Mosby; 2003. p. 1589–90.
53. Roland JT Jr, Fishman AJ, Waltzman SB, et al. Stability of the cochlear implant electrode array in children. Laryngoscope 1998;108:1119–23.
54. Zeitler DM, Budenz CL, Roland JT Jr. Revision cochlear implantation. Curr Opin Otolaryngol Head Neck Surg 2009;17(5):334–8.
55. Cohen NL, Kuzma J. Titanium clip for cochlear implant electrode fixation. Ann Otol Rhinol Laryngol Suppl 1995;104:402–3.
56. Balkany T, Telischi FF. Fixation of the electrode cable during cochlear implantation: the split bridge technique. Laryngoscope 1995;105:217–8.
57. Cohen NL, Hoffman RA, Stroschein M. Medical or surgical complications related to the Nucleus multichannel cochlear implant. Ann Otol Rhinol Laryngol 1988;97:8–13.
58. Niparko JK, Oviatt DL, Coker NJ. Facial nerve stimulation with cochlear implantation. Otolaryngol Head Neck Surg 1991;104:826–30.
59. Muckle RP, Levine SC. Facial nerve stimulation produced by cochlear implants in patients with otosclerosis. Am J Otol 1994;15:394–8.
60. Weber BP, Lenarz T, Dahm MC, et al. Otosclerosis and facial nerve stimulation. Ann Otol Rhinol Laryngol Suppl 1995;16:445–7.
61. Battmer R, Pesch J, Stöver T, et al. Elimination of facial nerve stimulation by reimplantation in cochlear implant subjects. Otol Neurotol 2006;27:918–22.
62. Nicholas J, Geers A. Expected test scores for preschoolers with a cochlear implant who use spoken language. Am J Speech Lang Pathol 2008;17:121–38.
63. Balkany TJ, Hodges AV, Buchman CA, et al. Cochlear implant soft failures consensus development conference statement. Otol Neurotol 2005;26:815–8.
64. Venail F, Sicard M, Piron JP, et al. Reliability and complications of 500 consecutive cochlear implantations. Arch Otolaryngol Head Neck Surg 2008;134:1276–81.
65. Brown KD, Connell SS, Balkany TJ, et al. Incidence and indications for revision cochlear implant surgery in adults and children. Laryngoscope 2009;119:152–7.
66. Cullen RD, Fayad JN, Luxford WM, et al. Revision cochlear implant surgery in children. Otol Neurotol 2008;29:214–20.
67. Lassig A, Zwolan T, Telian S. Cochlear implant failures and revision. Otol Neurotol 2005;26:624–34.
68. Cote M, Ferron P, Bergeron F, et al. Cochlear reimplantation: causes of failure, outcomes and audiologic performance. Laryngoscope 2007;117:1225–35.
69. Geers A, Brenner C, Davidson L. Factors associated with development of speech perception skills in children implanted by age five. Ear Hear 2003;24(Suppl 1):24S–35S.
70. Francis H, Buchman C, Visaya J, et al. Surgical factors in pediatric cochlear implantation and their early effects on electrode activation and functional outcomes. Otol Neurotol 2008;29:502–8.
71. Poetker DM, Runge-Samuelson CL, Firszt JB, et al. Electrosurgery after cochlear implantation: eighth nerve electrophysiology. Laryngoscope 2004;114(12):2252–4.
72. Antonelli PJ, Baratelli R. Cochlear implant integrity after adenoidectomy with Coblation and monopolar electrosurgery. Am J Otol 2007;28(1):9–12.
73. Labadie RF, Clark NK, Cobb CM, et al. Electroconvulsive therapy in a cochlear implant patient. Otol Neurotol 2010;31(1):64–6.
74. Roland JT Jr, Fishman AJ, Waltzman SB, et al. Shaw scalpel in revision cochlear implant surgery. Ann Otol Rhinol Laryngol Suppl 2000;185:23–5.
75. Roland JT Jr, Huang T, Cohen NL. Revision cochlear implantation. Otolaryngol Clin North Am 2006;39:833–9.

76. Laszig R, Ridder GJ, Aschendorff A, et al. Ultracision: an alternative to electro-cautery in revision cochlear implant surgery. Laryngoscope 2002;112:190–1.
77. Vallés Varela H, Royo López J, Abenia Ingalaturre JM, et al. Cochlear implants using the Ultracision harmonic scalpel. Acta Otorrinolaringol Esp 2005;56(10): 491–4.
78. Jackler R, Leake P, McKerrow W. Cochlear implant revision: effects of reimplantation on the cochlea. Ann Otol Rhinol Laryngol 1989;98:813–20.
79. Kang SY, Zwolan TA, Kileny PR, et al. Incomplete electrode extraction during cochlear implant revision. Otol Neurotol 2009;30(2):160–4.
80. Nadol JB Jr, Eddington DK. Histologic evaluation of the tissue seal and biologic response around cochlear implant electrodes in the human. Otol Neurotol 2004; 25:257–62.
81. Connell SS, Balkany TJ, Hodges AV, et al. Electrode migration after cochlear implantation. Otol Neurotol 2008;29:156–9.
82. Battmer RD, Backous DD, Balkany TJ, et al. International classification of reliability for implanted cochlear implant receiver stimulators. Otol Neurotol 2010; 31(8):1190–3.
83. Arnoldner C, Helbig S, Wagenblast J, et al. Electric acoustic stimulation in patients with postlingual severe high-frequency hearing loss: clinical experience. Adv Otorhinolaryngol 2010;67:116–24.
84. Talbot KN, Hartley DE. Combined electro-acoustic stimulation: a beneficial union? Clin Otolaryngol 2008;33(6):536–45.
85. Fitzgerald MB, Sagi E, Jackson M, et al. Reimplantation of hybrid cochlear implant users with a full-length electrode after loss of residual hearing. Otol Neurotol 2008;29(2):168–73.
86. Chung D, Kim AH, Parisier S, et al. Revision cochlear implant surgery in patients with suspected soft failures. Otol Neurotol 2010;31(8):1194–8.
87. Fayad J, Eisenberg L, Gillinger M, et al. Clinical performance of children following revision surgery for a cochlear implant. Otolaryngol Head Neck Surg 2006;134: 379–84.
88. Tambyraja RR, Gutman MA, Megerian CA. Cochlear implant complications: utility of federal database in systematic analysis. Arch Otolaryngol Head Neck Surg 2005;131(3):245–50.
89. Beadle E, McKinley D, Nikolopoulos T, et al. Long-term functional outcomes and academic-occupational status in implanted children after 10 to 14 years of cochlear implant use. Otol Neurotol 2005;26:1152–60.
90. Maurer J, Marangos N, Ziegler E. Reliability of cochlear implants. Otolaryngol Head Neck Surg 2005;132:746–50.
91. Parisier S, Chute P, Popp A. Cochlear implant mechanical failures. Am J Otol 1996;17:730–4.
92. Battmer RD, O'Donoghue GM, Lenarz T. A multicenter study of device failure in European cochlear implant centers. Ear Hear 2007;28(2 Suppl):S95–9.
93. Migirov L, Taitelbaum-Swead R, Hildesheimer M, et al. Revision surgeries in cochlear implant patients: a review of 45 cases. Eur Arch Otorhinolaryngol 2007;264(1):3–7.

Cochlear Implantation: Current and Future Device Options

Matthew L. Carlson, MD[a], Colin L.W. Driscoll, MD[a],*,
René H. Gifford, PhD[a], Sean O. McMenomey, MD[b]

KEYWORDS

- Cochlear implant(s) • Future designs • Deafness • Hearing
- Rehabilitation

"All of us in implant research have hoped that somehow we would hit upon an electrode configuration or external processing scheme that would suddenly give our patients normal hearing. This perfect device has eluded the many research teams that have formed around the world. Therefore, we have concentrated on determining whether one implant is a little better than another. However, differences in performance may be due as much to individual variation as to variations in the devices...

I am not discouraged. I am simply much wiser about cochlear implants. Twenty years ago I thought implants could be developed and widely applied in 4–5 years. Let us recognize that we have at least another 20 years of painful, step-by-small-step development if we are to continue to improve the cochlear implant."
—*William F. House, MD, 1986*[1]

Few modern medical advances better exemplify the success that can be achieved through synchronous technological and surgical innovations than the cochlear implant (CI). Despite early criticism from the scientific community, it was through persevering collaboration between pioneering surgeons, clinical scientists, and engineers that early prototype designs came to fruition. What once only provided individuals with

Financial & material support: No funding or other support was required for this study.
Conflicts of interest: Colin L.W. Driscoll, MD is a consultant for Cochlear Corporation and Advanced Bionics. The authors report no other conflicts of interest concerning the information presented in this article.
This article has not been previously published or submitted elsewhere for review.
[a] Department of Otolaryngology–Head and Neck Surgery, Mayo Clinic School of Medicine, 200 First Street Southwest, Rochester, MN 55905, USA
[b] Department of Otolaryngology–Head and Neck Surgery, Oregon Health and Science University, 3181 SW Sam Jackson Park Road, Portland, OR 97239, USA
* Corresponding author.
E-mail address: driscoll.colin@mayo.edu

Otolaryngol Clin N Am 45 (2012) 221–248
doi:10.1016/j.otc.2011.09.002
0030-6665/12/$ – see front matter © 2012 Elsevier Inc. All rights reserved.

the crude sensation of sound, allowing for improvements in lipreading ability, the majority of patients are now achieving more than 80% on open-set speech recognition tasks.[2] Today nearly 200,000 patients have undergone implantation worldwide,[3] and cochlear implantation has become the standard of care for hearing rehabilitation in patients with severe to profound sensorineural hearing loss (SNHL).

Despite tremendous progress over the last quarter-century there remains room for improvement. Looking forward, the ideal device should emulate natural hearing in both quiet and complex noise conditions, demonstrate safe long-term reliability, and overcome issues with user performance variance; the hardware package must be durable, energy efficient, and boast an inconspicuous design. In this article the authors provide a brief history of the development behind the CI, discuss the current state of available technologies, and review potential future directions both near-term and long-term.

HISTORY OF COCHLEAR IMPLANT DEVELOPMENT

In 1790, Allesandro Volta first discovered that electrical stimulation of the auditory system could create the perception of sound when he placed metal rods in his own ears.[4] After activating a ~50-V circuit he experienced the sensation of "une recousse dans la tete" ("a boom within the head"), followed by a sound likened to that of boiling thick paste. During the early 1900s, further research laid the theoretical groundwork for future implant development, realizing that electrical current may create auditory percepts through direct stimulation of the cochlear nerve.[5]

In 1957, a French otologist (Djourno) and physicist (Eyriés) provided the first detailed description of the effects of directly stimulating the auditory nerve in a deaf patient.[6] During a radical resection for extensive bilateral cholesteatomas the right cochlear and facial nerves were sacrificed. With a subsequent surgery aimed at grafting the severed facial nerve, an electrode was applied to the proximal auditory nerve stump. When a current was applied the patient was able to discern differences in intensity and frequency, and over time was able to appreciate environmental sounds and recognize several simple words.

In the early 1960s several independent groups in the United States began implanting patients with prototype CI designs. In 1964, Blair Simmons from Stanford University implanted 6 stainless-steel electrodes into the cochlear nerve through the modiolus.[7] William House in Los Angeles fortuitously learned of Djourno and Eyriés' earlier work when one of his patients provided an article describing their results.[8] Inspired by this account, in 1961 House implanted several gold electrodes, and in 1965 he teamed up with engineer Jack Urban to develop devices that might weather long-term use. In 1972, House introduced a commercially available implant with a wearable signal processor, platinum electrodes, and an induction coil system, and in 1973 he began the first phase of clinical trials.

Despite these early triumphs there was growing skepticism from other experts in the field, and the concept of achieving *meaningful* audiologic rehabilitation in deaf patients through electrical stimulation was condemned by the scientific community.[9] It was not until 1977, after a National Institutes of Health commissioned investigatory team evaluated the first 13 single-channel electrode implantees, that the concept of cochlear implantation became legitimized. In his report, Robert Bilger confirmed that CI technology could afford improved hearing with enhanced lipreading, recognition of limited environmental sounds, and improved control of voice modulation with minimal patient risk.[10]

During this time, Graeme Clark in Sydney, Australia developed a multichannel banded electrode and implanted his first patient in 1978, which afforded limited open-set speech recognition.[11] Early success prompted interest from the Australian national government and a partnership was formed between the University of Melbourne, the Australian government, and a medical equipment company, Nucleus Ltd, which led to the establishment of Cochlear Ltd.

Early CI commercial device development benefited from advancements in computer microcircuit fabrication and implantable pacemaker technologies. On November 26, 1984, the first single-channel CI (House/3 M) was approved by the Food and Drug Administration (FDA) for implantation in adult patients with profound postlingual deafness.[8] Owing to improved spectral perception and open-set speech recognition, the multichannel design soon replaced earlier single-channel devices.

Early innovations including the addition of the multichannel electrode and increasingly sophisticated signal-processing strategies have revolutionized the CI industry. However, within the last 10 years we have seen a plateau in speech recognition performance in quiet, and our attention has thus shifted toward overcoming more difficult listening tasks including performance in background noise, sound localization, and music appreciation, in the quest to more perfectly replicate normal hearing.

CURRENT IMPLANT SYSTEMS
Overview

There are currently 3 manufacturers of CIs that have FDA approval: Advanced Bionics Corporation (Valencia, CA, USA), Cochlear Corporation (Lane Cove, Australia), and Med-El GmbH (Innsbruck, Austria) (**Fig. 1**). Despite variations in component design and sound-processing strategies, device performance is generally comparable between all 3 implant manufacturers when evaluating present-day designs.[12]

Virtually all modern CIs share a set of common functional components. In its most fundamental form, the CI is a transducer that changes acoustic energy into an electrical signal, which is used to stimulate surviving spiral ganglion cells of the auditory nerve (**Fig. 2**). Despite the loss of stimulating inner hair cells from associated disease processes, the cochlea is able to preserve sufficient numbers of spiral ganglion cells, which are critical to successful implant stimulation.[13]

The external hardware comprises 3 separate components: the microphone, the sound processor, and the transmitter. The microphone is generally placed on or

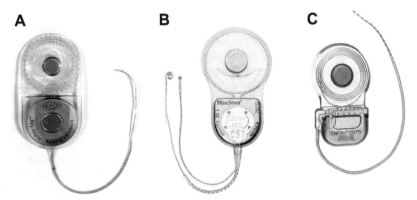

A   **B**   **C**

Fig. 1. Most recent cochlear implant models from the 3 major device manufacturers: (*A*) Advanced Bionics Corporation HR90 K; (*B*) Cochlear Corporation Nucleus 5; and (*C*) Med-El GmbH Sonata ti100. (*Courtesy of:* [*A*] *Courtesy of* Advanced Bionics, LLC, Valencia, CA. [*B*] Photo provided *courtesy of* Cochlear™ Americas, © 2011 Cochlear Americas. [*C*] *Courtesy of* MED-EL Inc, Durham, NC; with permission.)

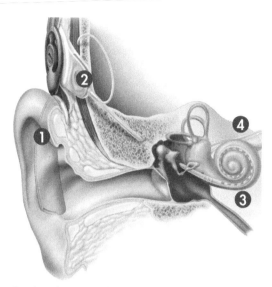

Fig. 2. The cochlear implant: how it works. (1) Sound is received by a microphone located on the behind-the-ear sound processor unit. The signal is then processed, coded, and sent via transcutaneous radiofrequency link to the (2) implanted receiver-stimulator package. Once received, the data are decoded and sent to individual electrodes along (3) an intracochlear multichannel array. Individual channels then electrically stimulate spiral ganglion cell populations within their vicinity and transmit the signal along (4) the auditory nerve for central processing. (Photo provided *courtesy of* Cochlear™ Americas, © 2011 Cochlear Americas.)

near the earhook; it receives natural acoustic information and converts it to an analog electrical signal that is subsequently sent to the behind-the-ear (BTE) sound processor. The sound processor in turn alters the signal to a format that is meaningful to the receiving cochlea and central nervous system through the processes of amplification, compression, and filtering. In modern digital sound processors, this process also involves an analog-to-digital conversion. The processed signal, which contains temporal and spatial patterns of stimulation, is then encoded and sent through a transcutaneous transmitter, generally by way of radiofrequency, to the implanted device.

The implanted package contains the magnet, telemetry coil, and a hermetically sealed electronics package. Once received, the data are decoded and can be sent to individual channels according to the signal processing strategy that is used. The fantail protects the transmitting electrodes as they exit the hermetically sealed housing. The active lead contains individual wires that transmit data for each respective channel along the implanted multichannel electrode, while a second extracochlear lead serves as the ground electrode and is only used with the monopolar electrode configuration (**Fig. 3**). Because the spiral ganglion cells located in Rosenthal's canal are the intended site of stimulation, the ideal electrode location is near the modiolus in the scala tympani.

Electrical stimulation of the auditory system requires the completion of a full circuit loop whereby one electrode along the implanted array serves as the "active" electrode and a second serves as the "inactive" or return electrode. Monopolar stimulation is the most commonly used strategy in modern CI designs and generally incorporates a remotely located extracochlear reference electrode, which is either located on the case of the receiver-stimulator package or placed under the temporalis muscle. In many cases, the current return path for the monopolar electrode configuration is divided equally between the case ground and the remote ground placed under the

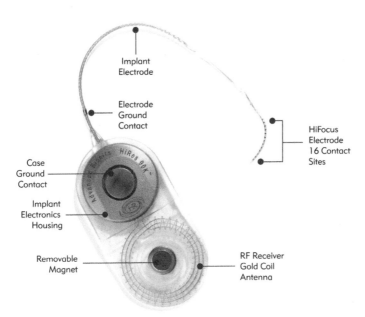

Fig. 3. Common internal device components: radiofrequency (RF) receiver, magnet, titanium electronic package housing, extracochlear ground electrode(s), and distal multichannel "active array." (*Courtesy of* Advanced Bionics, LLC, Valencia, CA.)

temporalis muscle. A pseudomonopolar electrode configuration can also be used, which allows for the most basal electrode, or band electrode (Advanced Bionics Corp), to serve as the ground. Bipolar stimulation, on the other hand, uses a neighboring electrode within the implanted array as the return. Monopolar stimulation has been found to perform on par or better than bipolar strategies while simultaneously providing more efficient power use and reducing the likelihood of exceeding the limits of voltage compliance for any given electrode along the array.[14,15]

Device Designs

This section provides a description of the most recent device and electrode designs available from the 3 major manufacturers (**Tables 1–3**), reviews several notable advances with respect to electrode design and use, and finally discussed potential future electrode design options. While there are multiple driving concepts that continually influence and shape the evolution of electrode design, for the sake of brevity the authors focus their discussion on the electrode-nerve interface and the incorporation of trauma-minimizing strategies.

Current device and electrode designs

The Nucleus 24 series devices (Cochlear Corp) all feature a single current source with 22 intracochlear electrode contacts housed within a silicone carrier. Electrode contacts are pure platinum with platinum-iridium wires, and the receiver-stimulator is housed in a hermetically sealed titanium case. The 24 M had a straight configuration and contained individual banded electrodes (exposed 360°) with 10 inactive proximal "stiffening rings" to facilitate insertion. The CI24RCS first introduced the curved or "perimodiolar" design and insertion stylet (Contour). It contained 22 half-band electrodes (exposed 180° facing the modiolar side); the 10 stiffening rings seen on the earlier 24 M model were replaced by 3 silicone rings. The Nucleus

Table 1
Specifications of the most recent receiver-stimulator package by implant manufacturer

Category	Subcategory	Advanced Bionics Corp: HR90K	Cochlear Corp: Nucleus 5	Med-El GmbH: Sonata ti100
Dimensions, mm (max. length × width × thickness)	Receiver-stimulator package (overall)	56 × 28 × 5.5	50.5 × 30.5 × 3.9	45.7 × 24.8 × 5.9
	Titanium housing	20 × 20 × 5.5	22.3 × 23.5 × 3.9	17.4 × 24.8 × 5.9
	Telemetry coil	28 × 28 × 3.0	28.2 × 30.5 × 3.3	28.3 × 24.8 × 3.7
Weight, g	Receiver-stimulator package	12	8.8	8.6
Case impact resistance, J	Receiver-stimulator package	Up to 6	Up to 2.5	Not available
Diagnostic testing	Impedance level testing	Yes	Yes	Yes
	Neural telemetry	Yes	Yes	Yes
	Electrically evoked stapedius reflex threshold	Yes	Yes	Yes
	Electrically evoked auditory brainstem response	Yes	Yes	Yes
Electronics platform	Maximum stimulation rate	Up to 83,000 pps	Up to 31,500 pps	Up to 50,700 pps
	Current range	0–1.75 mA	0–1.75 mA	0–1.2 mA
	Current source (simultaneous stimulation capable)	Multiple (Yes)	Single (No)	Multiple (Yes)

Table 2
Specifications of the most recent behind-the-ear sound processors from Advanced Bionics Corporation, Cochlear Corporation, and Med-El GmbH

Category	Advanced Bionics Corp: Harmony	Cochlear Corp: Nucleus 5 (CP810)	Med-El GmbH: OPUS 2
Dimensions, mm (max. height × thickness)	54 × 13	51 × 9	57.8 × 8.7
Weight, g (including lightest battery option)	13.5	10.9	10.1
Listening modes	BTE Omni Mic, T-Mic, Telecoil	BTE Omni Mic, SmartSound BEAM (adaptive [Focus] and fixed [Zoom] directionality), Telecoil	BTE Omni Mic, Telecoil
Frequency range, Hz	150–8000	100–8000	70–8500
Input dynamic range, dB	Up to 80	Up to 75	75
Number of programs that can be stored	3	4	4
Bilateral control with single remote	No	Yes	Yes
Water-resistant rating	No	Yes, IP44 & IP57	No

CI24RCA first used the Advance Off-Stylet (AOS) system and added a tapered soft tip (Softip) to decrease trauma during insertion (Contour Advance). The subsequent 24RE (ie, Freedom) device has a smaller size, but otherwise keeps a similar design to prior models. The recently added Nucleus 5 implant improves on the receiver-stimulator size in terms of both its overall footprint size and thickness, but again maintains an identical electrode design to previous generation implants. Cochlear Corp also manufactures a double array (Nucleus 24 Double Array) for use in patients with significant cochlear ossification; a basal array of 11 electrodes can be inserted through a standard cochleostomy location and a second apical array containing 11 additional electrodes can be inserted into the second turn of the cochlea. The previously mentioned thinner straight (ST) array remains available, and may be useful in patients with partially ossified cochleae or revision cases where a straight array was first used.

The HR90 K (Advanced Bionics Corp) implants similarly feature a hermetically sealed titanium housing and a telemetry coil encased in silastic. There are currently two electrode options, each incorporating 16 independent current sources corresponding to 16 intracochlear electrodes housed in a silicone carrier. The HiFocus Helix electrode uses a 24.5-mm perimodiolar design with stylet and houses 16 planar contacts arranged along the medial surface of the electrode. The HiFocus 1j uses a straight design, and is slightly thinner and longer than the HiFocus Helix. Both electrodes use a unique insertion tool to reduce trauma and decrease the risk of tip fold over and electrode buckling.

Med-El's Sonata ti100 also incorporates a titanium device housing and platinum-iridium electrode wires. The standard array incorporates 12 independent current

Table 3
Electrode specifications for conventional "long" and "short" electroacoustic designs

Feature	Conventional-Length Electrode Designs				
	Advanced Bionics Corp: HiFocus Helix	Advanced Bionics Corp: HiFocus 1j	Cochlear Corp: Contour Advance with AOS	Cochlear Corp: Straight Electrode (ST)	Med-El GmbH: Standard (H)
Number of active electrodes	16 half bands	16 half bands	22 half bands	22 full bands	12 paired (total 24)
Number of potential pitch percepts	460	460	161	161	Not available
Proximal array diameter, mm	1.1	0.8	0.8	0.6	1.27
Distal array diameter, mm	0.6	0.4	0.5 (Softip 0.2)	0.4	0.5
Recommended cochleostomy size, mm	1.2–1.6	1.5–2.0	1.2–1.5	1.0–1.4	1.3
Shape	Perimodiolar	Straight	Perimodiolar	Straight	Straight
Stylet incorporation	Yes	No	Yes	No	No
Total length, mm	24.5	25	17.8	23.9	31.5
Total length of active electrodes, mm	13	17	14.4	16.4	26.4
Spacing between contacts, mm	0.85	1.1	0.31–0.42	0.45	2.4
Approximate angular insertion depth	360°–420°	400°–500°	360°–450°	270°–390°	540°–630°

Electroacoustic (Short) Electrode Designs

Feature	Cochlear Corp: Hybrid S(8)	Cochlear Corp: Hybrid L	MED-EL GmbH: Flex^EAS
Number of active electrodes	6 Half bands	22 Half bands	7 Basal pairs + 5 single apical
Proximal array diameter, mm	0.4 × 0.25	0.55 × 0.4	0.8 × 0.78
Distal array diameter, mm	0.4 × 0.25	0.35 × 0.25	0.58 × 0.35
Recommended cochleostomy size, mm	0.5–0.7	0.6–1.0	0.8
Shape	Straight	Straight	Straight
Stylet incorporation	No	No	No
Total length, mm	10	16	26
Total length of active electrodes, mm	4.3	15	20.9
Spacing between contacts, mm	0.45	0.75	1.9
Approximate angular insertion depth	180°–205°	230°–290°	330°–390°

sources with 24 electrodes featured as 12 twin surfaces contained within a silicone carrier. Med-El also offers the Pulsar ti100 device, with an identical electronics package to the Sonata ti100, but uses impact-resistant ceramic casing with a smaller overall size and thickness (uniformly 4 mm thick). The most commonly used Standard (H) array uses a straight design with 2.4-mm spacing between the electrodes, which are distributed over 26.4 mm for an estimated insertion depth of 31.5 mm. Med-El also offers other additional electrode options; those currently with FDA approval include:

1. Medium (M), with the same 12-electrode configuration with 1.9-mm spacing over 20.9 mm, designed for those with considerable low-frequency hearing or in patients for whom a deeper insertion is not desired (eg, cochlear malformations)
2. Compressed (S), with the identical 12 paired electrodes but with 1.1-mm spacing between contacts along 12.1 mm, designed for patients with cochlear malformations or partial ossification
3. Split electrode array (GB), where one lead contains 5 electrode pairs and the other 7 electrode pairs each with 1.1-mm spacing, designed for patients with extensive cochlear ossification.

Minimizing trauma

With early CI systems it was believed that electrode insertion resulted in significant intracochlear trauma, thereby irreversibly destroying all residual hearing. However, over the last 2 decades we have witnessed improved rates of hearing preservation following implantation through the use of modified surgical techniques and electrode design.[16] Within last 10 years there has been a paradigm shift toward the development of minimally traumatic electrode designs and soft surgical techniques to improve performance and expand candidacy criteria.

There are at least 3 common mechanisms responsible for acute mechanical inner ear injury during electrode insertion. The electrode may be inserted through a cochleostomy created anteroinferior to the round window, or alternatively may be placed through the round window membrane. The round window membrane sits in close proximity to the vertically aligned osseous spiral lamina, and during electrode insertion it is possible to fracture the osseous spiral lamina or spiral ligament.[17] A second common method of injury involves traumatic abutment of the lateral scalar structures at the first basal turn of the cochlea and beyond.[18] Most electrodes demonstrate a relatively straight mid-scalar course down the basal turn of the cochlea. However, once reaching the first turn most electrodes abut the lateral wall and are forced toward the basilar membrane. This positioning may be true regardless of the type of electrode used, whether a straight or perimodiolar configuration. If continued force is applied, the electrode can displace the basilar membrane or fracture the interscalar partition, which can result in electrode excursion into the scala media or even the scala vestibuli. Finally, with today's designs there appears to be a limit as to how far an electrode can be inserted before substantial trauma is incurred. The deeper the insertion, the narrower the radius of turn and smaller the scalar cross section becomes, making it more difficult to traverse without incurring damage.[19]

Minimizing electrode-associated trauma during implantation offers several important advantages:

1. For patients with residual low-frequency hearing, limiting trauma can allow for the preservation of natural hearing, thereby permitting concurrent electric-acoustic stimulation (EAS) strategies[20] (see the section Electroacoustic Technologies)

2. Lessening intracochlear damage may limit the amount of intracochlear fibrosis and ossification, making revision surgery less problematic[21,22]
3. Limiting injury may permit patient participation in future developments such as cellular regeneration
4. Attenuating injury serves to reduce the risk of device-related otogenic meningitis[23]
5. There is evidence that patients with less intracochlear trauma following conventional length electrode insertion may perform better under the electric-only condition.[24] To this end, implant designs have adapted perimodiolar technologies with insertion devices,[18] and have explored shorter and thinner electrodes with more shallow insertion angles to reduce trauma and improve overall performance.[25]

A thinner and shorter electrode allows for a smaller cochleostomy and is less likely to cause damage when contacting the delicate scalar structures. On the other hand, with a deeper insertion there are more surviving nerve fibers or spiral ganglion cell populations available to stimulate, theoretically allowing for better frequency coverage. This factor then raises one of the most important questions in current CI electrode design: what is the ideal depth of insertion? During the Hybrid 10 clinical trial, two different implant designs were investigated. The initial 6-mm design allowed for excellent hearing preservation but had poor electrical stimulation such that patients only received on average a 10% improvement in Consonant-Nucleus-Consonant (CNC) monosyllabic word scores. However, when a longer 10-mm electrode was used, patients received on average a 40% gain in CNC word scores in the combined electric-acoustic mode.[26] Looking at the other end of the spectrum, what is too deep? In a study by Finley and colleagues,[27] the electrode scalar location, whether in the scala tympani or scala vestibuli, and angular depth of insertion were evaluated using high-resolution computed tomography in 14 CI recipients. Lower CNC word scores were found to be associated with greater insertion depths and more numbers of contacts located in the scala vestibuli. While most studies have demonstrated similar findings (less than 400°),[28,29] others have found no statistical correlation between insertion depth and monosyllabic word recognition.[30] Spiral ganglion frequency mapping suggests that to stimulate low tone frequencies (<1000 Hz), an electrode must be inserted over 500°; however, with the current electrode models it appears that achieving such a depth of insertion would be met with unjustifiable trauma.[19] Future technologies focusing on minimizing trauma beyond one and a half turns will be required if it is hoped to successfully use the full frequency spectrum of speech.

Improved electrode-to-nerve coupling

A second area of interest centers on optimizing the electrode-to-neuron interface through minimizing the distance between the stimulating electrode and the receiving neural cell groups. There are many theoretical advantages to perimodiolar positioning including lower energy requirements, a reduction in channel interactions, more discrete neural population stimulation, and less trauma during insertion.[28] Earlier designs aimed at improving electrode position used large space–filling designs or incorporated "positioner" components. However, such attempts resulted in substantial trauma and have since been abandoned.[31] One notable advance has been the introduction of precurved perimodiolar designs with accompanying insertion guides. Roland[18] demonstrated that in comparison with conventional insertion techniques, the use of the AOS technique combined with a tapered soft-tip modification resulted in less insertional force and intracochlear trauma (**Fig. 4**).

The early success of the multichannel electrode demonstrates the importance of improved spatial selectivity during stimulation. The number of largely independent

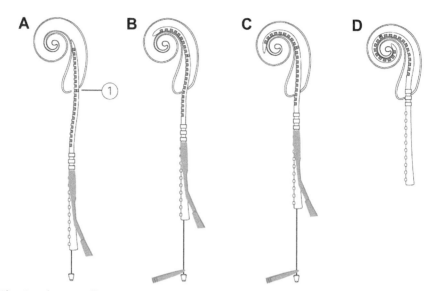

Fig. 4. Advance Off-Stylet technique. (*A*) The electrode is inserted until the marker "1" approximates the cochleostomy site. (*B*) The stylet is held in place as (*C*) the array is slowly advanced off of the stylet, and (*D*) removed from the field. (Photo provided *courtesy of* Cochlear™ Americas, © 2011 Cochlear Americas.)

filters used during normal hearing includes at least 28 for the frequency range covered by speech.[32] Although today's designs may include as many as 22 electrodes, the majority of users achieve less than 10 perceptually unique channels.[33,34] Factors including electrode design, signal processing strategy, distance between stimulating electrode and modiolus, number and spatial distribution of surviving spiral ganglion cells, and intracochlear fibrosis may all limit spatial specificity during stimulation. Therefore, even when a large number of electrodes are available for use, such factors may limit the maximal number of discrete spiral ganglion cell populations that can be stimulated. It is interesting, however, that under testing conditions many users are able to discern frequency/pitch differences with each successive electrode along an entire array (as many as 22 physical electrodes or more using "virtual channels").[15] However, during real-time sound-processor use, even the highest performing subjects peak on objective performance testing with use of less than 10 perceptually independent channels,[33,34] although more channels may permit improved subjective sound quality.

What does the future hold for electrode design? Drug-eluting designs[35] and micropump delivery systems[36] might allow for use of anti-inflammatory drugs that may lessen postimplant inflammation, reactive tissue formation, and neural-element degeneration. The use of neurotropic factors may prevent further neural degeneration associated with either electrode placement or progression of the underlying otologic disease, and may even allow for neural ingrowth allowing for improved electrode-to-neuron coupling.[37] Robotic electrode insertion with steerable electrode arrays may minimize insertion variability and more consistently reduce traumatic array placement.[38] There has been a renewed interest in intramodiolar electrode placement, with theoretical advantages including improved spatial resolution, lower energy requirements to achieve stimulus threshold, and a greater number of available stimulus sites.[39] Finally, the use of pulsed optical stimulation may overcome issues of current spread seen with electrical stimulation and improve the spatial selectivity of stimulation.[40]

Signal-Processing Strategies

Many of the performance improvements seen with conventional CIs over the last 2 decades can be directly attributed to the refinement of sound-coding strategies.[12] Signal processing extracts and refines acoustic information to provide meaningful neural stimulation patterns that are palatable to the diseased inner ear and central auditory system.

Two important operations used by all current sound processors include signal compression and bandpass filtering. Normal hearing permits an approximate 120-dB dynamic range of stimulus amplitude with the ability to discern alterations of less than 1 dB, whereas the electric dynamic range of implant users is generally between 6 and 15 dB.[41] Nonlinear signal compression seeks to reduce the output-to-input ratio, thereby narrowing the dynamic range to make it suitable for stimulation within the narrow spectrum of implant users. Bandpass filtering is another important processing step first introduced with multichannel implants. The frequency spectrum of interest for speech and other important environmental sound cues resides primarily between 100 and 8000 Hz. Selective frequency filtering removes unwanted information and allows for different frequencies to be applied to separate channels for independent processing along the corresponding neural frequency map of the cochlea (frequency-to-electrode matching).[42]

The first commercially available single-channel CI (House/3 M) used a solitary compressed sinusoidal current.[8] Early multichannel models subsequently adapted overlapping frequency bands with simultaneous stimulation. The next major development came from the discovery that formants, based on the resonance of the human vocal tract, could be selectively extracted and applied to specific electrodes corresponding to their matched modiolar frequency locations. The Nucleus Wearable Speech Processor was the earliest implant to implement formant use and adopted an F0F2 (F0, fundamental frequency; F2, second resonant frequency) strategy that provided more consistent open-set speech recognition.[43]

Today there are multiple commonly used signal processing strategies used by the 3 main CI manufacturers. All commercially available pulsatile strategies are based on the Continuous-Interleaved-Sampling (CIS) strategy, which was first described by Wilson and colleagues[44] in 1991. With CIS, a temporal envelope is extracted from several bandpass filters (5–20) and after nonlinear signal compression they are delivered to each electrode in nonoverlapping (or interleaved) pulses (>800 pulses per second per channel [pps/ch]). In other words, the pulse train is modulated with the temporal envelope of the incoming speech signal for any given filter bandpass. By using nonsimultaneous signal delivery, the CIS strategy is able to minimize problems associated with channel interaction. Advanced Bionics Corporation further developed several strategies based on the CIS blueprint. The Multiple Pulsatile Sampler (MPS), formerly known as the Paired Pulsatile Sampler (PPS), differs from the CIS strategy in that set electrodes pairs (1/5, 2/6, 3/7, 4/8) are designated so that the two electrodes within each pair stimulate in concert.[45] By choosing relatively distant electrodes for each pair, the strategy reduces concerns of current summation. The MPS strategy also uses a faster stimulation rate (1445 pps/ch).

The "n-of-m" strategy[46] is also based on the principles of CIS in that it uses bandpass filtering and temporal envelope extraction, but additionally integrates temporal frames lasting 2.5 to 4 milliseconds. Sound is sampled in sequential 2.5- to 4-millisecond intervals and is processed to several frequency bands. Within each interval, several bands with the highest envelope amplitude are selected and interleaved (~1000 pps/ch) between corresponding electrodes. The Spectral Peak (SPEAK)[47] and Advanced Combination Encoder (ACE)[48] strategies were subsequently adapted by Cochlear Corporation from the n-of-m strategy. The SPEAK strategy estimates the envelope amplitude of 20 bandpass filters, and uses 6 to 10 bands containing the largest amplitudes while using a relatively low rate of stimulation (180–300 pps/ch). The ACE strategy alternatively identifies a discrete number of bands, called maxima (generally ranging from 8 to 12), from 22 bandpass filters, and is capable of a much faster stimulation rate (250–2400 pps/ch).

With all CIS-based strategies described here, the channel stimulation rate is not varied across electrodes. Recently, however, there has been interest in developing methods to deliver "fine-frequency" cues that are lacking in current envelope extraction–based strategies in hopes of improving hearing performance in noise, music appreciation, and other more complex listening tasks. Med-El's Fine Structure Processing (FSP) strategy using FineHearing technology is based on envelope and fine-structure processing.[49] Timing of stimulation is used to code the temporal structure of the sound signal through the use of channel-specific sampling sequences in the low to mid frequencies (apical channels, typically 70–300 Hz). In the remaining channels, fine-structure coding is accomplished through the use of sequential "virtual channels"; bandpass filters use a bell-shaped frequency response allowing for a gradual transition from one electrode to a neighboring electrode, thereby creating intermediate pitch percepts that are different than those created from stimulating any one electrode alone. Though not yet available in the United States, the FS4 and FS4-p (parallel stimulation) coding strategies are two further refined versions that provide fine-structure processing on 4 channels ranging up to 1000 Hz.[50]

The current HR90 K implant system (Advanced Bionics Corp) implements another strategy called HiResolution Sound (HiRes).[51] The HiRes platform offers a wide programmable dynamic range (up to 80 dB) and is capable of rapid stimulation rates (up to 83,000 pps/ch). Each individual electrode is powered and controlled independently, allowing the system to operate under a simultaneous (ie, paired) or a nonsimultaneous (ie, sequential) CIS-based strategy. The HiRes Fidelity 120 (HiRes 120) is designed to further improve spatial resolution of stimulation using "current steering" (also called "virtual channel") techniques. By delivering simultaneous but varying amounts of current to neighboring electrode pairs, the number of stimulation sites can be increased beyond the actual number of discrete contacts (8 spectral bands assigned to 15 electrode pairs creating up to 120 spectral bands).[52] Though not yet available in the United States, Advanced Bionics Corporation is currently trialing a signal enhancement algorithm, "ClearVoice," built on HiRes Fidelity 120 technology.[53] With this strategy, speech is distinguished from unwanted noise by analysis of amplitude changes over time. When noise is added to speech, the amplitude changes (modulations) are flattened. The ClearVoice noise reduction algorithm estimates the noise level in each frequency band in sequential time frames (1.3 seconds) and reduces the gain in frequency bands containing less ideal signal-to-noise ratios (SNR), thereby emphasizing those frequencies containing meaningful sound cues (ie, speech).

Finally, Cochlear Corporation has introduced an approach termed MP3000 (previously referred to as Psychoacoustic Advanced Combination Encoder [PACE]; not yet available in the United States) aimed at improving spectral resolution, which was adapted from the previously described ACE strategy.[54] The MP3000 strategy differs from ACE and other related n-of-m strategies in that after selecting the largest envelope amplitudes, the masking pattern of the envelope is determined and the next largest acoustic component is used, thereby better emulating the masking capabilities of the normal hearing auditory system. The current Cochlear Corporation devices use a single current source and do not allow for simultaneous stimulation. Of note, in a white paper publication Cochlear Corporation demonstrated that sequential pulse pairs could create intermediate pitch percepts using the slopes from the overlapping of channel bandpass filters. In their study, up to 161 discernible pitches could be produced with a 22-electrode array.[55]

Back Telemetry and Device Fitting

Following implant activation, implant programs must be fitted (or mapped) to guarantee optimal safe electric performance. Today's processors can store multiple independent maps so that users can benefit from a choice of programs that are optimal for different auditory tasks in various environments. Programming is most time intensive during the first 3 to 6 months when regular corrections are required as the user adapts to electrical stimulation. The majority of adjustments involve correcting minimal threshold levels (T-level) and the maximum comfortable loudness levels termed the C-level (Cochlear Corp) or M-level (Advanced Bionics Corp and Med-El). The optimal dynamic range can be determined by setting current levels defining T- and C- or M-levels for each individual electrode.

The availability of objective internal device integrity and function testing remains critical for optimizing individual user outcomes. This aspect is especially crucial in young patients and those with poor language ability who are unable to communicate issues of abnormal sound perception or unpleasant nonauditory sensations. For these patients, telemetry testing may be the only method for screening electrode dysfunction. With earlier designs such as the Nucleus 22 device, acquiring averaged electrode voltage was the only objective means of assessing CI electrode integrity.[56] Now all device manufacturers routinely fit new-generation implants with impedance and neural response telemetry.

Impedance telemetry assesses the electrode-tissue interface by measuring the resistance met across a closed-circuit loop. Open-circuit failures result from damage to individual channel lead wires and are characterized by excessively high impedances. Short-circuit failures, on the other hand, occur when there is a breach of insulation between two separate wires, and are characterized by low impedance values. Faulty channels disrupt speech perception performance and may result in undesirable nonauditory stimulation (facial nerve or vestibular system activation, and pain), or in the case of a short circuit an aberrant pitch percept, and therefore should be selectively excluded from the fitting strategy. Studies have found that multiple individual electrode failures (greater than 3 or 5) within an array may be a sign of impending device deterioration requiring future revision surgery.[56]

First debuted in 1998 with FDA approval for the Nucleus 24 M implant (Cochlear Corp), Neural Response Telemetry (NRT) (Neural Response Imaging [NRI], Advanced Bionics or Auditory nerve Response Telemetry [ART], Med-El) is a tool used to measure electrically evoked compound action potentials (ECAP) after filtering out background artifact. ECAP thresholds generally lie between behaviorally measured T-levels and C-levels, and thus may be used to estimate initial settings or at least estimate the shape of the T- and/or C/M-level profile during fitting; however, behavioral-level testing remains the preferred method for those able to participate in testing.[57] Beyond ECAP thresholds, electrically evoked stapedius reflex threshold testing may be another objective method available in the future for determining appropriate C- or M-levels for mapping.[58]

In general, dynamic range determination and faulty channel exclusion are given the most weight during CI fitting while individualized frequency-to-electrode programming receives less attention. Current electrode designs and implantation strategies generally use a "one-size-fits-all" approach despite large variations in cochlear dimensions and angular insertion depth. At present, most implant users receive a default frequency-to-electrode allocation strategy that may result in considerable frequency mismatch, which could account for some of the variance seen between "star" implant users and those who perform poorly. Future approaches using novel software or imaging technologies may allow for customized frequency-to-electrode matching to improve speech perception performance.[59]

Device Reliability and Safety

Internal device failure requiring reimplantation occurs in approximately 3% to 6% of all implantees, and represents the most commonly reported significant postoperative complication.[56] Driving concepts of development may be at odds: electrodes must be durable and resist tip foldover, but at the same time should have a forgiving structure to allow for an atraumatic insertion; the internal device casing must be low profile and compact but at the same time must remain impact resistant and impervious to moisture. Enhanced device hermetics and design durability have resulted in an overall decrease in the frequency of spontaneous device malfunction[60]; however, the sheer number of implant surgeries performed every year ensures that device failure will remain a significant burden in the foreseeable future.

Whereas much attention has been given to device failures requiring reimplantation, few reports have investigated the incidence of individual electrode failures along an array. Because individual electrode anomalies generally do not require reimplantation and are simply managed by in-house channel deactivation, device reliability data generally fail to report such occurrences. Individual faulty electrodes can lead to deterioration in speech performance and unpleasant nonauditory stimulation, and may be a sign of impending total device failure.[56] While a general decline in the number of total device failures related to failing hermeticity has been seen,[60] the prevalence of individual electrode failures with successive implant models has not reliably declined.[56] Previous studies have shown that even with modern designs, approximately 10% of implanted arrays will experience at least one individual electrode circuit failure. Moving forward, universal reporting and use of standardized terminology is critical to improving device design.

Device safety must remain a high priority with all new CI designs. CI development has benefited from the advances seen in other implantable device technologies, and tissue incompatibility and device exposure fortunately remain relatively uncommon.[60] Beyond this, the CI carries a unique set theoretical concerns associated with intracochlear electrode placement and inner ear infection. The CI electrode traverses the middle ear space and enters the sterile environment of the inner ear. This process allows for the possibility of an ascending infection from the middle ear space to the cochlea, which could result in substantial loss of spiral ganglion cells and device-associated meningitis; this is particularly relevant in children in whom the incidence of otitis media is disproportionately high. There are many factors that may predispose implantees to meningitis including young age, dual-component electrodes, intracochlear trauma, cochleostomy design, and cochlear dysplasia.[23] From a practical standpoint, these variables can be divided into "controllable" and "uncontrollable" factors. While uncontrollable anatomic and physiologic patient factors will likely maintain an inevitable low baseline rate of meningitis even despite proper vaccination, improvements in surgical technique and device design may result in an overall decreased rate of meningitis.

In 1999, a two-part electrode containing an integrated positioning device (first with C1.2 and later with HiFocus II) was introduced onto the market and was found to be associated with a 4.5-times increased risk for developing meningitis; this model was voluntarily removed from the market in 2003 and replaced with a positioner-free version.[61] The increased risk with the positioner was attributed to greater intracochlear trauma and a larger cochleostomy requirement to accommodate the wider-diameter electrode. Cadaver studies demonstrated that the larger two-part electrode resulted in increased trauma to the osseous spiral lamina and modiolus,[31] and animal studies corroborated that such trauma increases the risk for otogenic meningitis.[62] It is now recommended that cochleostomy size and intracochlear trauma be minimized to decrease the risk of postimplant meningitis.[63]

RECENT ADVANCEMENTS
Bilateral Cochlear Implantation

One recent strategy for overcoming many of the limitations of traditional unilateral cochlear implantation has been achieved through the use of bilateral implants.[64] Simultaneous binaural electrical stimulation has demonstrated improved performance in speech perception (both in quiet and in noise) and enhanced sound localization compared with unilateral implantation. Interaural timing and level differences allow normal-hearing subjects to identify sound location when off midline in the horizontal plane (left-right discrimination); bilateral implantation is thought to at least partially restore this arrangement and permits many bilateral users directional awareness.

Dual-ear stimulation also allows the majority of users to take advantage of the physical phenomenon of the head shadow effect on both sides. This effect occurs when the patient's head and shoulder mass acts as an acoustic barrier, effectively shielding one ear from contralateral competing background noise. In such cases, bilateral CI recipients may be able to preferentially use the ear with the more optimal SNR to improve overall speech understanding in noisy environments. Unilateral CI recipients may also benefit from the head shadow effect, but are more limited in that the competing signal must come from the side of the nonimplanted ear.

To a lesser degree, bilateral implantation may improve performance in hearing in noise through binaural summation and squelch. Binaural summation occurs when identical acoustic sounds processed from both ears provide overlapping central stimulation. Binaural squelch allows listeners to discriminate sound streams using interaural timing, level, and spectral differences between the intended speech source and competing background noise. To date, only a single study has demonstrated binaural squelch effects for bilaterally implant recipients, and it was present only after at least 1 year of experience with bilateral stimulation.[65]

Finally, the use of two independent implant systems can effectively double the number of functional electrodes and spiral ganglion populations stimulated. In addition to additive gains, it is possible that during bilateral stimulation, one implant might compensate or "fill in" for contralateral frequency gaps resulting from asymmetric loss of spiral ganglion cell population.[52]

Electroacoustic Technologies

There remains a population of patients who have sufficient low-frequency hearing to disqualify them from traditional cochlear implantation, yet have insufficient hearing to profit from conventional hearing-aid amplification. In 1993 Lehnhardt[66] from Hannover, Germany first described soft surgical techniques for cochlear implantation, recognizing the importance of minimally traumatic technique in preserving any residual hearing. The concept of combining simultaneous electric and acoustic stimulation with the goal of improving hearing was first realized by von Ilberg and colleagues from Frankfurt, Germany, in 1999.[67] After appreciating the potential for electroacoustic hearing in patients with residual low-frequency hearing and descriptions of surgical techniques designed to minimize trauma, the next logical step was the development of shorter electrode arrays. A shorter, more slender electrode combined with minimally traumatic insertion techniques may be able to adequately rehabilitate mid- to high-frequency SNHL through electrical stimulation of the basal cochlea, and preserve any remaining low-frequency hearing by reducing distal injury. While there have been several published designs, the most well-described models include the Hybrid S8,[20] Hybrid L,[68] and Flex^{EAS}[69] electrodes (see **Table 3**).

Electric-only stimulation provides adequate levels of speech understanding in quiet backgrounds for the majority of CI users; however, it is currently limited in its ability to provide sufficient frequency resolution, which appears to be critical for speech recognition in background noise. Combining acoustic and electrical stimulation has demonstrated improved speech understanding both in quiet and in the presence of competing background noise, and has resulted in enhanced music appreciation.[70] In addition, when combining gains from ipsilateral EAS with contralateral hearing-aid amplification, patients receive a binaural advantage that facilitates sound localization.[71]

In a review of the Hybrid 10 clinical trial, more than 90% of patients were able to maintain low-frequency pure tone thresholds within 30 dB of preoperative levels at initial activation. Although there was some delayed hearing loss seen, more than 70% maintained less than a 30-dB threshold shift at the conclusion of the trial.[20] In the Hybrid L clinical trial, 95% of patients were able to maintain low-frequency thresholds within 30 dB of preoperative levels at 6 months following implantation, and 94% at 1 year.[68] In both studies, patients received substantial postoperative speech-performance benefit in the EAS mode compared with preoperative aided performance and postoperative electric-only performance. These results compare favorably with those of studies reporting hearing preservation rates among conventional-length electrode recipients. Although it is somewhat difficult to compare across studies given differences in definitions, length of follow-up, and the surgical techniques used, the rate of at least partial hearing preservation among conventional length electrode users ranges from approximately 50% to 90%.[16]

Preprocessing Strategies and External Accessories

Most CI improvements aimed at enhancing speech recognition have focused on signal-processing strategies and electrode design. Directional and remote microphone technologies improve signal quality by optimizing the acoustic signal before sound processing, and have demonstrated enhanced sound quality and background noise reduction.[72,73] The use of remote microphones (frequency modulated [FM] and infrared) and directional microphones with hearing-aid amplification has been extensively described; however, their application to CI technologies has received less attention.

Several studies have demonstrated the benefit of remote microphone application in both pediatric and adult CI users.[72,74–76] Fitzpatrick and colleagues[72] evaluated 15 adult unilateral CI users under the CI-only and CI plus remote microphone conditions. These investigators found that in quiet, patients experienced an approximate 15% improvement on AzBio sentence scores using the FM device. With increasing SNRs, more benefit was realized using the remote microphone system (17.5% mean improvement at +5 SNR, 20.4% mean improvement at +10 SNR). Additionally in their study, they demonstrated the benefit of remote microphone use with television viewing, with up to a 22% improvement when using the CI plus remote microphone in comparison with the CI-only mode.

In 2005, Cochlear Corporation debuted a monaural 2-microphone adaptive beam-former, termed "BEAM," aimed at improving preprocessing signal quality.[77] The beamformer combines a directional microphone located on the front of the BTE processor and a second omnidirectional microphone located on the rear. The 2-micro-phone beamformer consists of a fixed spatial preprocessor and an adaptive noise cancellation stage (see Spriet and colleagues[77]). In 2009, Gifford and Revit[78] evaluated 20 postlingually deafened adult Nucleus Cl24 series (Cochlear Corp) implant recipients using adaptive speech reception thresholds (SRT) with Hearing in Noise Test (HINT) sentences. Subjects were tested using the Revitronix R-SPACE environmental stimu-lation system (emulating semidiffuse high-level background noise environments) in both their preferred listening and preprocessing strategy, as well as with the addition of the Focus program (BEAM with autosensitivity and adaptive dynamic range optimi-zation preprocessing strategies). The mean improvement over the patients' preferred everyday strategy in the SRT for all subjects was 3.9 dB when using the Focus program. Cochlear Corporation now incorporates BEAM in the Nucleus 5 CP810 processor with the choice of either adaptive directionality (Focus) or fixed directionality (Zoom), which can be set in individual programming slots.

A novel external accessory developed by Advanced Bionics Corporation is the T-Mic auxiliary microphone, designed to improve speech recognition in noise.[78] The T-Mic consists of a conventional omnidirectional microphone strategically placed just lateral to the opening of the external auditory canal. Such a location allows users to take advantage of the natural amplification and frequency adaptation afforded by the shape and forward-facing position of the pinna. The T-Mic also has the added benefit of allowing implantees the option of more natural telephone receiver and headphone/ear-bud usage. In the previously described study, Gifford and Revit[78] further evaluated 14 adult Advanced Bionics device recipients (HR90 K and CII implant types) and compared performance using the BTE microphone or in the T-Mic setting. The mean SRTs for the BTE microphone and the T-Mic systems were 14.6 and 10.2 dB SNR, respectively demonstrating a mean 4.4 dB improvement when the T-Mic was used.

DEVELOPING STRATEGIES AND TECHNOLOGIES
Cochlear Implantation for Unilateral Deafness

Over the past 3 years, several groups have reported on the use of cochlear implanta-tion in subjects with unilateral deafness who otherwise have intact cochlear nerves and patent cochleae.[79,80] Subjects with unilateral deafness have more difficulty with sound localization and the understanding of speech in noisy conditions than do normal-hearing peers. Traditionally, patients with unilateral deafness who desire rehabilitation have been managed with contralateral routing of signal (CROS) aids or Bone-Anchored Hearing Aids (BAHA). Recently, Arndt and colleagues[79] reported their experience of implanting 11 subjects with unilateral deafness who failed traditional CROS or BAHA rehabilitation. The investigators found that unilateral electrical stimu-lation did not interfere with speech understanding in the normal-hearing ear, and patients achieved improved speech understanding and sound localization compared with CROS, BAHA, and unaided conditions. Their results also corroborate previous reports demonstrating the utility of electrical stimulation in suppressing tinnitus.[81] Common strategies for tinnitus therapy include masking and retraining. Unfortunately these approaches rely on acoustic input and therefore are useless in patients with severe SNHL. Van de Heyning and colleagues[81] reported a significant and consistent reduction in tinnitus in 21 of 22 subjects (95%) with concurrent unilateral deafness and severe tinnitus following implantation.

Totally Implantable Cochlear Implants

Conventional CI designs require the use of a separate external component containing a microphone, battery, sound processor, and transcutaneous transmitting coil to relay data and power to the implanted receiver-stimulator package. An externally worn component precludes CI use in certain environments including water sports, bathing, and during sleep. In addition, even with newer systems the external device can be cumbersome and is highly visible, particularly in patients with shorter hairstyles. "Invisible" hearing rehabilitation using a totally implantable cochlear implant (TICI) could potentially mitigate the social stigma associated with a visible hearing appliance and more effortlessly integrate users with their hearing peers.

With such theoretical advantages, the development of a TICI is appealing.[82,83] Unfortunately, with today's designs it is not uncommon to require external device upgrade and component exchange of faulty external wires, sound processors, or transmitter coils. Given the inaccessible nature of a totally implanted system, great care must be taken to minimize the chance of component failure. Before such technologies become a mainstream reality, there are several hurdles that must be overcome. (1) The battery should be rechargeable, compact, safe (impact resistant, minimal heat production, leakproof), provide reasonable battery life (minimum of 10+ hours using the maximal stimulation rate), and support reliable long-term performance (large number of charge cycles). (2) To avoid issues with implant exposure, skin irritation, and water contamination, the microphone must either use direct transcutaneous sound transmission or take advantage of tympanic membrane or ossicular vibration. (3) The sound processor unit must be small, energy efficient, and capable of dampening electrical and body noise that might be associated with a subcutaneous microphone. (4) Finally, the TICI must take into account that even with the most ideal design, failure is inevitable whether from battery expiration or component failure. In such circumstances, the device should be capable of providing the user the option of simply using an external sound processor as with current technologies, or perhaps have an integrated modular system that would allow for battery exchange without complete device replacement.

Recently Briggs and colleagues[82] published the results of the first clinical trial using the experimental TICI developed by Cochlear Corporation and the Cooperative Research Center for Cochlear Implant and Hearing Aid Innovation. This device used a rechargeable lithium battery and internal device mounted microphone. The implant was capable of "invisible hearing," using only the implanted components and also the conventional configuration using an external ESPrit 3 G sound processor; packaging technology and electrodes were identical to those found in other commercial Cochlear Corporation devices. No surgical or device complications were noted, and all subjects were able to use both implant modes. Speech perception scores were unanimously improved in all subjects over preoperative levels; however, implantees performed nearly twice as well at 12 months on speech-recognition tasks (CNC word scores 77% vs 33%; City University of New York sentence scores in multitalker babble noise [+5 to +6 dB SNR] 72% vs 34%) when using the external processor on comparison with the invisible hearing mode. Furthermore, when using the invisible hearing mode, subjects noted audible body noises such as breathing and swallowing that interfered with perceived sound quality. Although clearly there are limitations with the tested prototype, this study demonstrates that with future refinement the TICI might be a safe and feasible option.

Integrated Drug-Delivery Systems

There is growing interest in direct pharmacologic applications for reducing or even reversing neural tissue loss and intracochlear fibrosis.[35,36] Immediate mechanical trauma and delayed events such as fibrosis, ossification, and activation of proapopto-tic pathways may lead to segmental loss of spiral ganglion cell populations, particu-larly in the basal turn of the cochlea.[21,84] An integrated drug delivery system may allow for a steady infusion of anti-inflammatory and antimicrobial therapies to resist untoward postimplant tissue formation. Furthermore, the neuroprotective effect of electrical stimulation[85] combined with the application of neurotropic factors might reduce the loss of peripheral dendritic appendages and spiral ganglion cells.[37]

Minimally Invasive and Robot-Assisted Cochlear Implantation

Minimal-access surgical procedures are becoming more common in all surgical fields, with otolaryngology being no exception. The evolution of improved anesthetic tech-niques, novel surgical instrumentation, and image navigation systems have allowed surgeons to perform operations with greater accuracy through limited access. Theo-retical advantages include improved cosmesis, attenuated surgical morbidity, decreased operative time, and more rapid convalescence; all of which may improve patient satisfaction and confer potential cost savings.

To date, several implant centers have demonstrated through graduated experi-ments that image-guided surgical systems may perform percutaneous postauricular transmastoid access to the basal turn of the cochlea for implantation.[86,87] While traditional access through a postauricular incision is generally very well tolerated with minimal cosmetic concerns, percutaneous CI surgery may decrease overall surgical time and associated costs even when comparing the results against expe-rienced surgeons.[88] Furthermore, studies have demonstrated that with traditional cochlear implantation, over one-fourth of electrode insertions might result in elec-trode placement outside the scala tympani either through inadvertent direct place-ment in the scala vestibuli or as a result of traumatic interscalar excursion[89,90]; even experienced implant surgeons may have a difficult time detecting early resis-tance during electrode insertion and, despite careful attention, severe trauma is not uncommon with larger electrode designs.[28,91] Automated determination of optimal drilling trajectories could identify which candidates might be most amenable to percutaneous implantation based on variations in anatomy, and may allow for more consistent scala tympani access.[92] After accessing the cochlea, it may be possible to integrate a robotic insertion tool system with haptic control and force-sensing capabilities for safe, minimally traumatic electrode insertion.[38] In the future, percutaneous implantation systems may allow the clinician to perform office-based outpatient cochlear implantation under local anesthesia, which may be particularly beneficial to high-risk surgical patients through avoidance of a general anesthetic. Over time such technologies may offer the benefits of cochlear implanta-tion through telesurgery to populations in developing countries where highly trained otologic surgeons may be unavailable.

FUTURE CHALLENGES
Issues of Outcome Variability

Moving forward, one of the chief obstacles we face lies in the tremendous perfor-mance variability seen among implantees; patients implanted with the same system by a single surgeon can have a tremendous range of outcomes.[93] As it stands, device systems generally use a "one-size-fits-all" paradigm. While many patients score at or near 100% on standard sentence in quiet recognition tests, there remains a group of poor-performing users who have limited or no open-set recognition; performance disparity becomes even more pronounced under difficult testing conditions.

Differences in the number and distribution of surviving spiral ganglion cells, electrode position in relation to the modiolus, degree of incurred electrode insertion trauma, cognitive ability (learning and memory), language capacity, and condition of the central auditory processing system are some of many potential factors that may account for the discrepancy between poor performers and star users.

Much effort has been devoted to identifying prognostic indicators that might presage user performance. Multivariate regression analysis has demonstrated that duration of deafness and preoperative speech-perception scores can predict 80% of the variance seen among CI recipients.[94] This finding suggests that prolonged auditory stimulus deprivation and associated deterioration of central auditory processing capacity may be largely responsible for poor user performance.

To improve outcome consistency, over time we will see the adoption of more individually tailored strategies. High-resolution imaging may allow us to choose the most appropriate electrode design (size, length, number of electrodes), determine the ideal insertion depth, and select the best surgical approach (round window vs cochleostomy). Implant fitting will likely progress beyond behavioral dynamic-range testing, and include objective and automated fitting strategies and customized frequency-to-electrode allocation to limit frequency-electrode mismatch.[59] Finally, customized postsurgical rehabilitation may help overcome some of the deficits associated with prolonged central auditory deprivation and cognitive impairment.[52]

Future Sustainability

In the early 1980s, implant eligibility was limited to postlingual profoundly deaf adults, and in the United States only approximately 25,000 patients were potential implant candidates.[95] With improving outcomes, candidacy criteria have expanded and the number of patients eligible for implantation has grown exponentially; today approximately 70,000 people within the United States have received implants[3] while still nearly an estimated 1 million individuals may benefit from surgery.[95]

There is growing concern that the current medical infrastructure, with a limited number of qualified personnel and poor reimbursement plans, will be unable to meet the rising demand. It has been calculated that the societal economic burden for an individual with prelingual deafness exceeds $1 million over a lifetime.[96] Unfortunately, monetary savings accrued by early implantation and mainstream societal integration is seldom seen in reimbursement schemes. Implantees require support far beyond surgery and initial activation; after the initial postoperative fitting phase, recipients may require periodic program adjustments and invariable replacement of failing external components. Finally, there is a shortage of audiologists trained in CI rehabilitation, and poor reimbursement threatens to only further inhibit adequate audiological staffing needs.[95]

With the limits imposed by our current health care system, we must look for ways to streamline care delivery, and CI manufacturers must work to provide affordable devices with easy-to-use software to facilitate long-term maintenance. One viable option for CI fitting might be met through remote audiology.[97,98] McElveen and colleagues[97] recently reported on the results of a pilot program in which patients underwent early-implant programming using a virtual private network; the 12-month speech perception scores for individuals who received remote consultation were similar to those that underwent in-house evaluation. With this approach, large specialized centers could facilitate efficient programming schedules to lighten patient load on understaffed CI programs, and may be particularly helpful in servicing patients in underserved areas. With the increased number of households having personal computers and improving population computer literacy, perhaps a final avenue for future support might be met through automated or self-servicing software programs[59] for basic programming and maintenance, requiring only periodic professional consultation.

SUMMARY

The healthy cochlea contains roughly 3000 inner hair cells that transmit data along 30,000 auditory neurons, while today's CIs use 12 to 22 electrodes to stimulate a reduced number of spiral ganglion cell populations.[12,99] The ability to restore normal hearing following partial or complete sensorineural deafness continues to elude us. However, we must remain encouraged that even with such crude stimulation strategies, a majority of patients are achieving tremendous hearing rehabilitation, and we continue to see steady progress with each successive implant design and processing strategy. Recent paradigm shifts including hearing preservation with EAS and bilateral cochlear implantation have afforded implant users improved speech recognition in noise, musical appreciation, and enhanced sound localization. Future developments will likely continue to focus on overcoming limitations of spatial resolution and issues pertaining to variability of user performance. The momentum of innovation is truly tremendous, and the future of cochlear implantation, both near and far, promises to be extraordinary.

REFERENCES

1. House WF. Cochlear implants present and future. Otolaryngol Clin North Am 1986;19:217–8.
2. NIH Consensus Conference. Cochlear implants in adults and children. JAMA 1995;274:1955–61.
3. Implants. C. National Institute on Deafness and Other Communication Disorders (NIDCD, NIH). Available at: http://www.nidcd.nih.gov/health/hearing/coch.asp. Accessed November 5, 2010.
4. Volta A. On electricity excited by the mere contact of conducting substances of different kinds. Phil Trans 1800.
5. Jones RK, Stevens SS, Lurie MH. Three mechanisms of hearing by electrical stimulation. J Acoust Soc Am 1940;12:281–90.
6. Djourno A, Eyries C, Vallancien B. Electric excitation of the cochlear nerve in man by induction at a distance with the aid of micro-coil included in the fixture. C R Seances Soc Biol Fil 1957;151:423–5 [in French].
7. Simmons FB, Epley JM, Lummis RC, et al. Auditory nerve: electrical stimulation in man. Science 1965;148:104–6.
8. House WF, Berliner KI. Safety and efficacy of the House/3M cochlear implant in profoundly deaf adults. Otolaryngol Clin North Am 1986;19:275–86.
9. Kiang NY, Moxon EC. Physiological considerations in artificial stimulation of the inner ear. Ann Otol Rhinol Laryngol 1972;81:714–30.
10. Bilger RC, Black FO. Auditory prostheses in perspective. Ann Otol Rhinol Laryngol Suppl 1977;86:3–10.
11. Clark GM, Tong YC, Martin LF. A multiple-channel cochlear implant: an evaluation using open-set CID sentences. Laryngoscope 1981;91:628–34.
12. Zeng FG. Trends in cochlear implants. Trends Amplif 2004;8:1–34.
13. Blamey P. Are spiral ganglion cell numbers important for speech perception with a cochlear implant? Am J Otol 1997;18:S11–2.
14. Bingabr M, Espinoza-Varas B, Loizou PC. Simulating the effect of spread of excitation in cochlear implants. Hear Res 2008;241:73–9.

15. Zwolan TA, Kileny PR, Ashbaugh C, et al. Patient performance with the Cochlear Corporation "20 + 2" implant: bipolar versus monopolar activation. Am J Otol 1996;17:717–23.

16. Balkany TJ, Connell SS, Hodges AV, et al. Conservation of residual acoustic hearing after cochlear implantation. Otol Neurotol 2006;27:1083–8.

17. Briggs RJ, Tykocinski M, Xu J, et al. Comparison of round window and cochleostomy approaches with a prototype hearing preservation electrode. Audiol Neurootol 2006;11(Suppl 1):42–8.

18. Roland JT Jr. A model for cochlear implant electrode insertion and force evaluation: results with a new electrode design and insertion technique. Laryngoscope 2005;115:1325–39.

19. Rebscher SJ, Hetherington A, Bonham B, et al. Considerations for design of future cochlear implant electrode arrays: electrode array stiffness, size, and depth of insertion. J Rehabil Res Dev 2008;45:731–47.

20. Gantz BJ, Hansen MR, Turner CW, et al. Hybrid 10 clinical trial: preliminary results. Audiol Neurootol 2009;14(Suppl 1):32–8.

21. Roland PS, Wright CG. Surgical aspects of cochlear implantation: mechanisms of insertional trauma. Adv Otorhinolaryngol 2006;64:11–30.

22. Briggs RJ, Tykocinski M, Saunders E, et al. Surgical implications of perimodiolar cochlear implant electrode design: avoiding intracochlear damage and scala vestibuli insertion. Cochlear Implants Int 2001;2:135–49.

23. Cohen NL, Hirsch BE. Current status of bacterial meningitis after cochlear implantation. Otol Neurotol 2010;31:1325–8.

24. Carlson M, Gifford R, Tombers N, et al. Hearing conservation with conventional cochlear implantation. Presented at the 2010 American Academy of Otolaryngology-Head and Neck Surgery Annual Meeting and Oto Expo, Otology/Neurotology Section. Boston, September 29, 2010.

25. Woodson EA, Reiss LA, Turner CW, et al. The Hybrid cochlear implant: a review. Adv Otorhinolaryngol 2010;67:125–34.

26. Gantz BJ, Turner C. Combining acoustic and electrical speech processing: Iowa/Nucleus hybrid implant. Acta Otolaryngol 2004;124:344–7.

27. Finley CC, Holden TA, Holden LK, et al. Role of electrode placement as a contributor to variability in cochlear implant outcomes. Otol Neurotol 2008;29:920–8.

28. Wardrop P, Whinney D, Rebscher SJ, et al. A temporal bone study of insertion trauma and intracochlear position of cochlear implant electrodes. I: Comparison of Nucleus banded and Nucleus Contour electrodes. Hear Res 2005;203:54–67.

29. James C, Albegger K, Battmer R, et al. Preservation of residual hearing with cochlear implantation: how and why. Acta Otolaryngol 2005;125:481–91.

30. Lee J, Nadol JB Jr, Eddington DK. Depth of electrode insertion and postoperative performance in humans with cochlear implants: a histopathologic study. Audiol Neurootol 2010;15:323–31.

31. Aschendorff A, Klenzner T, Richter B, et al. Evaluation of the HiFocus electrode array with positioner in human temporal bones. J Laryngol Otol 2003;117:527–31.

32. Moore BC. Coding of sounds in the auditory system and its relevance to signal processing and coding in cochlear implants. Otol Neurotol 2003;24:243–54.

33. Friesen LM, Shannon RV, Baskent D, et al. Speech recognition in noise as a function of the number of spectral channels: comparison of acoustic hearing and cochlear implants. J Acoust Soc Am 2001;110:1150–63.

34. Fishman KE, Shannon RV, Slattery WH. Speech recognition as a function of the number of electrodes used in the SPEAK cochlear implant speech processor. J Speech Lang Hear Res 1997;40:1201–15.

35. Clark G. The multi-channel cochlear implant: past, present and future perspectives. Cochlear Implants Int 2009;10(Suppl 1):2–13.
36. Hochmair I, Nopp P, Jolly C, et al. MED-EL cochlear implants: state of the art and a glimpse into the future. Trends Amplif 2006;10:201–19.
37. Pettingill LN, Richardson RT, Wise AK, et al. Neurotrophic factors and neural prostheses: potential clinical applications based upon findings in the auditory system. IEEE Trans Biomed Eng 2007;54:1138–48.
38. Zhang J, Wei W, Ding J, et al. Inroads toward robot-assisted cochlear implant surgery using steerable electrode arrays. Otol Neurotol 2010;31:1199–206.
39. Middlebrooks JC, Snyder RL. Intraneural stimulation for auditory prosthesis: modiolar trunk and intracranial stimulation sites. Hear Res 2008;242:52–63.
40. Littlefield PD, Vujanovic I, Mundi J, et al. Laser stimulation of single auditory nerve fibers. Laryngoscope 2010;120:2071–82.
41. Fu QJ, Shannon RV. Effects of dynamic range and amplitude mapping on phoneme recognition in Nucleus-22 cochlear implant users. Ear Hear 2000;21:227–35.
42. Sridhar D, Stakhovskaya O, Leake PA. A frequency-position function for the human cochlear spiral ganglion. Audiol Neurootol 2006;11(Suppl 1):16–20.
43. Clark GM, Tong YC, Dowell RC. Comparison of two cochlear implant speech-processing strategies. Ann Otol Rhinol Laryngol 1984;93:127–31.
44. Wilson BS, Finley CC, Lawson DT, et al. Better speech recognition with cochlear implants. Nature 1991;352:236–8.
45. Loizou PC, Stickney G, Mishra L, et al. Comparison of speech processing strategies used in the Clarion implant processor. Ear Hear 2003;24:12–9.
46. Wilson BS, Finley CC, Farmer JC Jr, et al. Comparative studies of speech processing strategies for cochlear implants. Laryngoscope 1988;98:1069–77.
47. Skinner MW, Clark GM, Whitford LA, et al. Evaluation of a new spectral peak coding strategy for the Nucleus 22 Channel Cochlear Implant System. Am J Otol 1994;15(Suppl 2):15–27.
48. Kiefer J, Hohl S, Sturzebecher E, et al. Comparison of speech recognition with different speech coding strategies (SPEAK, CIS, and ACE) and their relationship to telemetric measures of compound action potentials in the nucleus CI 24M cochlear implant system. Audiology 2001;40:32–42.
49. Arnoldner C, Riss D, Brunner M, et al. Speech and music perception with the new fine structure speech coding strategy: preliminary results. Acta Otolaryngol 2007; 127:1298–303.
50. Opus 2 Processor: Audio Processor for MAESTRO CI System. Med-EL. Available at: http://www.medel.com/data/downloads/MAESTRO/20324_OPUS2_Factsheet_English.pdf. Accessed November 15, 2010.
51. Firszt JB, Holden LK, Reeder RM, et al. Speech recognition in cochlear implant recipients: comparison of standard HiRes and HiRes 120 sound processing. Otol Neurotol 2009;30:146–52.
52. Wilson BS, Dorman MF. Cochlear implants: current designs and future possibilities. J Rehabil Res Dev 2008;45:695–730.
53. Buechner A, Brendel M, Saalfeld H, et al. Results of a pilot study with a signal enhancement algorithm for HiRes 120 cochlear implant users. Otol Neurotol 2010;31:1386–90.
54. Buchner A, Nogueira W, Edler B, et al. Results from a psychoacoustic model-based strategy for the nucleus-24 and freedom cochlear implants. Otol Neurotol 2008;29:189–92.
55. Pitch steering with sequential stimulation of intracochlear electrodes (FUN656). Lane Cove (Australia): Cochlear Ltd; 2006.

56. Carlson ML, Archibald DJ, Dabade TS, et al. Prevalence and timing of individual cochlear implant electrode failures. Otol Neurotol 2010;31:893–8.
57. Seyle K, Brown CJ. Speech perception using maps based on neural response telemetry measures. Ear Hear 2002;23:72S–9S.
58. Caner G, Olgun L, Gultekin G, et al. Optimizing fitting in children using objective measures such as neural response imaging and electrically evoked stapedius reflex threshold. Otol Neurotol 2007;28:637–40.
59. Jethanamest D, Tan CT, Fitzgerald MB, et al. A new software tool to optimize frequency table selection for cochlear implants. Otol Neurotol 2010;31:1242–7.
60. Tambyraja RR, Gutman MA, Megerian CA. Cochlear implant complications: utility of federal database in systematic analysis. Arch Otolaryngol Head Neck Surg 2005;131:245–50.
61. Reefhuis J, Honein MA, Whitney CG, et al. Risk of bacterial meningitis in children with cochlear implants. N Engl J Med 2003;349:435–45.
62. Wei BP, Shepherd RK, Robins-Browne RM, et al. Effects of inner ear trauma on the risk of pneumococcal meningitis. Arch Otolaryngol Head Neck Surg 2007; 133:250–9.
63. Cohen N, Ramos A, Ramsden R, et al. International consensus on meningitis and cochlear implants. Acta Otolaryngol 2005;125:916–7.
64. Dunn CC, Tyler RS, Oakley S, et al. Comparison of speech recognition and localization performance in bilateral and unilateral cochlear implant users matched on duration of deafness and age at implantation. Ear Hear 2008;29:352–9.
65. Eapen RJ, Buss E, Adunka MC, et al. Hearing-in-noise benefits after bilateral simultaneous cochlear implantation continue to improve 4 years after implantation. Otol Neurotol 2009;30:153–9.
66. Lehnhardt E. Intracochlear placement of cochlear implant electrodes in soft surgery technique. HNO 1993;41:356–9 [in German].
67. von Ilberg C, Kiefer J, Tillein J, et al. Electric-acoustic stimulation of the auditory system. New technology for severe hearing loss. ORL J Otorhinolaryngol Relat Spec 1999;61:334–40.
68. Lenarz T, Stover T, Buechner A, et al. Hearing conservation surgery using the Hybrid-L electrode. Results from the first clinical trial at the Medical University of Hannover. Audiol Neurootol 2009;14(Suppl 1):22–31.
69. Gstoettner W, Helbig S, Settevendemie C, et al. A new electrode for residual hearing preservation in cochlear implantation: first clinical results. Acta Otolaryngol 2009;129:372–9.
70. Gantz BJ, Turner C, Gfeller KE, et al. Preservation of hearing in cochlear implant surgery: advantages of combined electrical and acoustical speech processing. Laryngoscope 2005;115:796–802.
71. Dunn CC, Perreau A, Gantz B, et al. Benefits of localization and speech perception with multiple noise sources in listeners with a short-electrode cochlear implant. J Am Acad Audiol 2010;21:44–51.
72. Fitzpatrick EM, Seguin C, Schramm DR, et al. The benefits of remote microphone technology for adults with cochlear implants. Ear Hear 2009;30:590–9.
73. Chung K, Zeng FG. Using hearing aid adaptive directional microphones to enhance cochlear implant performance. Hear Res 2009;250:27–37.
74. Schafer EC, Thibodeau LM. Speech recognition abilities of adults using cochlear implants with FM systems. J Am Acad Audiol 2004;15:678–91.
75. Schafer EC, Thibodeau LM. Speech Recognition in noise in children with cochlear implants while listening in bilateral, bimodal, and FM-system arrangements. Am J Audiol 2006;15:114–26.

76. Wolfe J, Schafer EC. Optimizing the benefit of sound processors coupled to personal FM systems. J Am Acad Audiol 2008;19:585–94.

77. Spriet A, Van Deun L, Eftaxiadis K, et al. Speech understanding in background noise with the two-microphone adaptive beamformer BEAM in the Nucleus Freedom Cochlear Implant System. Ear Hear 2007;28:62–72.

78. Gifford RH, Revit LJ. Speech perception for adult cochlear implant recipients in a realistic background noise: effectiveness of preprocessing strategies and external options for improving speech recognition in noise. J Am Acad Audiol 2010;21:441–51 [quiz: 87–8].

79. Arndt S, Aschendorff A, Laszig R, et al. Comparison of pseudobinaural hearing to real binaural hearing rehabilitation after cochlear implantation in patients with unilateral deafness and tinnitus. Otol Neurotol 2011;32(1):39–47.

80. Buechner A, Brendel M, Lesinski-Schiedat A, et al. Cochlear implantation in unilateral deaf subjects associated with ipsilateral tinnitus. Otol Neurotol 2010; 31:1381–5.

81. Van de Heyning P, Vermeire K, Diebl M, et al. Incapacitating unilateral tinnitus in single-sided deafness treated by cochlear implantation. Ann Otol Rhinol Laryngol 2008;117:645–52.

82. Briggs RJ, Eder HC, Seligman PM, et al. Initial clinical experience with a totally implantable cochlear implant research device. Otol Neurotol 2008; 29:114–9.

83. Cohen N. The totally implantable cochlear implant. Ear Hear 2007;28:100S–1S.

84. Eshraghi AA. Prevention of cochlear implant electrode damage. Curr Opin Otolaryngol Head Neck Surg 2006;14:323–8.

85. Leake PA, Hradek GT, Snyder RL. Chronic electrical stimulation by a cochlear implant promotes survival of spiral ganglion neurons after neonatal deafness. J Comp Neurol 1999;412:543–62.

86. Majdani O, Rau TS, Baron S, et al. A robot-guided minimally invasive approach for cochlear implant surgery: preliminary results of a temporal bone study. Int J Comput Assist Radiol Surg 2009;4:475–86.

87. Balachandran R, Mitchell JE, Blachon G, et al. Percutaneous cochlear implant drilling via customized frames: an in vitro study. Otolaryngol Head Neck Surg 2010;142:421–6.

88. Labadie RF, Noble JH, Dawant BM, et al. Clinical validation of percutaneous cochlear implant surgery: initial report. Laryngoscope 2008;118:1031–9.

89. Aschendorff A, Kromeier J, Klenzner T, et al. Quality control after insertion of the nucleus contour and contour advance electrode in adults. Ear Hear 2007;28: 75S–9S.

90. Radeloff A, Mack M, Baghi M, et al. Variance of angular insertion depths in free-fitting and perimodiolar cochlear implant electrodes. Otol Neurotol 2008;29:131–6.

91. Eshraghi AA, Yang NW, Balkany TJ. Comparative study of cochlear damage with three perimodiolar electrode designs. Laryngoscope 2003;113:415–9.

92. Noble JH, Majdani O, Labadie RF, et al. Automatic determination of optimal linear drilling trajectories for cochlear access accounting for drill-positioning error. Int J Med Robot 2010;6:281–90.

93. Wilson BS, Lawson DT, Finley CC, et al. Importance of patient and processor variables in determining outcomes with cochlear implants. J Speech Hear Res 1993;36:373–9.

94. Rubinstein JT, Parkinson WS, Tyler RS, et al. Residual speech recognition and cochlear implant performance: effects of implantation criteria. Am J Otol 1999; 20:445–52.

95. Parisier SC. Cochlear implants: growing pains. Laryngoscope 2003;113:1470–2.
96. Mohr PE, Feldman JJ, Dunbar JL, et al. The societal costs of severe to profound hearing loss in the United States. Int J Technol Assess Health Care 2000;16: 1120–35.
97. McElveen JT Jr, Blackburn EL, Green JD Jr, et al. Remote programming of cochlear implants: a telecommunications model. Otol Neurotol 2010;31:1035–40.
98. Wesarg T, Wasowski A, Skarzynski H, et al. Remote fitting in Nucleus cochlear implant recipients. Acta Otolaryngol 2010;130:1379–88.
99. Rubinstein JT. How cochlear implants encode speech. Curr Opin Otolaryngol Head Neck Surg 2004;12:444–8.

Index

Note: Page numbers of article titles are in **boldface** type.

A

Adolescents, with congenital long-term deafness, cochlear implantation in, 60–61
Advanced Bionics, programming platforms for cochlear implants, 116–118, 227–230
Alport syndrome, 31
Auditory processing pathways, peripheral and central, 81–82

B

Binaural hearing, 161
Binaural squelch, 83
Binaural summation, 82–83
Biotinidase deficiency, 31
Brachio-oto-renal syndrome, 29

C

Children, acquired hearing loss in, bacterial meningitis and, 9
   cochlear implantation in. See *Cochlear implantation, pediatric.*
   residual hearing in, cochlear implantation and, 158
   with cochlear implants, rehabilitation and educational considerations for, **141–153**
   with hearing loss, from bilingual families, 151
   with multiple disabilities, hearing loss in, 150–151, 161–163
Cholesteatoma(s), cochlear implants and, 207–208
   pediatric cochlear implantation and, 56–57
Cochleae, dysplastic, cochlear implantations in, 98–106
      electrode choice and programming in, 104–105
      evaluation for, 99
      facial nerve in, 104
      outcomes of, 105–106
      posterior tympanotomy in, 100
      surgical technique for, 99–102
      transmastoid labyrinthotomy in, 100–102
   CSF leaks and, 102–103
   internal auditory canal implantation in, 103
  obstructed and malformed, implanting of, **91–110**
  ossified, cochlear implantations in, auditory brainstem implant in, 97–98
      double/split-array implantation for, 95–97
      preoperative planning for, 92–93
      scala tympani insertion in, 93–95
      scala vestibuli insertion in, 95

Otolaryngol Clin N Am 45 (2012) 249–255
doi:10.1016/S0030-6665(11)00213-1
0030-6665/12/$ – see front matter © 2012 Elsevier Inc. All rights reserved.
oto.theclinics.com

Moving?

Make sure your subscription moves with you!

To notify us of your new address, find your **Clinics Account Number** (located on your mailing label above your name), and contact customer service at:

Email: **journalscustomerservice-usa@elsevier.com**

800-654-2452 (subscribers in the U.S. & Canada)
314-447-8871 (subscribers outside of the U.S. & Canada)

Fax number: **314-447-8029**

Elsevier Health Sciences Division
Subscription Customer Service
3251 Riverport Lane
Maryland Heights, MO 63043

*To ensure uninterrupted delivery of your subscription, please notify us at least 4 weeks in advance of move.

ELSEVIER

Printed and bound by CPI Group (UK) Ltd, Croydon, CR0 4YY

03/10/2024

01040455-0008